HEALING AND PREVENTING AUTISM

ALSO BY JENNY McCARTHY

MOTHER WARRIORS:

A Nation of Parents Healing Autism Against All Odds

LOUDER THAN WORDS:

A Mother's Journey in Healing Autism

LIFE LAUGHS:

The Naked Truth About Motherhood,

Marriage, and Moving On

BABY LAUGHS:

The Naked Truth About the First Year of Mommyhood

BELLY LAUGHS:

The Naked Truth About Pregnancy and Childbirth

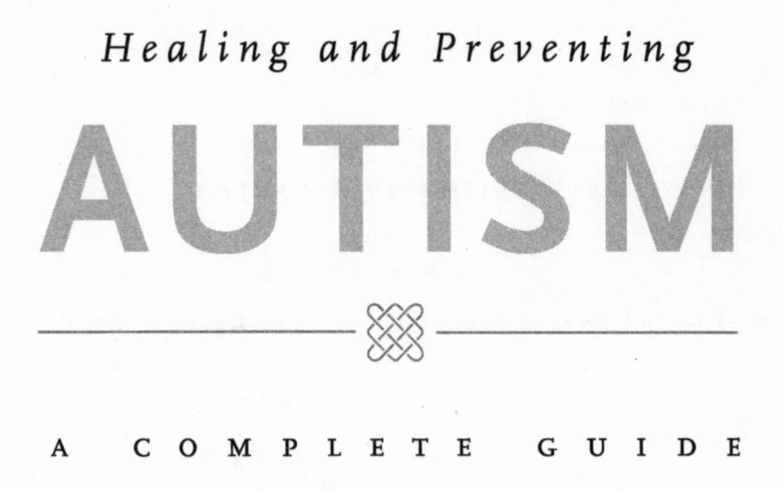

Healing and Preventing AUTISM

A COMPLETE GUIDE

Jenny McCarthy
and Jerry Kartzinel, M.D.

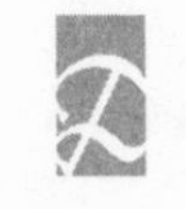

DUTTON

DUTTON
Published by Penguin Group (USA) Inc.
375 Hudson Street, New York, New York 10014, U.S.A.
Penguin Group (Canada), 90 Eglinton Avenue East, Suite 700, Toronto, Ontario M4P 2Y3, Canada (a division of Pearson Penguin Canada Inc.); Penguin Books Ltd, 80 Strand, London WC2R 0RL, England; Penguin Ireland, 25 St Stephen's Green, Dublin 2, Ireland (a division of Penguin Books Ltd); Penguin Group (Australia), 250 Camberwell Road, Camberwell, Victoria 3124, Australia (a division of Pearson Australia Group Pty Ltd); Penguin Books India Pvt Ltd, 11 Community Centre, Panchsheel Park, New Delhi—110 017, India; Penguin Group (NZ), 67 Apollo Drive, Rosedale, North Shore 0632, New Zealand (a division of Pearson New Zealand Ltd); Penguin Books (South Africa) (Pty) Ltd, 24 Sturdee Avenue, Rosebank, Johannesburg 2196, South Africa

Penguin Books Ltd, Registered Offices: 80 Strand, London WC2R 0RL, England

Published by Dutton, a member of Penguin Group (USA) Inc.

First printing, April 2009
10 9 8 7 6 5 4 3 2 1

LIBRARY OF CONGRESS CATALOGING-IN-PUBLICATION DATA
has been applied for.

ISBN 978-0-525-95013-2

Printed in the United States of America
Set in Scala
Designed by Katy Riegel

A Formless Art Publishing book

To the brave doctors, scientists,

and therapists who have fought so hard to

heal our children.

We, the parents, thank you.

CONTENTS

HEALING AND PREVENTING AUTISM

INTRODUCTION

Jenny McCarthy

MOST PEOPLE IN THE AUTISM COMMUNITY have heard my story of how I fought to get my son back from autism. For those of you new to my story, I'd like to share with you the events that led us down this path that an increasing number of families are experiencing right now.

Evan was two and a half years old when I found him in his crib convulsing and struggling to breathe. I had no idea it was a seizure until the paramedics began talking about how to stop it. I was hoping it was a fluke, but my nightmare had only just begun. Three weeks later Evan started seizing again, but this time he wasn't struggling to breathe. His body just lay lifeless, as foam started to come out of his mouth. I prayed to God to make it stop, but it didn't. Minutes later his body went blue and his eyes dilated. I knew he had just gone into cardiac arrest. As I begged God to bring him back to me, I felt this overwhelming feeling of calming energy. If it could have spoken, it would have said, "Everything is going to be okay." I trusted this energy. I felt that this experience happening before my very eyes had a purpose. After two minutes the paramedics revived him. The "calming energy" was right. He came back. Everything seemed okay. Unfortunately, it was short lived. Evan seized on and off for the next seven hours. The doctors didn't know what to make of it; they told me he had epilepsy. But I knew there was more to it. Everything in my mommy radar was screaming, "Keep looking, there's more." So, I hunted for the very best neurologist, someone who would give me insights into my unanswered questions. He took one look at Evan and said, "I'm sorry; your son has autism."

I died in that moment. All of my future images of Evan getting married or hugging me on his way to college broke into a million pieces. I recalled all of the oddities Evan had that had led up to this point. I had thought the flapping of his hands or staring out the window for hours made him "special." I had no idea it was autism. When I asked if there was anything that could be done, the doctor had little hope to offer me. "Some progress is being made with some speech and behavioral therapies, but that's about all," he said. I didn't want to hear that. I wanted to know WHY he had autism and I wanted to know HOW to get him completely back. Leaving the doctor's office that day, I knew I was about to embark on the biggest mission of my life. I was going to get my boy back. I had no idea how, but I trusted my instincts and knew they would always point me in the right direction.

I went online and learned about the gluten-free, casein-free diet. I listened to my instincts and started Evan on it, along with some vitamins. Within two weeks of implementing the diet and vitamins, his eye contact was better and his language doubled! I was out of my mind with joy. It was working! But when I called Evan's doctor to tell him about the progress, he told me it was all a fluke—that diet and vitamins don't really have an effect. I was shocked. I had just told him that I was witnessing huge progress without having implemented any other therapies. He ignored my findings, but I didn't care (yet). I kept digging and found communities that were healing kids with autism. I found a doctor who specialized in healing kids through diet, detox, and supplements. His name was Dr. Jerry Kartzinel. I contacted him and begged him to take my son as a patient. He had no idea that I had any celebrity status. He was taking me on only as a mom of a child with autism.

Within a year of following Dr. Jerry's protocol and intensive behavioral and speech therapies, Evan recovered from autism. I learned that not all kids recover, but MOST of them improve dramatacially from treatment. And I learned there are simple things we can all do to prevent this from happening in the first place.

Since I began this journey, I have spoken to nearly 100,000 moms face-to-face and have received letters and e-mails from around the world. We all have the same story of how our children regressed into autism. How could I possibly stand back from this day forward and be a witness to what's happening to our kids in our lifetime? I can't. I walk through grocery stores and airports where mothers approach me with tears in their eyes as they talk to me about their autistic children. The day Evan had that seizure and went into cardiac arrest, I knew that I had a mission in this lifetime and I wasn't going to stop until the calming energy was right. "Everything is going to be okay." That's my mission now. To make sure ALL of our children are going to be okay.

INTRODUCTION

Jerry Kartzinel, M.D.

MY WIFE AND I had three very healthy boys but felt that one more would complete our family. We decided to adopt a special child who may have had a difficult time being adopted due to the fact that his biological mother was a drug abuser. I knew there were going to be medical problems just because of her methamphetamine (along with other substances) usage. But I'm a pediatrician. Who would be better suited to take care of a child with this kind of background?

We wanted to be, in some small way, helpful to this world. It reminds me of the story where there were thousands and thousands of starfish that had just washed up on shore and this little boy was on the beach throwing each starfish that he could back into the water. A man came up to him and said, "Son, it's not going to impact this whole huge beach. This is not going to have any effect on this big group of starfish." And the little boy looked at him and said, "You might be right, but it affects this starfish." And he threw it back into the ocean. I know I can't take care of all of the world's children, but I can take care of at least this one. Joshua is our starfish.

Joshua was developing and thriving normally until I gave him his

MMR (measles, mumps, and rubella) vaccine. You see, as a pediatrician, I felt it was very important to vaccinate children against diseases. I made sure that Joshua received, in a timely manner, all of his vaccines, starting right after birth with the hepatitis B vaccine. He was around four months of age when he started getting ear infections, rashes, and even required a spinal tap to make sure he did not have spinal meningitis (he was really sick!)—and all of this followed his four-month vaccines. I was still clueless that his immune system was slowly breaking down. His ear infections continued to come and go. Then, at fourteen months of age, while he was coming off of an antibiotic, I gave him his MMR. Over the next two weeks he lost everything. My wife was the one who saw the change. She said, "You know, he's not been the same since you gave him the MMR." I gave the typical male response: "What?" And then I started to think about it and realized that she was right. This was 1997. I had no clue this was autism. Pediatricians in general had no clue. Very little was written about these kids in the early 90s and certainly nothing had been written in the 80s.

Josh developed some serious medical consequences following the MMR. He had large amounts of foul-smelling diarrhea going up his back and down his legs, he lost eye contact, he no longer listened, and his nights became sleepless. He also didn't respond to behavioral correction. You could not keep him out of the dog's water. There was no connection with us or with anything that mattered. He was cranky and nothing pleased him. Transitions became difficult . . . even transitioning from sleep to wakefulness! Over the course of eight weeks, he lost all of his language.

He developed obsessive-compulsive behavior, which was primarily the urge to look into other people's garages. So he would figure out a way to escape the house, but he would run only as far as the next open garage, not into traffic, thank God. He would just sit there rocking, looking at the garage's contents until we realized he was missing.

Two months after the MMR shot I had a clue it was autism. I

didn't want to share it with my wife at that point because I was trying to figure out if it was a late manifestation of the drug exposures that he'd had in utero from his birth mom. But I knew what was going on and then I finally shared it with my wife.

She said, "That's very interesting. What are *you* going to do about it? Obviously, it was from the vaccine because prior to the MMR, he was doing just fine." And then, she landed the bomb: "You broke him, you fix him!" I replied, "Well, dear, we really don't know how to fix this." And she said, "Well, you'll figure it out. Go for it." Now realize, she said a whole lot more, and there were some significant emotions shared at that time. . . . Need I say more?

The medical community doesn't get that these kids have medical complications such as ongoing bowel issues that present with chronic constipation, chronic diarrhea, and reflux. They are quick to label the symptoms they see, such as the constipation as "willful stool withholding behavior" or the diarrhea as "toddler's diarrhea." It seems that excuses are far easier to come by, especially if you only have a ten-minute appointment. But basically, it boils down to this: Doctors (and teachers, I might add) are being taught today about autism from textbooks that are outdated. They have not been able to keep up with the current trends. In fact, the American Academy of Pediatrics released a report/toolkit called *Caring for Children with Autism Spectrum Disorders: A Resource Toolkit for Clinicians* for the first time in November of 2007! There had never been a tool like this for doctors. In other words, they finally caught on to the fact that their board-certified pediatricians had no clue how to diagnose and manage autism.

Today, the number of children being affected by autism is staggering. It is going to require a major paradigm shift of thought for the medical community to consider that it may have caused, through mandatory vaccine programs, a massive iatrogenic (medicine-induced) disease called autism and most probably contributed to the huge increase in children being diagnosed with attention deficit disorder, allergies, asthma, and learning disorders, to name just a few.

It completely violates the "first, do no harm" mentality that is ingrained in most physicians. They have literally exchanged one possible epidemic (such as pertussis or measles) for this very real, lifelong epidemic of autism. It is just too horrible to consider. So it isn't. Those who do know about this at the CDC—and I believe there are those who really do know—will, well, have to answer eventually to a higher authority.

Other people take their children to the doc and they can blame somebody. Moms will say, "It was that stupid doctor's fault." And then they could follow that with, "I should have known better." But I'm actually the one who slipped the needle into my son. I did it to him. I changed his life forever in doing that. But you can't go through life regretting things. You can't go through life being angry with yourself and telling yourself, "I shouldn't have done it," because it doesn't help things. We've all wished we could roll back the clock so we didn't do this or that or another thing, but we can't. I've always been a positive person. The glass has always been half full not empty in my eyes. So, since I'm stuck with this, how do I make the best of it? Not only did I want to make the most of Josh's life, I wanted to learn how I could help other children with autism. And that's where we're at today. How can I help other people? I have to walk this road, anyway, with Josh and I'm going to do it hand in hand with him. But if I'm going to go down this road, I'm not going to be angry and upset with myself. I'm going to use my energy to make the best of my situation and help other people who have been pushed down this road unwillingly.

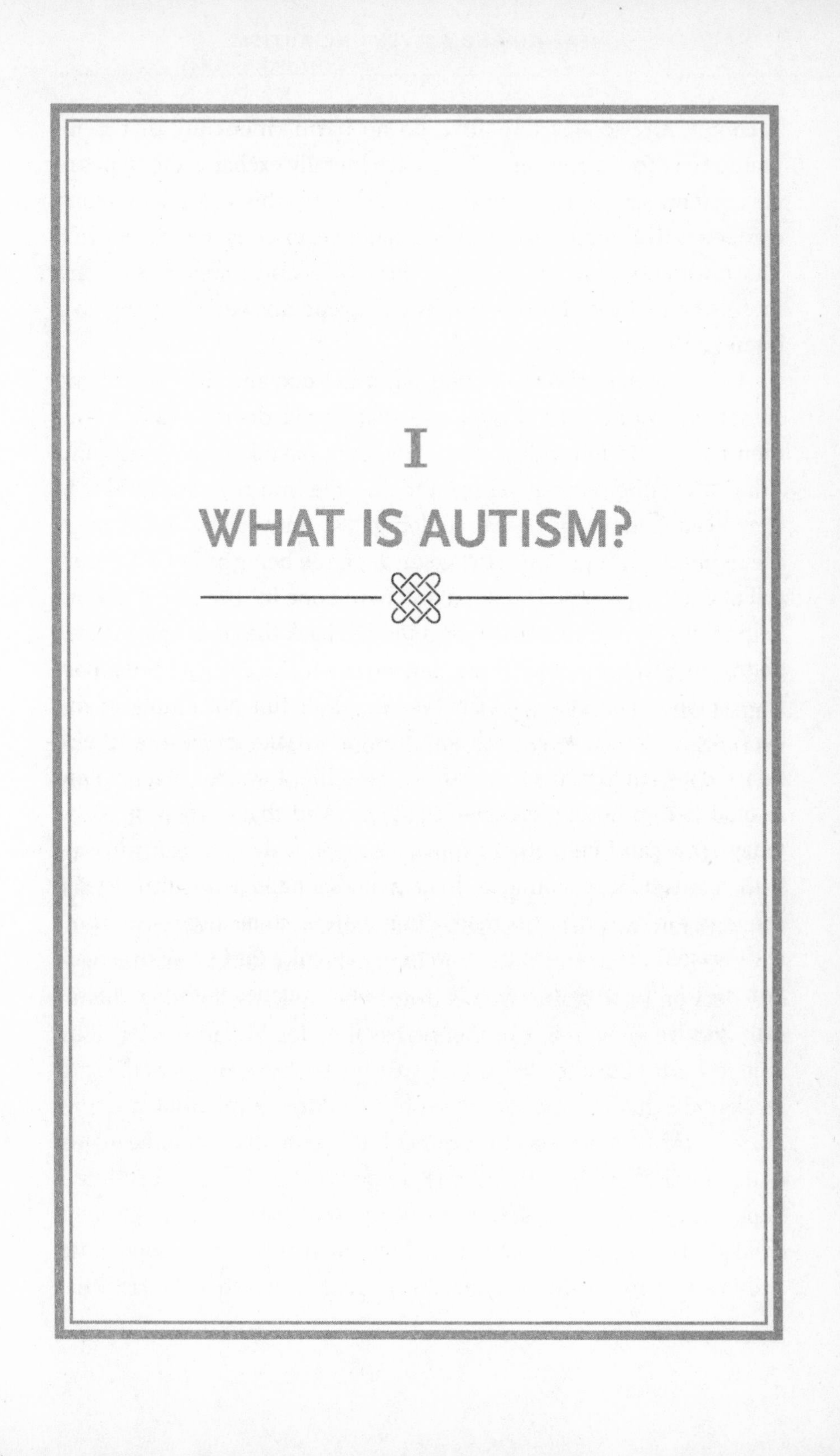

I
WHAT IS AUTISM?

EVERYONE HAS THEIR OWN DEFINITION of what autism is. Neurologists will call it a genetic neurological disorder. I call it a toxic overload. Gastroenterologists, gut doctors, might call it a viral issue. Immunologists will say it's only an immune issue. I believe in some way we are all correct. I only wish each "side" would open up to examine the possibilities that autism can happen in many different ways. I have been pleading with the American Academy of Pediatrics for years now to at least recognize that autism can be triggered by environmental assaults. Why is it so hard to believe that toxins can have an effect on your brain? We get dizzy when we smell strong chemicals, and we know many of them cross the blood-brain barrier. Why is it so hard to acknowledge that viruses, bacteria, or yeast that are stuck in the gut or brain can cause severe neurological problems? I'm not a doctor, so it's been a little difficult to speak up against the giants of the medical establishment to prove our claims. In the meantime I hope more and more parents speak up loudly when they see their child go from normal to sick in the first few years of life. I hope more and more parents investigate WHY their children have asthma,

WHY their children have severe allergies, WHY their children have seizures, WHY their children have developed autism! We must not settle for the diagnosis alone. We must question it, and then find a solution. Parents have been healing their children for years. I learned from them how they helped their children. I learned from them how to prevent further harm, and now Dr. Kartzinel and I are going to share information that could help heal many children. It's up to YOU now to do the work. Get your highlighters ready!!!

DEFINITION OF AUTISM

JENNY: What is your definition of autism?

DR. JERRY: There is a formal definition of autism, which usually coincides with meeting certain criteria as set forth by what is called the Diagnostic and Statistical Manual of Mental Disorders, version 4 (DSM IV). But autism is simply the abnormal response to everyday stimuli. These stimuli are routine, such as a child not responding when his name is called, not responding appropriately to the senses (for example, a high pain threshold), not responding to hunger, thirst, danger, etc. This is, as you can see, a potentially very long list. As the child improves medically, abnormal responses diminish. In addition, there is a whole host of medical conditions that truly need to be addressed as well. Also, I would like to mention that until recently an autism diagnosis usually came from the mother-in-law, the speech therapist, the school nurse, or the next-door neighbor—anybody but the pediatrician, which I always thought was funny.

JENNY: That's absolutely true. Numerous parents have told me how they demanded their pediatrician give them a referral to a diagnostic clinic and the pediatrician always tried to talk them out of it, claiming the child would "catch up to the other children soon." I still don't believe pediatricians can catch it before the parents can.

SIGNS OF AUTISM

JENNY: What are some behavioral signs early on a parent might notice that they should bring up to their pediatrician?

DR. JERRY: This is an interesting concept. There are two forms of regression. The first one, which is more obvious, is the loss of a particular skill or skills. The second form of regression may be a little more difficult to conceptualize. The fact that the child is not acquiring a particular trait in the same time period as his neurotypical peers is, too, a regression. Let's use language as an example. The child may have three, four, or five words, and four months later he should have two hundred words but does not. He still has only three, four, or five words. That's really a regression even though, technically, the child never lost words. It's a failure to keep up with his peers. Normal and predictable behaviors "regress" into abnormal behaviors.

JENNY: What are some other behaviors?

DR. JERRY: Children with autism have a tendency to develop stereotypical repetitive behaviors (stimming), like moving their arms, their hands, flapping, odd movements and gestures. They do not develop normal toy play. They become very repetitive and then they can be very obsessive-compulsive, perseverative, and anxious.

Stimming

JENNY: Evan was addicted to opening and closing drawers and doors. He also loved ceiling fans and escalators. Sadly that's all he ever wanted. He never even wanted to go to the park or play with toys.

DR. JERRY: This is called perseverating. These kids perseverate on ceiling fans. They're also turning on lights, turning off lights, rewinding movies, watching the movie credits over and over again. The list of repetitious and perseverative behaviors that these children can exhibit is quite long. There just seems to be an abnormal fascination with some sort of controlled repetitive behavior.

OCD

JENNY: Let's talk about some obsessive-compulsive behavior issues. Evan would drive me crazy with wanting his chair in the perfect position. He would also scream until I put his food on his Nemo plate and it couldn't be the Nemo with the mouth open, it had to be the Nemo with the mouth closed. I would lose my mind every morning hearing him scream, so I would just give in and let him eat on the Nemo plate that had the closed-mouth Nemo.

DR. JERRY: Yes, and if Mom parts her hair to the left one day, the child will scream until she moves it to the right. If the windows are up in the car, they have to be down. Sometimes these children have to get in the car a certain way. They also make Mom turn the car a certain direction. And on and on and on and on it goes. It's just a huge, long list.

JENNY: I've heard some parents say their kids are just "perfectionists," but really anytime things need to be that drastically perfect and with the same everyday ritual, it is considered obsessive-compulsive disorder.

DR. JERRY: People who specialize in making formal diagnoses will focus in on only psychiatric types of behaviors: OCD, sterotypia (stimming), anxiety DMS IV criteria such as a lack of socialization, lack of eye contact, and nonpurposeful play. Of course, these behaviors are seen, but we must also include the self-injurious behaviors, allergies, gastrointestinal inflammatory processes, constipation, diarrhea, recurrent bacterial infections (like ear infections), etc., just to name a few of the medical conditions that must eventually be addressed. Many times, these physical signs and symptoms are dismissed as just being a part of "autism." If you have a child who is autistic and she breaks her arm, you fix it. If you have a child who's autistic and she happens to have inflammatory bowel disease, you fix it; or constipation, you fix it. And when you do so, all of a sudden the child who wasn't sleeping through the night is now a great sleeper, or who was a screamer is no longer tantruming. In other words, when the underlying medical conditions are addressed, autistic behaviors improve dramatically.

SIGNS OF AUTISM

What you'd expect:

- Loss of skill set
- Not hitting language development marks
- Normal, predictable behaviors regress into abnormal behaviors
- Odd movements, gestures that fascinate them
- Not developing normal play with toys
- Repetitive, obsessive behaviors
- Abnormal levels of anxiety
- High pain threshold
- Lack of eye contact
- Lack of response to vocal commands

What you wouldn't expect:

- Allergies
- Reflux
- Gastrointestinal inflammatory processes
- Constipation
- Diarrhea
- Recurrent bacterial infections (like ear infections)
- Not sleeping properly

Comorbid Conditions: Multiple Secondary Disorders

JENNY: I recently learned a big, fancy medical term called "comorbid conditions."

DR. JERRY: That's what we are talking about here. Comorbidity describes a situation where there are one or more disorders in addition to the primary disorder occurring simultaneously.

JENNY: So comorbid conditions means those that exist with a diagnosis of some sort. Like migraines would be a comorbid condition with depression?

DR. JERRY: Yes, and if you treat the migraine, sometimes the depression will subside or go away. Now, did you cure depression? No, you healed the comorbid condition, which lessened the depression to the point of not having anymore "episodes." But what if you looked deeper and found that the depression and the migraines were hormonal in nature and you treated that? Then, while you managed the hormones, you cured the depression and migraines.

JENNY: Can you name as many comorbid conditions that you can think of that go with autism? Not behavioral ones, just medical symptoms?

DR. JERRY: Oh, Jenny, the list is so long, but here is a partial inventory:

Headaches, visual disturbances, auditory disturbances, oral sensory disturbances, numerous dental issues, frequent infections (ears, sinuses, bowels, "colds"), immune system dysfunction, allergies, sleep disturbances, gastrointestinal diseases such as reflux esophagitis, gastritis, inflammatory bowel disease, constipation, diarrhea, malabsorption, maldigestion, and dysbiosis.

Then there are neurological conditions that include seizures, hypotonia, and abnormal gait. Hypotonia is low muscle tone of the upper body, lower body, or trunk. It can be characterized by weak, stooping shoulders, an inability to hold even light objects like a pencil or having difficulty walking upstairs. Signs of an abnormal gait are not having a normal arm swing while walking, or running in a strange or awkward way. We also need to include dermatological manifestations (rashes, eczema), and problems with focus, concentration, obsessions, compulsions, anxiety, aggression, sleep disruption, just to name a few. This could be a whole medical textbook unto itself.

AUTISM AND COMORBID CONDITIONS

Headaches
Visual disturbances
Auditory disturbances
Oral sensory disturbances
Numerous dental issues
Frequent infections (ears, sinuses, bowels, "colds")
Immune system dysfunction
Allergies
Candida
Sleep disturbances
Gastrointestinal disease (reflux, esophagitis, gastritis, inflammatory bowel disease, constipation, diarrhea, malabsorption, maldigestion, dysbiosis)
Seizures
Hypotonia (low muscle tone)
Abnormal gait (awkward walking or running)
Rashes, eczema
Problems with focus, concentration
Obsessions
Compulsions
Anxiety
Aggression

But let's consider that perhaps these are NOT comorbid conditions. That is, they are not disease states coexisting together but are all a part of the same disease state. Consider that all these conditions are the result of a toxic insult so large that there are multiple metabolic and immune system failures. This is what my friend Dr. Haley refers to as a "metabolic train wreck." And finally, what if this train wreck is due, in part, to the cumulative exposures to vaccines?

JENNY: That makes so much sense to me. As you know, Evan lost his diagnosis after we treated his comorbid condition, which was candida. So parents really need to understand that we are not curing autism, we are only healing the comorbid conditions, which then helps the child's autism to some degree.

DR. JERRY: Thinking of each set of symptoms as part of a disease process gives physicians the ability to come up with treatment plans for each comorbid condition. As each issue, such as reflux, is erased from the child's list of things that are wrong, the child improves.

WHAT WORKS FOR ONE CHILD MIGHT NOT WORK FOR ANOTHER

JENNY: Many parents hope so much for a recovered child that when they don't get one, sometimes they'll go out to the rest of the community and say that biomedical treatments don't work because they didn't work for their child.

DR. JERRY: There are children who have had biomedical interventions and did not respond; it just flat out did not work. It is rare that medical interventions do not seem to bring about any positive changes. The inclination for that parent is to announce that they tried "everything" and it does not work. As you can imagine the parents are devastated, and will share this experience with the community. The experience of one child should not influence another parent's approach, except to reinforce the concept that nothing is 100 percent sure in medicine. If that were true, nobody would attempt chemotherapy for the treatment of cancer—there are many for whom chemo does not work. Along the same lines, hope must always prevail, whether treating cancers, strokes, or, in this case, our children who have been damaged and diagnosed with Autism Spectrum Disorder.

JENNY: Then there are the parents—and I'm guilty of this—who say, "Try this, it worked on my kid, it must work on yours, too!"

DR. JERRY: Yes, we all can be guilty of that and it is easy to understand why. You were excited that Evan improved and you wanted to share it with the world. We have many parents who try a particular treatment and want to tell everyone, and parents who hear of this marvelous treatment start it on their own children. Like with everything else, some children respond, some do not.

EXPERIENCE AND CAUSES OF AUTISM

JENNY: What do you think autism feels like?

DR. JERRY: Many of the children are in physical pain because of their comorbid conditions. This pain can be from headaches, tummy aches, self-inflicted, and possibly in other sites we just do not know about. Many children also suffer with mental pain, frustration, and not being able to live up to, or even understand, others' expectations. Another source of pain can include the irrational fears generated by distorted interpretations of information brought to them by their senses, resulting in covering their ears, pacing, running, and tantruming. The interpretations from their senses can be incredibly unsettling for them and can greatly contribute to their behaviors in a particular setting.

Let's explore this a little deeper with an example. When a child enters one of those *BIG* stores, like Home Depot, and hears the buzzing of those big lights that are up in the ceiling or the echoing of sound throughout the rafters, they can go into a panic mode (full "flight or fight"). A lunchroom at school can be a huge problem for these kids due to the intense sounds generated. I have children who are very sensitive to fluorescent bulbs and they just go ballistic in a fluorescent-light environment. We have to be mindful and sensitive to what's going on with these children both externally and internally, and never forget their medical problems.

GENETICS

JENNY: What about the doctors who say it's genetic, it's genetic, it's genetic.

DR. JERRY: Well, there is certainly a genetic model. You can be born allergic to cats and if you're never around cats, you're just fine. It's only when you're exposed to cats that your genetic manifestations show up. I think some of the biochemical pathways that these kids have are either broken or weak. They would have been fine if they hadn't been exposed to certain toxins or environmental conditions. It's the same thing as if you gave everybody a shot of penicillin. You'll find, if you will, the genetic weakness in those certain individuals who have an anaphylactic reaction, like my wife, who would be dead in five minutes. Is it genetic? Well, sort of, because it's been programmed in there. But if I never give my wife a shot of penicillin, she will never have a major problem.

JENNY: I use the diabetes analogy. If you become obese, you might trigger diabetes.

DR. JERRY: That's right. Health risks (as in your example, being overweight) may unmask preprogrammed genetic weaknesses. And that's why you'll hear people talking about this set of children as the canaries in the coal mine. They're the ones who are not going to do well when exposed to a certain amount of environmental toxins. And we're going to find them very quickly.

TRIGGERS

JENNY: There's not just one way to get to autism. There are a few different side streets to get to the highway.

DR. JERRY: Yes, and the analogy I would use is this:

Let's say I have four children in my office with a cough. Everybody recognizes that they have coughs—even people on the streets can point and say, "Oh, look, those children have coughs." But one child is coughing because he's having an asthma attack.

And another child is coughing because he has a cold. Another child, maybe a two-year-old, is coughing because he swallowed a little toy part and it went down into his lungs. But the final common diagnosis, if you will, is a cough. Autism is much the same way. We can look at these kids and they can go and get formally evaluated at a major medical institution, and they say, "Yes, they have autism." But the underlying mechanism is totally different from one child to another. And one learns no more from this diagnosis of autism than one learns from "cough" in my example.

JENNY: Damn! That's a kick-ass analogy.

DR. JERRY: (Laughs) I promised my wife there will be no swearing in this book.

JENNY: So I can swear, but you can't?

DR. JERRY: (Laughs) Or both of us can try to not swear.

JENNY: Well, that's no fun, but okay. I'll try really really hard. Let's talk about pesticides. They can trigger autism, too, right?

DR. JERRY: I think we need to take a long, hard look at the environmental toxins in general. We have to consider that the pesticides, along with other environmental exposures, may truly be affecting our developing children (from the point of conception on). But what we do know is that the human body does a whole lot better with the least amount of toxins, so it would be wise for all of us not to poison our bodies.

JENNY: So Mom should be cautious of her environmental toxins before and during pregnancy?

DR. JERRY: Everybody has a certain capacity to detoxify their body. It would be wise not to exceed this inborn capacity to detoxify. I am concerned that this is exactly what we are doing with some of our children and this is accounting for the huge surge in autism, along with the increasing diagnosis of mental illness, asthma, and allergies.

Let's think of this in a different way. Consider that we are all born with a garbage can that we can dump our toxins into. As long as the can has room, toxins can be dumped into it. But what if the can is full? The toxins will build up outside the can and can cause disease. Two more variables to consider here: One is that we are all born with different-sized garbage cans, some bigger and some smaller. The next is how efficiently we can dump our garbage can so it can accept more toxins. Now it becomes easy to understand how our children with autism can develop symptoms at different times following different exposures. They are just indicating to us when their "garbage container" began to overflow along with the severity.

VACCINE DAMAGE TO THE IMMUNE SYSTEM AND SIGNS OF A DAMAGED IMMUNE SYSTEM

JENNY: Do you think these kids come into this world with a broken immune system or do you think vaccines damage the immune system from being able to detoxify future toxins?

DR. JERRY: It can be both. The immune system can be damaged because of toxins. Furthermore, the immune system is initially modified by vaccines and their contents, for better or for worse.

The most common outward manifestations of a damaged immune system seen in our clinic are recurrent ear infections and sinus infections. Being that 80 percent of the immune system is involved with the gastrointestinal tract, it is not surprising to know that chronic diarrhea, chronic constipation, and recurrent abdominal pain are other common outward manifestations of a damaged immune system. Another sign that the immune system is not working properly is the development of hypersensitivity to allergens in our environment. You'll see these kids walking around with dark circles under their eyes, bright red cheeks, and bright red ears. These are just examples of what the children "look" like. An evaluation of the immune system in the laboratory (more blood work) will show us why.

JENNY: So autism really is a toxic overload.

DR. JERRY: It certainly appears that a toxic overload impacts the body's defense systems with the total end result being a child who cannot appropriately manage everyday stimuli.

Mercury

JENNY: Let's talk about mercury. Everyone believes it was completely removed out of vaccines because it's what doctors and news reporters are saying, which isn't true. It was only reduced. Why did they ever think mercury was okay to give to humans?

DR. JERRY: Well, they've never really done studies on it. It's one of those things that we've always used because it's a cheap preservative. It's always been okay.

JENNY: Wasn't the only real test for mercury in humans done sometime in 1930?

DR. JERRY: No safety data have been done. There was a trial of mercury used on patients already dying. This trial looked to see if mercury hastened death.

JENNY: Hastened death? Do you mean they were just seeing if it killed you quickly?

DR. JERRY: Yes. In 1938, researchers found serious vascular damage from mercury exposure. We have to understand that it's well accepted that mercury is one of the most toxic substances known to man on this planet. So how can they justify giving even a small amount of mercury to a pregnant woman in the form of a flu shot in her sixth month or in giving it to a newborn in the form of hepatitis B? Why would we inject anything that we know is a deadly toxin? It just doesn't make sense.

And it's not even a very good preservative. It doesn't really do a good job. Put another way, do you think they could do safety studies of thimerosal in vaccines given to newborns today? Not in the United States.

But a lessened deadly toxin is still a deadly toxin. And we talk about exquisitely small amounts and say, "Well, it's a very small amount." But you don't need anything but a very small amount to do damage. Mercury has a tremendous affinity for brain tissue, so even small amounts can potentially end up in the brain.

JENNY: Because the brain is fatty and metals store inside fat?

DR. JERRY: There are a lot of theories as to why mercury is drawn to the brain. It currently is believed that mercury is drawn to areas where there is intense growth (metabolism). The brain in the growing infant certainly meets this requirement, and different areas of the brain are rapidly developing, while others may be growing nominally. So, timing of the environmental insult (in this case, the exposure to mercury) will affect the area of the brain that happens to be really turned on to growth at that particular instant. This may help us understand why we have so many variations in our children with autism. Removing a neurotoxin, such as mercury, from our vaccine supply, was an excellent decision, but has been painfuly slow.

JENNY: In 2002 they said they were going to remove mercury from vaccines and right around that time they added the flu shot to the schedule, which has mercury in it. Are they that stupid? Wait, of course they are.

DR. JERRY: In 2002 the manufacturers changed the formulations of the contents of vaccines, namely decreasing the thimerosal (notice LOWER dose of thimerosal) and increasing the aluminum. The warehouses full of the thimerosal-containing vaccines continued to ship out, as scheduled, over the next two to three years. There is serious concern over the persistence of mercury in the vaccines, which includes many of the flu shots.

JENNY: I include a vaccine schedule at the end of the book, along with a list of shots that still contain mercury. (See page 304.)

GENETIC VULNERABILITY

JENNY: As you know, Doc, many neurologists and scientists are all looking for the one autism gene, but our autism community has always said it's because of a genetic vulnerability. What exactly is this genetic vulnerability? Is it a little gene? Could it be an autoimmune gene? Does it simply mean more vulnerable to toxins?

DR. JERRY: Our genes are the blueprint of how everything in our body functions. Everything.

Genetic vulnerability refers to a weakness or susceptibility that an individual may possess that may put one at risk for disease if certain conditions are met. This vulnerability can be determined by multiple areas on our individual blueprints. We are protected with lots of backup systems that can function to take over if there are some genetically "corrupted" pathways. One such pathway, labeled the methylation pathway, seems to be an area of concern in children on the autistic spectrum.

CONVINCING YOUR DOCTOR

JENNY: How do you emotionally deal with the medical community and the scientists who say, "This is all witch stuff"?

DR. JERRY: I present the child with autism as a child who is ill. We explore the concept of treating many of the conditions we have already outlined in this book.

For example, if I'm trying to illustrate that these children have chronic inflammatory bowel disease, I may present many different cases with photomicrographs, pathologists' reports showing that these kids have inflammatory bowel disease, along with the histories that the parents give. Bottom line: I break the autism down into "medical compartments" and say, "Let's look at the disease the child has, not autism; forget autism."

INFORMED CONSENT

JENNY: Was it hard to continue vaccinating kids in your practice?

DR. JERRY: Oh, I had to stop. Absolutely, I had to stop. Once I realized that vaccines were triggering autism I started phasing them out, for example, the hepatitis B. At this point in my career, there was a huge push to have all the kids vaccinated. One day, I was called by a school nurse saying that she was going to turn me into the medical board because I wasn't vaccinating teenagers with the hepatitis B vaccine. But I wanted the parents to know what was being given to their kids so that they could make an intelligent decision. I explained all of the good stuff about the hepatitis B, but I also explained all of the potential consequences of the hepatitis B and they were electing not to get it. I told this to the school nurse and she said, "Oh, don't tell them about the bad parts of it. Just tell them about the good parts."

JENNY: Did she actually say that?

DR. JERRY: Yes, and I told her, "Well, that's not really informed consent." And she said, "You don't have to do informed consent." So I realized, *Okay. We really have a problem here.*

JENNY: So, after seeing the effect of the vaccines on your son Josh, you began informing people of the consequences.

DR. JERRY: Yes, I was actually providing parents with true information prior to obtaining their written consent. In other words, before the parents actually accepted the shot, they knew why we were doing it, what we were using, and the consequences that had been associated with it.

JENNY: What would they usually say?

DR. JERRY: They were shocked most of the time. They would say, "Really? My child has a chance of having seizures or other side effects?"

Upon hearing all of the potential side effects, many did elect to postpone the vaccines. Some would get the vaccines, but at least with true medical informed consent. I believe parents have the right to raise their kids the way they want to raise them, even if it is to fully vaccinate them.

JENNY: Are you pretty impressed with this generation of parents who are proactive?

DR. JERRY: I'm amazed by most parents. They are so well educated and really want a physician who is willing to work with them and to explain what we do and do not know. In fact, they often come in and they'll tell me what the diagnosis is (and will be right on!), which is pretty cool. I'll say, "You figured that out on your own? Cool! What do you need me for?"

MOMMY RADAR

JENNY: One of the best tools God has given us mothers is instinct. It's like we have this built-in radar device buried deep within us that guides us while we raise our children. Evan is where he is today because I followed my instinct. Can you confirm that mommy radar ROCKS?

DR. JERRY: Mommy radar is phenomenal. I think we, as a medical community, have always underestimated mommy radar on how the kids are doing. And I can tell you, maybe because my lovely wife beat this into me, that she really does know what's going on. Mothers do possess an excellent skill set and instinctively know when their children are not "quite right."

JENNY: Well, I think it's time we get it on and give these moms out there some amazing direction on how to heal autism.

DR. JERRY: And dads! You can't forget about the dads!

JENNY: Who? Ha, ha. Just kidding!

YOUR DIARY: THE TOOL YOU'LL NEED TO MANAGE YOUR CHILD'S HEALING

JENNY: Now, I know we've just thrown a lot at you moms and dads, but in order to get started on this book, you're going to have to take a lot of notes—not on the book but on every single thing that goes into and out of your child, his behavior, his health, his sleep, his meds, his supplements, everything. Without this, you won't know what's working and what isn't, and without this, your doctor will have a hard time collaborating with you in the recovery of your child. Dr. Jerry gave me a great idea for tracking Evan's progress. It's something he gives all his patients and now we're going to share it with you. So, before you do anything else, get a notebook, and get ready to track the following EVERY SINGLE DAY:

DAILY DIARY

(scale of 1–4, where 4 is most intense or highest)

Bowel movement (frequency and size, scale of 1–4)
Supplements (dosage and frequency)
Food diary (yes, you need to write down everything he or she eats)
Sleep (hours, naps, and nighttime)
Rashes (describe color, size, and location; whether larger or smaller than previous day)
Self-injurious behavior (frequency during the day, or scale of 1–4)
Evenness of temperament (scale of 1–4)
Irritability (scale of 1–4)
Staring off into space (duration)
Flexibility versus rigidity (scale of 1–4)

DR. JERRY: Jenny, I'm glad you brought this up. I started using this for my son Josh and it was the diary, for instance, that made me realize my son didn't do well on a supplement called GABA. He'd lose language and start crawling around on the floor. Because I could see from the diary that the behavior began when I started him on the supplement and that it was the only new thing I'd introduced, I realized right away that it was the culprit. So I removed GABA and he was fine. A supplement is easy to track. Some of these other things can creep up on you and you won't notice little changes each day, say in sleeping or eating. But when you look at how the weeks and months shape up, it'll be easier to spot patterns and triggers. Or for example, I had a bunch of kids have difficulty during December. There was nothing different in their diaries, but there was a difference in their environments: Christmas trees, and the mold that comes with it. So you have to look at everything in order to become partners wth your physicians to heal your kids.

2

DIET
Where to Begin

Doc, I heard that if I try and change some foods in his diet, his behavior might improve.
Don't start with that! I'm tired of you moms coming in here thinking food and vitamins will help. Only Prozac helps behavior.

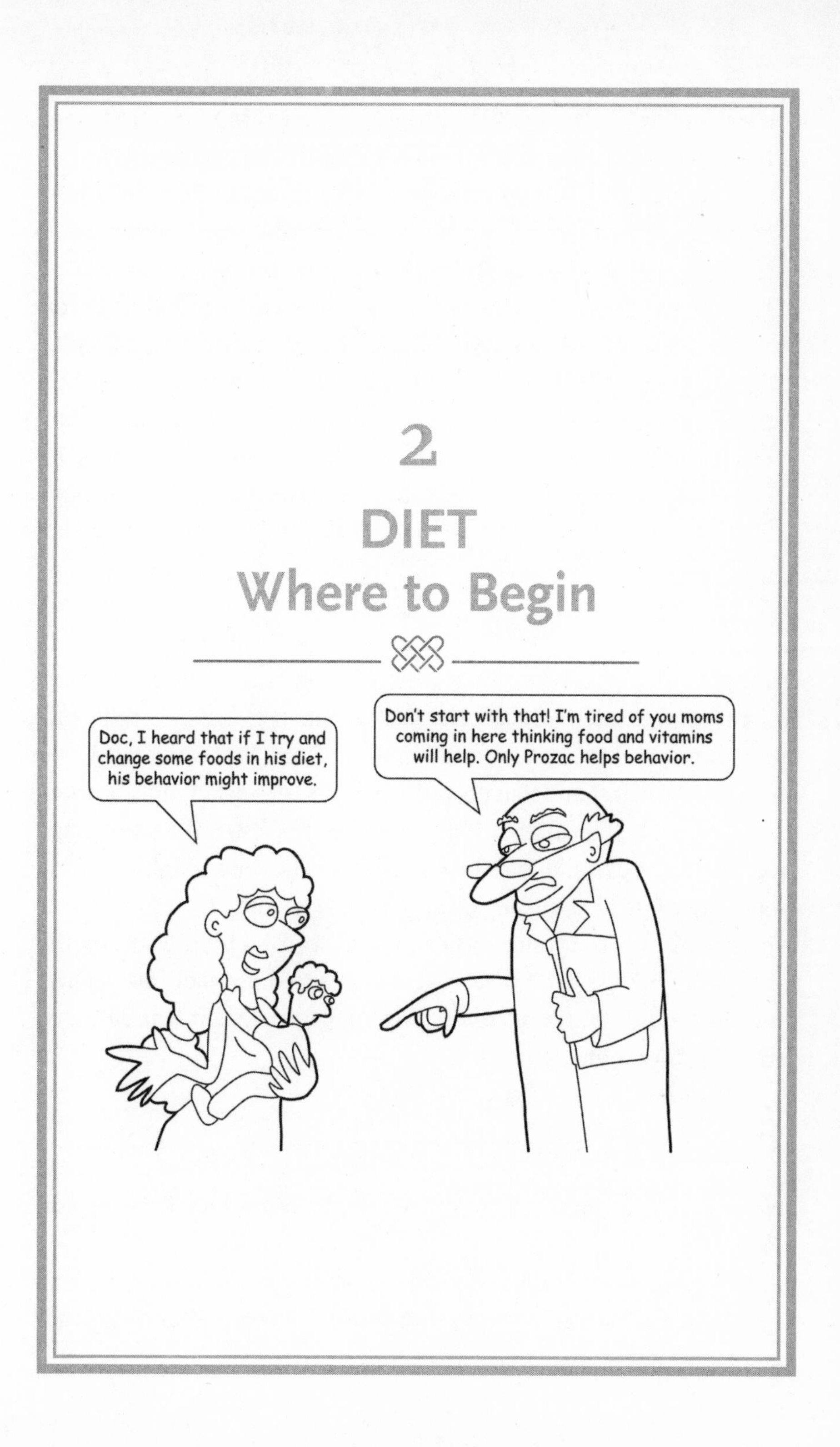

ONE OF THE FIRST THINGS I tell parents is that the gluten-free and casein-free diet, which removes wheat, rye, barley, spelt, and other grains, and the casein found in dairy, is the first thing to try, because it's the safest and usually gives parents the instant gratification that diets can help heal their kids. There may be other diets more appropriate for your child, but the GFCF diet is the one I highly recommend right out of the gate. Once I educated myself on WHY it is beneficial, it made it much easier to stick to. Watching Evan utter a four-word sentence after a few weeks on the diet made me realize what we put into our kids' mouths is vitally important. I urge every parent to at least give it a try!

GLUTEN AND CASEIN

JENNY: Can you explain why diet seems to be so beneficial to our kids?

DR. JERRY: We have found that gluten and dairy seem to affect a lot of our children with autism and thus we see a lot of children respond terrifically when these are removed from the diet. The goal behind changing diets is to remove chemicals, toxins, and potential neurotransmitters, which are liberated when foods are broken down (in the process of digestion). These substances could be toxic for the brain and cause behavioral trouble in kids who are sensitive to them—whether it is gluten, dairy, phenols (which are chemicals found in food), salicylates (found in foods), rice, corn, or others. Whether kids test as allergic or not, often they are causing a negative effect on the child, and they must be removed. Each child has his or her own set of sensitivities that he or she can't deal with properly. When we change their diets, 80 percent of the kids with autism seem to respond.

JENNY: That's a pretty big percentage. Are they actually allergic to wheat and dairy? Is this why they have a reaction?

DR. JERRY: Not necessarily. If they are allergic, it can cause inflammation from just eating them and that is one response. Another response would come from the partial breakdown of gluten (from commonly used flours) and casein (from dairy) into neurotransmitters that act like opiates (morphine-like substances) in our children's brains. So it is not that they're allergic to these foods, but there is a morphine-like substance that's affecting the brain.

JENNY: So to break that down a little more, you're saying that even if the child's allergy test does not come up as allergic to wheat or dairy, it's essential to remove these things because sometimes they make our kids drunk or stoned from the opiates that are being created when these kids eat them.

DR. JERRY: That's correct. And if you look at opiates, one of their hallmarks is constipation. So a lot of these kids have a lot of constipation problems. Another use of opiates in medicine is to block pain. And as we discussed, many of our children have a very high threshold to pain.

Opiate Effect of Gluten

JENNY: That's so true. So many parents have the same story of their kid being able to withstand a hard fall or even break a bone without sometimes crying. That makes sense that the opiate would act like a painkiller.

DR. JERRY: Another characteristic of opiates is that they are very addictive. And what do these kids do? They will crave the foods that contain gluten and dairy. This can explain why they gravitate to these foods and why it is so difficult to remove them.

JENNY: One of the biggest things I hear from parents is, "But all my child drinks is milk. And all he eats is cheese. If I take those away, he won't eat anything." I try to explain to them it's because they are addicted to them. And that it's even more proof that they need to be removed from the diet immediately.

DR. JERRY: When you remove them, kids will commonly find the other sources that have wheat or dairy in them. I have had several children eating out of a dog food bag because one of the major ingredients in that dog food was gluten. I've had kids lick the floor because the floor cleaner that was used had gluten in it. They can smell this gluten and we can't. They know where it is.

I remember when we went gluten-free for the first time with my son Josh. We were all at a restaurant watching him eat a gluten-free meal, but his attention was on the two-week-old soda cracker that was on the floor. My wife and I could tell that he was trying to figure out how to drop his napkin on the floor so he could reach down and get that piece of old soda cracker without us noticing.

JENNY: The same thing with Evan. I caught him one time in the pantry on the top shelf just sitting there eating a loaf of bread.

Opiate/Gluten Withdrawal Symptoms

DR. JERRY: That is why the withdrawal symptoms are so bad with these kids.

JENNY: Yeah, let's talk about the withdrawals these kids experience.

DR. JERRY: Sometimes you may feel like checking them into "Betty Ford." You're taking a drug away from an addict. They can be irritable, cranky. Their noses can get red and run. They can be more stimmy and throw more tantrums. These things could last for two weeks. Obviously, it's easier to manage a two-year-old who is going through withdrawals than, say, a twelve-year-old. If you're going to do it, don't wait. It's just going to get harder years from now.

JENNY: And would you suggest to parents to take their child off dairy or gluten first?

DR. JERRY: Well, I remember when I first started doing this, I was very adamant that gluten and dairy be removed at the same time and I actually almost put one kid in the hospital. He just about went catatonic. He was on the couch and wouldn't move. He would not eat. He would not drink. He would have rather died than not get his gluten or dairy. I don't mean that figuratively. I mean that literally. He was not going to eat or drink. So much so that I actually had to put him on gluten and dairy to rehydrate him to get his energy level up.

I learned then that slow withdrawal works best. I now recommend removing dairy first. Get your child used to being dairy-free. And then slowly think of different foods that can replace the gluten. For example, if he's used to eating chicken nuggets from a fast-food place, learn how to make GFCF ones or buy them premade. Some moms use their favorite potato chips and then roll the potato chips with a rolling pin, dip the chicken in egg, and then "bread" it with the crushed potato chips. But some kids will not touch that. If it's not McDonald's, they don't want it. Even if you put that in a McDonald's box, they know really quickly it's not gluten. So it can be difficult. You should include a list of Web sites that have GFCF recipes so moms will know how to cook these things on their own.

JENNY: Great idea! I'll post them at the end (see page 341). I started Evan on the GFCF diet a few weeks after his diagnosis. I'd read about it online, before you became Evan's doctor, and I took him off both at the same time. He didn't have huge tantrums like I hear about from other moms, but he did refuse to eat all the GFCF foods I put in front of him. I didn't know what to do, so my mom gave me some great advice. She told me to pull the food away and not replace it with another meal. If he wouldn't eat breakfast, then wait until lunch, and if he didn't eat lunch, offer him dinner. She said he wasn't going to starve to death. By the time lunch came around the next day he was never so happy to eat GFCF nuggets. Other moms since then have told me they had to do the same thing. I guess in that other little boy's case it could be more severe, but I encourage parents to not give up too easily.

GOING CASEIN-FREE: HOW TO IDENTIFY DAIRY HIDDEN IN PRODUCTS

DR. JERRY: So now I recommend removing dairy first. That's easier. Moms and dads can wrap their heads around what dairy products are. They have to learn all the little code names for what dairy is.

JENNY: "Casein." That's the word that took me three months to figure out. Packages might say "dairy-free," but there could still be casein in the ingredients. Casein is milk. Rice milk and almond milk are not.

DR. JERRY: Yes, rice milks and soy milks are not milks. Rice does not have boobies. You cannot milk them. Neither do the soybeans. The only reason they say "milk" on the containers is because it's a marketing term to make moms think that they're getting something like milk. It's just sugar water derived from rice or almonds or potatoes, depending on what you use. It's a medium to get supplements in. It's something to cook with, like making gluten-free pancakes or in GFCF cereals. But it's not "milk," so it's safe to use these products—just watch the sugar content!

JENNY: So many moms have said to me, "But how will they get their calcium if they don't drink milk?"

DR. JERRY: Give them vitamins and minerals, which of course include calcium.

JENNY: We'll discuss supplements next. What about soy? I've noticed a lot of these kids can't have soy and I've also read that soy is not so good.

DR. JERRY: Yes, 50 to 60 percent of the kids who can't tolerate dairy can't tolerate soy as well. So I don't even go to soy milk or soy cheese.

HOW TO READ A LABEL

If you want to get your child off dairy and gluten, you'll have to become an expert at reading labels. It's not always obvious. Read the allergy alerts on packages that tell you whether or not what you're buying was produced on machines that also process dairy or gluten. If it doesn't say, call the manufacturer.

Label Alerts

Remember, "dairy-free" does not always mean "dairy-free." Look for the word "casein" in the ingredients. If there's casein, don't buy it. Hidden dairy ingredients: casein

Remember, "wheat-free" does not mean "gluten-free." "No gluten ingredients" also does not mean "gluten-free." You have to know the manufacturing process. Hidden gluten ingredients: starch, vinegar

Gluten-containing products other than bread and pasta: soy sauce, ice cream, many over-the-counter medicines in tablet form, some miso paste, some sushi rice

GOING GLUTEN-FREE WHETHER YOUR CHILD TESTS POSITIVE FOR THE ALLERGY OR NOT

JENNY: Let's talk about gluten, which is in wheat, rye, barley, spelt, and perhaps oats as well.

DR. JERRY: Gluten is derived from the Latin word "glut," which means "glue." It is a small piece of a protein that gives flour its elastic consistency when baked. Commonly used flours that contain gluten are wheat, oats, barley, and rye. So, the protein that gives pizza dough the ability to be tossed into the air and formed, or the bagel that is so chewy, is gluten. That's why these guys can throw the stuff up in the air and it comes down like rubber. That's the elastic gluten that's holding it together.

In the old days people would mix water and flour together and put up wallpaper. The flour and its "gluten" was the glue!

JENNY: That's gross. I have a gluten allergy and it really does feel like glue when it's going through my intestines.

DR. JERRY: This gluten, which holds baked goods together, is what is actually being turned into the morphine-like substance. We call it gliadorphin (or gluteomorphin). It is this small protein (seven amino acids), and because kids with autism can't break down this protein, it acts up in our children's brains. It reacts with the opiate receptors in their brains. It acts like a narcotic. We can even measure the gliadorphin in the urine. Just like you can go into a job interview that requires urine "drug" testing, we can measure the opiates in our children's urine.

Now, we know that the kids aren't doing morphine, so if it is positive, the urine can be further fractionated to determine the derivative source of the positive "morphine test." The test will identify the source as dairy, gluten, or both. Some parents need this information prior to embarking on a gluten-free, dairy-free diet—especially the dads. "Why do we need to do this diet? Prove it to me." So I run the tests and show them that there are a lot of morphine-like substances in the urine.

JENNY: I'm glad you just said that because I want to reiterate that a lot of people say, "Well, my husband made me test for an allergy and there wasn't any."

DR. JERRY: A good example for this might be potatoes. You can test negative for a potato allergy/sensitivity, but every time it is eaten by the child, it makes him very obsessive-compulsive. So, even though a child isn't allergic to potatoes, it can absolutely cause behavior problems for that child.

JENNY: It's amazing to me that gluten could be hidden in so many foods, like soy sauce.

DR. JERRY: That is why it is imperative to check labels!

SPECIFIC CARBOHYDRATE DIET

JENNY: So let's move on to another popular diet, which is the Specific Carbohydrate Diet. The Specific Carbohydrate Diet is another limiting/removal diet. This diet consists of meats, eggs, vegetables, nuts, and low-sugar fruits while avoiding starches, grains, pasta, legumes, and bread. I know that carbs can aggravate existing bacteria in the gut, which is why so many moms prefer this diet over GFCF. Are you a big fan of the Specific Carbohydrate Diet?

DR. JERRY: Yes, this is a popular diet. But remember, whether a diet works or does not work depends on the child. What a diet really means is the removal of specific things that may be toxic for that particular child. I have kids who are like fruitaholics. They're eating fruit all the time. They'll eat eight apples a day. They'll eat five bananas a day. They'll be drinking juice and eating fruit all day. I'll say, "You know, he's so stimmy, he's so irritable—let's take him off fruit for a week and see what happens." All fruit, anything that's fruit-derived. Nothing with fruit in it passes through the mouth of a fruit addict. And they go on what I call a fruit-free diet. What I'm doing is asking, "Is there something in the fruit adversely affecting this child? Is there something in the fruit that's messing up this kid?"

JENNY: But the Specific Carbohydrate Diet has so much to do with eliminating carbs, right?

DR. JERRY: In this diet, we are asking the question whether or not certain carbohydrates are messing this child up. This diet tests to see if the child does better with monosaccharides—or very simple sugars such as glucose and fructose, which are readily absorbed by the digestive tract—rather than di- or polysaccharides (complex carbohydrates found in refined sugar), which require digestion and potentially foster the growth of harmful bacteria and yeast in the gut. This diet consists of meats, eggs, vegetables, nuts, and low-sugar fruits and eliminates starches, grains, pastas, legumes, and breads.

JENNY: So, parents really have to do a trial-and-error when it comes to some diets. There's not a blood test that can say, "Oh, this is going to work or this one is not going to work."

I've noticed that most parents are doing trial-and-error, anyway, because they can't get into a biomedical doctor fast enough. It's a year to a year and a half wait for many, so they go, "I'm going to take medicine into my own hands, as best as I can," which is why we're doing this book.

DR. JERRY: The reason we try this particular elimination diet is to see if a child improves after we eliminate certain carbohydrates from the diet. As we've explained, when disaccharides and polysaccharides are not digested properly, they pass down the digestive tract and become food for yeast and probably some unhealthy bacteria. By removing these carbohydrates, the children don't have to break them down and they're deleting the food source for yeast to grow. At least, that's the idea. We often hear that when you're on this diet, you can't grow yeast. And yeast, when overgrown, can cause havoc within the body. But the bottom line is some of the kids do really improve and it is worth a try. There are some other problems that are alleviated with this diet, such as exposure to potential pesticides found in grains. So, this is a rational diet to try. Essentially, it is a meat, fruit, nut, and veggie diet. All fresh.

JENNY: What do people do, then, to make muffins or chicken nuggets if you can't use GFCF flour?

DR. JERRY: GFCF flour is usually made up of rice, so moms should use nut flour. They'll take almonds or they'll take pecans and grind them into flour. Then your breads, your coffee cakes, your muffins, whatever, are now nut-based. The problem with that is that some of our kids are so allergic to things in the environment that when you constantly give them a nut-based carbohydrate, they're going to become allergic to the nuts. And we need to be sure that they are gluten-free nuts. Check the manufacturing.

JENNY: Oh, nuts!

DR. JERRY: Good one! Moving on, Elaine Gottschall basically brought the Specific Carbohydrate Diet into existence. She was treating inflammatory bowel disease, before autism was even on the radar. It was good for inflammatory bowel disease. And it's good for a lot of our kids. Remember, many of our children do have a form of inflammatory bowel disease, currently called autistic enterocolitis.

JENNY: Well, when I toured the country and talked to mom after mom, I was really blown away by how many parents said they saw great things from doing the Specific Carbohydrate Diet. People would applaud in the audience whenever I said the name. Parents really believe in it, but it takes real warrior parents to make the commitment because it's so limiting.

LOW OXALATE DIET

JENNY: I've also heard of some parents doing the Low Oxalate Diet. I read that oxalates are molecules that, if crystallized, can cause some problems. Is this correct?

DR. JERRY: Oxalates have been observed to increase oxidative stress and decrease glutathione levels. Remember that glutathione is one of the most important antioxidants our body makes. Oxalates also enhance the inflammatory response, which can harm tissues in the body. So, to answer your question, yes, the crystal formation can be a source of pain. Oxalates are very poorly absorbed in the digestive tract but can more easily be absorbed in the presence of a leaky gut. In this case, removing foods known to have elevated levels of oxalates has been beneficial because these foods cause inflammation, they decrease the production of glutathione and harm the immune system. There are published lists that describe which foods are high in oxalates and thus easily avoided.

JENNY: Yes, I included a link at the end of this chapter (see page 51). What kind of problems can occur with this diet?

DR. JERRY: One problem that occurs is when parents try to implement different diets at the same time. For example, if one selects the Specific Carbohydrate Diet, in which the carbohydrates are nut-based, and then concurrently selects the Low Oxalate Diet . . . there go the nuts, as they are high in oxalate content, and now the parent faces the problem of not being able to offer any baked products.

JENNY: What are some of those remarkable changes that are common amongst our kids after implementing a diet?

DR. JERRY: The first thing that diets tend to help with is sleeping through the night. Other benefits include language, connectedness, eye contact, and a sense of calming with a decrease in stimming behavior. A sense that the child is now comfortable in the skin he's in.

JENNY: Have you heard of or seen kids who have recovered from diet alone?

DR. JERRY: Actually, I have had children who go on a gluten-free, dairy-free diet and are essentially cured of their autistic traits. And that's what I've called the "lotto" winners of autism. It's not common, but we rejoice and we're thrilled for those families. But for me, in what I do, this diet intervention is just the beginning. Mostly, these children's roadway to recovery is in steps. And the things that we do may take five steps or require ninety-five steps to recovery.

JENNY: What about the nonresponders? I hear parents say, "It didn't work, we tried it and saw nothing."

DR. JERRY: What is a nonresponder in my book? A nonresponder in my book is somebody who has been gluten-free, dairy-free 100 percent for at least three months with NO, and I mean NO, discernable changes or improvements. Keep in mind that you can't be 90 percent gluten-free and say, "He's a nonresponder." The fact is, there is enough gluten in one crouton to mess up a child (who would be a responder, like my son) for two weeks. So they have to be 100 percent. And they have to make sure that they really did try, and they really did tell me, "I knew all the hidden gluten names, I knew all the hidden dairy names. The kid was just eating meats and fruits and vegetables, nothing packaged. He did that for three months. His urine was normal. There's nothing there." That's pretty rare. But if they truly did not respond, then we move on to the next biomedical intervention to try to heal them.

GOING ORGANIC

JENNY: I want to talk about how important organic foods are for our kids. Can you get into it a little?

DR. JERRY: One of the things that I have found across the country right now is that we have a generation of moms and dads I lovingly refer to as "baking impaired." They did not grow up with a mom (or a dad!) at home showing them how to cook. They do not know how to measure; they don't even know what a cup is or how many ounces are in a cup. They truly are baking impaired. Fortunately, there are enough options in the marketplace today where one can purchase 80 percent of GFCF meals already done, but this can be prohibitively expensive because they are found only in health food stores. In an attempt to LOWER the grocery bill, we do have to make things from scratch again, like many of our grandparents did. We also have to make the food as organic and as fresh as possible. Not from a box. When you ask a group of people why we should eat organic foods, the number one reason they say is because they don't have pesticides in them. And that's true and that's very important. But what's even more important is that if a piece of broccoli or a strawberry is going to grow in the wild, so to speak, without the aid of pesticides, it has got to be really tough! And what God gave these foods to keep from being bored into by worms or eaten by mold or whatever are the nutrients that we also need to keep us healthy and cancer-free. These nutrient-dense foods are required to keep our immune system healthy. If a piece of food can survive in the field without the aid of pesticides and come to the marketplace and be healthy enough for you to buy, then it's going to have a lot more nutrients provided in each bite compared to "conventionally grown" produce. It may even contain nutrients that have not yet been discovered.

JENNY: You know, I've read this report about how the AAP [the American Academy of Pediatrics] had come out saying that they had done a double-blind study. I don't know if you saw that about the artificial coloring, the red dye, and in their double-blind test for these ADHD, attention deficit/hyperactivity disorder kids, they confirmed that diet did make a difference. It proved that removing artificial colors and flavors decreased the behaviors associated with ADD, attention deficit disorder, and ADHD.

DR. JERRY: Every schoolteacher knows that the kids are just atrocious after Halloween and after Easter because of all the sugar, food colorings, and the dyes. And it took the AAP until now to come out with something like that?

Avoid Dyes in Foods!

JENNY: I know. It's just crazy. Can you explain why red dye affects our kids? Because Evan is psychotic if I give him a Pedialyte red Popsicle.

DR. JERRY: Dyes are biologically active. They are generally derived from petroleum and coal tar. They are known to cause hyperactivity, eczema, loss of focus and concentration, allergic reactions, and even cancer.

High-Fructose Corn Syrup

JENNY: And let's talk about the food Satan, which is also known as high-fructose corn syrup.

DR. JERRY: High-fructose corn syrup use has steadily increased since 1966. It is derived from cornstarch, whose sugar is glucose. This glucose is enzymatically acted upon and forms the fructose/glucose syrup. This type of sugar promotes the formation and storage of triglycerides, which have a tendency to lay fat around the belly. It is estimated now that 40 percent of our sugar intake is from high-fructose corn syrup, which causes the body changes like the poochy belly we are seeing in our teens.

JENNY: I've noticed that twenty-year-olds all have this pooch.

DR. JERRY: That may very well be the high-fructose corn syrup found in mostly all sodas and in many foods. It preferentially deposits fat in a woman between the belly button and pubic bone. Even though they have never had a baby, they look like they've had a little baby.

JENNY: Yeah, baby pouch.

DR. JERRY: It also seems to impact behaviors that include loss of concentration, increase in activity—not being able to sit down because they are so hyper—especially in our autistic population. So, this is one sugar source quickly nixed out of the diet.

JENNY: I go crazy when I see parents give their kids soda.

DR. JERRY: Sometimes I see it in baby bottles.

JENNY: No!

DR. JERRY: As a pediatrician, I have seen chocolate milk in baby bottles and I have even seen soda in baby bottles. And you look at people nowadays and you see what's happening. We've changed our food, and our population is getting more and more obese. It's time to take the reins of what we put into our bodies!

So we talk about vaccines, but it's vaccines AND foods AND environmental toxins. The stuff Mom ate for twenty years now that has been stored in her body. Mom is now giving many of these substances to the baby. So there are a lot of things that have changed from when I was a kid growing up. This was in the late 50s and early 60s. We had Pepsi every other Friday night. We had one bottle that we shared. And if we went to McDonald's, we had to drive really far and it was a special treat. Looking at different polls, it appears that two to three nights out of seven, families are eating prepared foods found in all those freezer cases that you see in the grocery store (just go into the Walmart or Costco freezer sections and see how much prepared food is available), or they're eating out. It's not the fresh foods anymore.

JENNY: I also want to bring up artificial colors, artificial flavors, artificial preservatives, and nitrates. I don't give anything to Evan that has nitrates, but I still don't know what a nitrate is. I just know it's bad.

Nitrates and Nitrites

DR. JERRY: We are trying to recover these children's brains, so we do not want to dump any more chemicals into their bodies. We want their diets to be as pristine as possible because we are trying to return all of their cycles that are currently vicious to their original, pristine functions. We want all of their biochemical functions to work, without any hindrance. So why would you dump soda or any other chemical into a kid whose brain is trying to recover? That just doesn't make sense. It's not a treatment, it's a toxin.

JENNY: What are sodium nitrates?

DR. JERRY: Sodium nitrates are preservatives that enhance the color of meats so they can be refrigerated and look pretty. Otherwise, these uncooked meats would be the color of cooked hamburger. Thus, in the refrigerator section, these nitrate-treated meats look healthy and nutritious. So nitrates are added as a preservative so that the "pinkness" of the meat stands out. There is a lot of science of the mind here. It is well understood which colors appeal best to consumers, and in this case, pink appears "healthy." (Check out the signs in the refrigerator case of salmon next time you are in the supermarket. . . . You'll see they add red/pink coloring to the fish!) We know that when nitrates are exposed to stomach acids, they are converted to nitrosamines, which are associated with cancer in animals.

Bottom line: The best preservative I know of is called the freezer!

HOW LONG DO YOU KEEP YOUR CHILD ON ANY DIET?

JENNY: I know I will always have Evan eat organic only and additive-free, with no artificial anything, but will he ever be able to go off the GFCF diet?

DR. JERRY: Our goal, especially for our young children, is to make it so that by the time they're teens, they can eat pizza with their buds. And unless they were born allergic to a specific food, they should be able to handle a more liberal diet. They may not be able to drink a glass of milk and dunk Oreos, but they can occasionally have one of the two. I know we will need to heal the gut (see Chapter 11), with biomedical interventions, so we can introduce these foods later. The good news is that many patients I have been working with for years and years are now able to consume a gluten and dairy diet.

JENNY: Why is that?

DR. JERRY: Their guts are healing from their immune systems becoming disregulated due to vaccines or other bacteria/viruses/fungi. Their gut is now doing what it was programmed to do in the first place before we interfered. The gut is 80 percent of the immune system! So my son Josh, for example, after ten years of gluten- and casein-free foods, is now eating gluten and dairy once a week.

JENNY: Many parents say, "My kid will only eat four things. How am I supposed to get him to change his eating when he barely eats to begin with?"

DR. JERRY: There can be a lot of complications involved with a child who severely self-limits. If the foods tend to be dairy and gluten (like macaroni and cheese), then we are back to talking about the addictive nature of these foods. But, there can be a severe obsessive-compulsive component to these behaviors that may actually cause the child to compulsively eat only certain foods and may even require a short course of medication to alleviate obsessive-compulsive disorder. Keep in mind, there can also be a severe sensory and behavioral component intertwined in the appetite center. So, the practitioner has to consider all these issues when composing a treatment plan.

JENNY: And isn't it true that if you eat the same thing every day, you can become allergic to it?

DR. JERRY: Our children can certainly become sensitized to the same foods consumed every day. Again, if the leaky gut, which consists of holes in the intestinal walls, is passing the same proteins over and over again, the immune system will make antibodies to these "foreign" proteins and there will be an immune response. This is why the children who have enough foods in their repertoire are encouraged to rotate the diet.

JENNY: Another thing I hear is, "There is no way in hell my kid will ever eat a vegetable." If that's the case for these parents, what do you do?

DR. JERRY: What do you do as far as giving vegetables to Evan?

JENNY: Well, he doesn't like them, so I juice them.

Juicing

DR. JERRY: That's perfect. Juicing is a great way to get those vegetables down.

JENNY: I bought a juicer from Target and threw a bag of organic spinach in there, after being washed really well, with one apple, and it tastes pretty good to me!

DR. JERRY: Does Evan like it?

JENNY: No, I usually just chase him with a giant syringe (no needle of course!) of it every day and he gets it down. The chasing has gone down to about two minutes now. I know it doesn't taste bad, but the color freaks him out. We've also done kale and beets; it's so good for our bodies that I started juicing every day, too. This way, Evan learns by example.

DR. JERRY: I recommend juicing especially if you can do organic. But, even if you can't afford organic produce, or if it is not available, conventionally grown produce will do fine; just wash it really well before juicing. If you have a child who will drink juiced veggies and fruits, this is a far better way to introduce vitamins and minerals into the diet than, say, many of the supplements available. Another potential source, especially if your child is open to smoothies, is the Garden of Plenty meal-replacement formula specifically blended for patients who are not able to eat or digest fruits and vegetables (www.kartnerhealth.com). With that said, one of the reasons we are giving them supplements is because they won't eat anything green. And they won't drink any of this wonderful juice. So, plan B: Supplement with vitamins, minerals, and oils.

JENNY: Any final words about changing the food?

DR. JERRY: Yes, our job is to recover these children so they are not lifelong dependents on family or on society. We are fighting for their lives, their independence, and if there is a food problem, just get rid of it—the stakes are too high. I do see a difference when it comes to removing certain foods and I urge parents to go into this 100 percent. Food affects behavior. That's a fact!

ADVICE

Start the GFCF diet. Avoid casein (dairy) and gluten (wheat). Things might say "wheat"-free but that does NOT mean gluten-free. Also, products might say, "lactose"-free but that does NOT mean casein-free. Look for rice milk or almond milk as alternatives to dairy. Use brown rice noodles and brown rice bread as noodle and bread substitutes. And don't forget to track food intake in your daily diary.

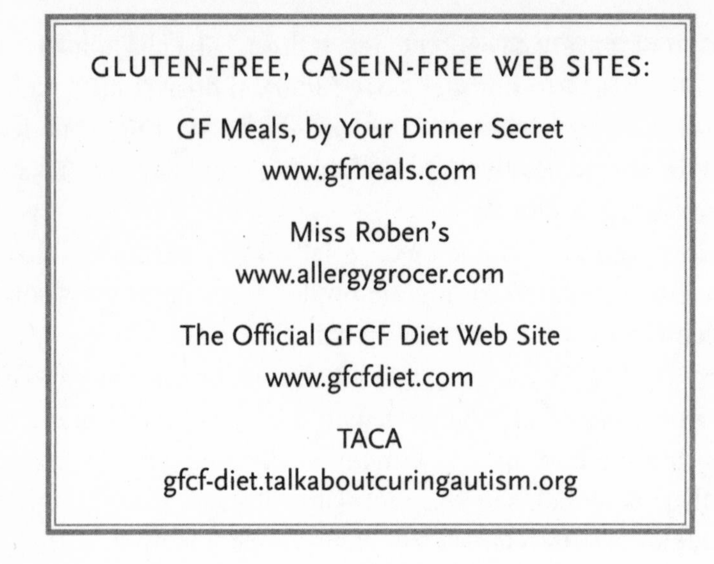
GLUTEN-FREE, CASEIN-FREE WEB SITES:

GF Meals, by Your Dinner Secret
www.gfmeals.com

Miss Roben's
www.allergygrocer.com

The Official GFCF Diet Web Site
www.gfcfdiet.com

TACA
gfcf-diet.talkaboutcuringautism.org

The GFCF Diet Web Site Suggests for Meals

Sample breakfast

Gluten- and casein-free cereal and milk. There are many different kinds that the health food stores carry. Milk is substitutable by potato milk, almond milk, rice milk, or soy milk.

Ener-G and Kinnikinnick mail orders carry GFCF donuts. (Make sure you specify GFCF when ordering.) Several companies make GFCF English muffins.

Eggs are a great source of protein; bacon and sausage can be bought nitrate-free; and rice or millet toast with CF margarine and low-sugar jelly.

There are many GFCF muffin mixes available and several health food stores carry fresh-baked versions and there are recipes for lots of flavors in cookbooks mentioned in this book.

Mail order and local health food stores carry GFCF bagels or you can make them yourself with GFCF ingredients and freeze them.

GFCF waffles are available at many stores. Van's products or other GFCF mixes are available at health food stores, by mail order, or from recipes you make from scratch. Both GFCF pancakes and GFCF waffles are a snap, and freeze well.

Millet or rice bread make excellent GFCF French toast. Mix GFCF vanilla and eggs and potato milk. (Potato milk may be deleted.)

Potato milk, soy or rice milk, and watered-down juices are fine.

Sample lunch (See list of acceptable products for more selection.)

Boar's Head lunch meat (some are not GFCF—see list)

Lay's potato chips

Fritos corn chips

Tostitos tortilla chips

Fruit juice http://gfcfdiet.com/Beverages.htm

Hot Dogs (Ball Park, Kahn's, Hebrew National Reduced Fat), no bun needed but available (see below)

Peanut butter and jelly

GFCF Breads (health food stores) Kinnikinnick and Glutino (www.kinnikinnicks.com; www.glutino.com)

Cascadian Farms French fries (see list)

Fruit leathers (read ingredients)

Fresh fruit and vegetables

With millet or rice bread, sandwiches are a snap.

GFCF mayonnaise and GFCF lunch meats, nitrate-free of course (Example: Applegate Farms is nitrate-free), and their favorite toppings make for seamless substitutions. Peanut butter and jelly sandwiches are easy, too. If GFCF bread is inaccessible, rolled cold cuts and GFCF crackers or rice cakes are okay.

Of course, dinner leftovers like GFCF soups, GFCF spaghetti with GFCF meatballs, meat and rice, etc. work well.

100 percent juices and CF milks are all easy and can go to school as well.

Sample dinner

Meat

Potatoes (no prepackaged with mixes) cooked to GFCF standards

Rice (no prepackaged with mixes) cooked to GFCF standards

Rice spaghetti noodles (health food stores and online purchase—see Appendix)

Vegetable (fresh is best, but frozen without any added ingredients is acceptable)

Earth Balance or Fleischman Light (read labels!) for "butter substitute" (see Appendix)

Dinner is the easiest meal, generally. A plain cooked piece of meat with potato or rice and vegetable always works.

Freeze meats individually so they are quicker to defrost. Cook a chicken breast in a little corn oil or GFCF breadcrumbs and bake.

Meatloaf with GFCF crumbs goes well for the whole family.

Also, cook GFCF meatballs in large batches and freeze them to use as needed.

Rice or potatoes or even GFCF pastas work well as sides.

GFCF pizza can be made several ways:

Get a GFCF flatbread, top with GFCF pizza sauce and melt Soymage, SLOWLY.

You can also make your own crusts from scratch or mixes that are GFCF.

Snacks and desserts (Though the children love these, they can be very high in sugar and MUST be limited!)

Nana's cookies (flavors include: ginger, chocolate chip, lemon, and more)

Specific Carbohydrate Diet: Remove ALL complex carbohydrates such as pastas, breads, and potatoes. Think of it as a meat-, veggies-, and nut-only diet.

Two good books to learn more about the Specific Carbohydrate Diet are: *Breaking the Vicious Cycle,* by Elaine Gloria Gottschall, and *Healing Foods,* by Sandra Ramacher.

RECIPES AND INFORMATIONAL SITES FOR THE SPECIFIC CARBOHYDRATE DIET:

www.scdiet.org/
www.scdrecipe.com/home/

To find a comprehensive food list of oxalate content, GFCF status, and SCD status, please go to http://lowoxalate.info/

Remove artificial coloring, flavors, high-fructose corn syrup, and sugar, immediately! ALWAYS check labels to find out if you see these ingredients. Avoid them the best you can!

Go completely organic, if possible. No preservatives!

Use the least-processed food possible. Try to stay away from packaged and prepared food. They have more chemicals in them that could be damaging your child.

3
SUPPLEMENTS

But I've read studies that inflammation can be decreased by using cod liver oil.
Haven't you learned anything? Vitamins and supplements don't work! Besides, we can't make any money off of them. Whoops! Did I just say that last sentence out loud?
BIG PHARMA
MED SCHOOL

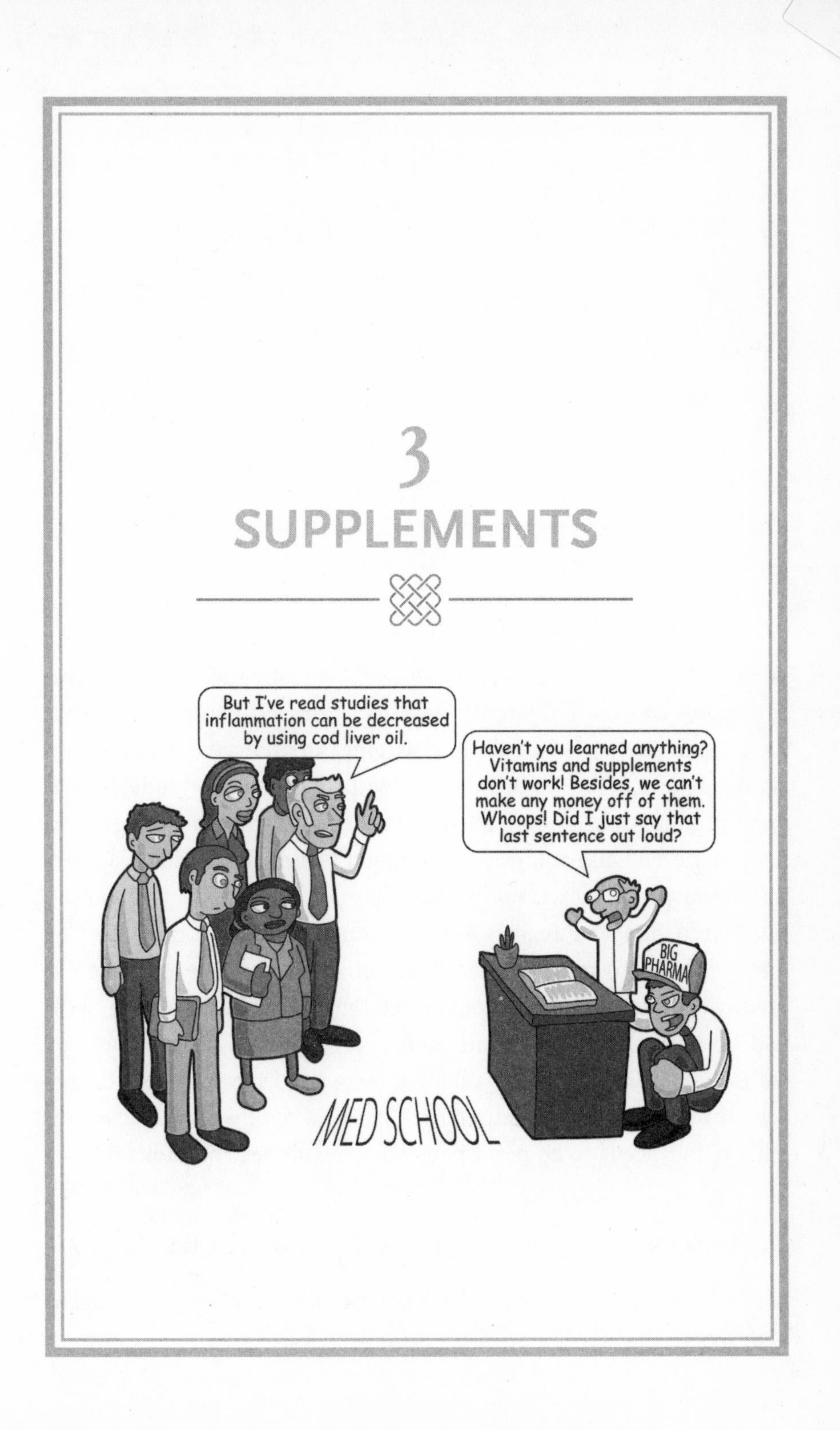

WAY BACK IN THE OLDEN DAYS of 1974, my mom used to give my sisters and me Flintstone vitamins as dessert because we didn't have much money for anything else. Her intentions were good—she wanted to supply her four little girls with vitamins—but today's generation of kids needs even more vitamins and minerals in order to help them heal and achieve overall good health. Today, food is overprocessed and filled with preservatives, so it doesn't give the body as much nutritional value as it needs. Along with the fact that many of our children are picky eaters, it becomes an absolute must to fill them with proper nourishment. You'll know what to give them, why, and how much to give them, even if your doctor doesn't know or completely believe in their value. Dr. Jerry and I have witnessed miracles because of them. Supplementation is a must for recovering autism and needs to be part of everyone's daily regimen for life!

VITAMINS AND WHY YOUR CHILD NEEDS THEM

JENNY: Why do we have to give so many vitamins and supplements to our kids?

DR. JERRY: They have such limited diets by the time they come to see us. They're not going to get their vitamins, minerals, and oils naturally from the foods they eat. Many children have a history of antibiotic use, and have chronic diarrhea, or they can be constipated. They're not digesting well. They're failing to thrive. Bottom line here is that these children, by history, have major nutrient deficiencies. These deficiencies can all be substantiated by laboratory evaluations, and supplementation is supported by published studies.

JENNY: So what do these vitamins, minerals, and oils specifically do?

DR. JERRY: Vitamins are essential for growth and development. Minerals help the vitamins do their job. Some minerals are iron, selenium, zinc, and calcium. Oils such as omega-3s can dramatically help maintain better brain health and cell function.

JENNY: Supplements come in powders, liquids, and different flavors, so which ones do we choose? Which ones are best?

DR. JERRY: Anything your child will take is the first consideration. Some children do great with powders dissolved in their drinks, some better with the liquids placed in a needleless syringe and gently administered into the mouth. For some children, any supplement can be a challenge.

JENNY: Ha, ha! That shouldn't scare too many people.

DR. JERRY: Many of these supplements don't taste that great but are essential for the healing process to work. Many taste fine, but our children can be most finicky.

B_{12}

JENNY: Can we get a little bit more into B_{12} since parents love to talk about B_{12}?

DR. JERRY: Vitamin B_{12} therapy has been an exciting addition in the treatment of autism. Vitamin B_{12} is utilized in almost every cell in the body and has a tremendous impact on the normal functioning of the nervous system, the gastrointestinal system, as well as some of the biomedical pathways already described. Dietary sources of

B_{12} may have a hard time being absorbed naturally as they require the proper stomach acidity (pH). In addition, the glycoprotein called intrinsic factor joins to the B_{12} in the stomach and allows absorption of the B_{12} in the last part of the intestines, called the terminal ileum—the exact same place shown to be markedly inflamed by GI endoscopy and biopsy. There are different forms of B_{12}, but the one that seems to work best for our children is called methyl B_{12}. It also appears that the small injection, called a subcutaneous shot, works best. In this case, the parent actually gives a small painless injection into the child's bottom periodically . . . from every other night to once monthly, depending on how the child responds. It is a matter of education for many families, as there is an innate fear of giving this medication because it's a small injection.

JENNY: Very small.

DR. JERRY: It's very small and it has a very small amount of fluid in it. They have developed a very short, thin needle that makes this a painless injection. The preferred site is on the upper buttocks, but it could literally be given just about anywhere. You're not going into the deep fat tissue or into muscle tissue. By doing it just under the skin you can't get into a vein or a nerve or an artery. Since this preparation is kept in the refrigerator, rolling the syringe between the palms of the hands for a few minutes will warm it up, also allowing the fluid to enter under the skin undetected.

JENNY: I've heard so many different opinions on which angle to put the needle in. Do you go in sideways or straight on?

DR. JERRY: All you're trying to do is get it under the skin. However you give it under the skin is just fine, as long as it's quick and the needle actually goes in. Then all you have to do is give a little squish on the plunger, and you're back out. It's over within a second. We can also give it to our children when they're sleeping. If you have a child who does not sleep well, you can do it after bath time, when Mom is rubbing the child down and has the towel over the kid's head and she's just fluffing him up and Dad comes behind and gives him a quick zap.

JENNY: Some other good advice I'd like to tell parents is to do it on themselves for a while so they can get used to it. I was always needle phobic and I had to force myself to get used to it by injecting myself. I would just twist around, grab some butt fat, and inject. It didn't hurt at all. Mosquito bites actually hurt more. The only thing I *did* notice that could hurt was when they combined folic acid with the B_{12} shot.

DR. JERRY: When combined very carefully by a compounding pharmacy, this combination of methyl B_{12}, folic acid, and N-acetyl-cysteine is painless. If combined *not* so carefully, you are right, it will sting bigtime! In my clinic, we use the combined product: methyl B_{12}, folic acid, and N-acetyl-cysteine. A direct benefit of this is that there are three fewer supplements we have to give orally. The next huge benefit is that it just seems to work much better than when given orally. Again, as with everything we do, there may be a component in this trio that does not go well for the child. Folic acid can be a double-edged sword. It really can make some kids go nuts, so we have to be very careful with folic acid. It can burn certain kids; it shouldn't, but it can. Some parents will tell me, "Look, I give this with the B_{12} and folic acid, he screams. I give B_{12} only, no screaming, doesn't even feel it." It's coming from the same company; they're pH balancing it just perfectly, but for whatever reason, it hurts. Again, if you listen to the child, you will know what is working and what is not.

JENNY: So many parents along this journey have talked about the B_{12} shots triggering a burst in language. It happened with Evan. He was at UCLA autism school at the time and they said, "What did you just do? What did you just do recently? He just had a burst of language."

And I said, "B_{12} shots."

DR. JERRY: This form of therapy seems to really allow a bloom in language, concentration, and focus in many children.

B_{12} Dosage

JENNY: I've met a lot of parents who say, "Oh, my God, it increased speech and he was doing great in school and then it went away after two days. A week later I gave him his next B_{12} shot and he spoke really well and then it just went away." Why does it go away?

DR. JERRY: If we have a child who does great on weekly injections of B_{12}, but it is noted that two days later following the injection his performance and his ability to speak or understand seem to diminish, then we have the perfect example of "listening" to the child! In this case he is saying, "You know, this stuff is good, but I need it twice a week or four times a week." I have some very big children on one shot a month and that's all they need. And I have some really tiny little peanuts who need an injection every day. A point here is to know that B_{12} is a pretty deep magenta color, and every now and then when a child goes tinkle there's a little bit of the magenta color in the urine, and it's not blood, but it's the magenta color being excreted by the body because we are giving the child a lot of B_{12} and we may need to decrease the dosing.

JENNY: When moms go to the pediatrician's office and they really want to try the B_{12} or other supplements, for that matter, can they get tested for B_{12} deficiency?

DR. JERRY: There are different ways to measure different chemical substances in our body. It can be helpful to measure the blood level of B_{12}. This is a blood level, and does not necessarily reflect accurately what is going on *inside* the cell. If the level is low, this will be easy to convince the doctor to institute replacement therapy. We can also have a B_{12} level that's normal in our body while being very low in the cells. Now, this type of testing of intracellular B_{12} levels is difficult. There can be a problem with getting the B_{12} actually inside the cell where it works. By giving large doses of B_{12}, as with every-other-day injections, we are creating a situation that favors more B_{12} to cross the cell membrane despite whatever is hampering its movement into the cell. These larger doses of B_{12} easily exceed the minimum daily requirements, but for each child, we are trying to find the *optimum* daily requirement.

JENNY: B_{12} is not a dangerous shot, right? If our bodies have too much, they will get rid of it, so to speak. Can you say that in pretty doctor words?

DR. JERRY: B_{12} is not a dangerous shot.

JENNY: Ha, ha. You didn't turn that into pretty doctor words at all.

DR. JERRY: B_{12} is a water-soluble vitamin that, if the level becomes too high, will be washed out in the urine. Rare but reported side effects would include rash and itching.

JENNY: There ya go! I knew you had it in you!

DR. JERRY: There are certain vitamins, for example, that can accumulate to toxic levels, such as vitamins A, D, E, and K. The B vitamins do not build up to toxic levels in the body. We may have some side effects from giving too much of a B vitamin, such as tingling or an arm feeling like it's asleep, but that's really when we're giving elevated doses. And generally, B_{12} is well tolerated.

JENNY: Supplements are not that exciting to talk about.

DR. JERRY: Maybe you should do one of your cartoon drawings and make a supplement do something funny.

JENNY: Like make cod liver oil wear a bikini?

DR. JERRY: That would be pretty funny.

JENNY: Done.

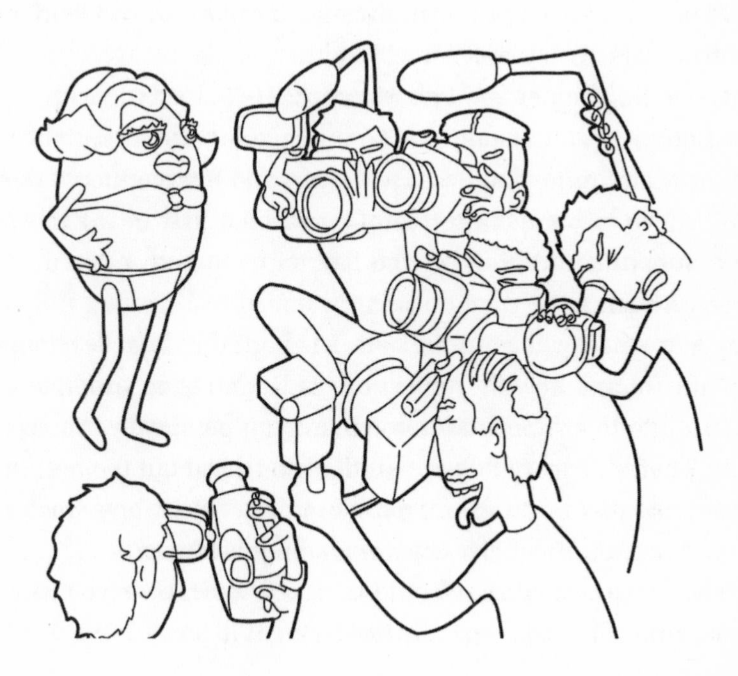

How to Pick a Supplement Brand

JENNY: Please tell parents the importance of choosing the right ingredients for their supplements.

DR. JERRY: It is very important to select manufacturers that understand our children with autism, as these children have unique metabolic needs and sensitivities. The supplements must have quality ingredients that are gluten-free, dairy-free, soy-free, and corn-free.

JENNY: When I heard you were developing your own line of high-quality supplements for our kids, called Kartner Health, I was so proud to help out and be an investor in it. So many times you have to trust what the manufacturers are saying by their word. I'm happy to know you are personally formulating them and ensuring the highest quality products because there is no one I trust more with our kids than you. Other brands that have done a great job are Kirkman Labs and Klaire Labs.

DR. JERRY: Yes, those are great labs also. I partnered with Dr. Bo Wagner, who has been formulating vitamins and supplements for thirty years, to create Kartner Health.

JENNY: Dr. Bo Wagner and I go way back. He helped me with my own gut problems and taught me so much about the importance of vitamins and minerals. Because of him and his products I was able to believe in biomedical treatment when I first heard about it in the autism community, so the fact that you both created Kartner Health makes me want do a happy dance!

DR. JERRY: And I will continue to learn about the latest developments in autism and how they affect our kids, and to incorporate what I learn into this supplement line that I can personally oversee.

JENNY: There is a lot of talk out on the Internet about the best time to give vitamins or supplements. Some say "must give this at bedtime" or "you must give this on an empty stomach."

DR. JERRY: In most cases, I would say just give it when you can. Let's not artificially make this any harder than it is.

Kartner Health (Dr. Jerry's supplements)	www.kartnerhealth.com 866-960-9251
Brainchild Nutritionals	www.brainchildnutritionals.com
Kirkman Labs (Super Nu-Thera)	www.kirkmanlabs.com 800-245-8282
Klaire Labs	www.klaire.com 888-488-2488

Parents need to know that getting vitamins "down" is easier said than done with many children. I like to use the supplements that have the least taste "footprint." That is, selecting supplements that are the most difficult for the child to detect.

JENNY: I would also recommend that parents not start off with a full dose. Start off with an itsy-bitsy-bitsy drop on the child's tongue with some apple juice mixed in it and then expand as the week goes on.

DR. JERRY: I think that's a good point. Sometimes parents will give too many things at once. They get really excited and start all the vitamins and minerals at once." And the kids can get really sick. So I like your idea that you start with one thing at a time and start a smaller dose than suggested! Wait a couple of days. Just keep in mind that any one of these supplements can cause significant side effects that include hyperactivity, irritability, staring spells, whining, abdominal pain, and not sleeping.

JENNY: Can you give me an idea of some supplements you can recommend for parents to get started?

DR. JERRY: Let us start with the multivitamins first. There are many companies that provide excellent quality vitamins: Kartner Health has their vitamin and mineral supplement (www.kartnerhealth.com); Klaire Labs has their VitaSpectrum (www.klaire.com); Kirkman Labs has their Super Nu-Thera line (www.kirkmanlabs.com); Brainchild Nutritionals has theirs as well (www.brainchildnutritionals.com).

JENNY: Great, what's next?

Two Essentials: Zinc and Selenium

DR. JERRY: We have to work on replenishing the minerals next. We again will need to add a multi-mineral supplement as well. The greatest need in these children is for zinc and selenium.

JENNY: That's great information!

DR. JERRY: So if we're really limited in what we can get into our kids, those two are an absolute must.

A safe starting point for zinc is 20 mg per day. Selenium is measured in micrograms, abbreviated "mcg," and, depending on weight, can be added anywhere from 50 mcg to 100 mcg per day. We can get blood levels very easily, and they should be monitored periodically.

Also, since we're putting the kids on a dairy-free diet, it's good to supplement them with calcium.

Calcium and Magnesium

DR. JERRY: Calcium is in the multi-mineral preparations. It is important to add magnesium to the calcium, as it aids in calcium's absorption. Now here is where we have to jump back to vitamins. Vitamin D (1,000 IU per day) is essential for calcium to be absorbed as well. Vitamin D levels (the blood test is called 25 OH vitamin D) are commonly very low in children with autism. Higher daily doses of vitamin D may be recommended, but it is necessary to follow the vitamin D levels so they do not get too high.

Fatty Acids

JENNY: And what about fatty acids?

DR. JERRY: Fatty acids are commonly referred to as omega-3s (usually along with omega-6 and omega-9). These omega-3 fatty acids have many benefits, and the biggie would be that they are anti-inflammatory. The omega-3 oils are incorporated into the cell's membrane, which is crucial for proper cell functioning. If you think about it, the building blocks that will eventually become proteins, enzymes, hormones, etc., have to travel through the cell membrane for proper assembly. Once the products are made in the cell, they have to leave the cell, again through the membrane. If the membrane is not constructed with just the right lipids (fats), these processes can be expected to be hindered. I start my patients right away with cod liver oil for several reasons. Dr. Mary Megson has demonstrated that cod liver oil is beneficial for eye contact and focus and that the vitamin A in cod liver oil is in a very special form that the body can use readily.

JENNY: I was so grateful when you told me to start Evan on cod liver oil because his weird eye movements went away. He would always look at toys out of the corner of his eye. Not anymore!!

We should also mention that people should only use mercury-free fish oils.

DR. JERRY: Yes! Mercury-free. Again, it is important to stress purchasing fish oils from companies that specialize in optimizing this product for our children with autism. Cheaper oils may be partially rancid or may have higher levels of contaminants. The companies that pay more attention to providing a really clean cod liver oil, like Kartner Health (www.kartnerhealth.com or call 866-960-9251), Nordic Naturals (www.nordicnaturals.com or call 800-662-2544, ext. 3), and Carlson (www.carlsonlabs.com or call 888-234-5656), are the companies that send the oil out for laboratory testing to ensure that the oil does not have contaminants.

Digestive Enzymes and Protein

JENNY: I'm just understanding the importance of enzymes for the first time; digestive enzymes in our kids help so much!

DR. JERRY: Digestive enzymes are responsible for breaking down the foods that we eat. Proteins are broken down to amino acids. Fats are broken down to fatty acids, and carbohydrates are broken down to sugars. It has been demonstrated that children with autism may not be generating enough of their own digestive enzymes and may require additional supplementation. I recommend starting with 1/2 to 1 capsule *with* each meal. Let me emphasize here that digestive enzymes must be given with the meal or ten to fifteen minutes before. They do not work if given later. If your child ate a cupcake at school and needs help digesting it, giving her a digestive enzyme hours after the fact won't help. The digestive enzyme is very important to add to this list of "must have" supplements. There are several good brands available: Kartner Health (www.kartnerhealth.com, Kirkman Labs (www.kirkmanlabs.com), and Klaire Labs (www.klaire.com).

JENNY: I know some parents who have kids who don't eat protein. Do you think it's a good idea to supplement that also?

DR. JERRY: Absolutely! I like to use rice-based protein supplements if the child is not allergic to rice. We'll talk more about allergy testing later. For now, keep in mind that there are other sources of protein supplements: Soy, milk, and fish are the most common.

JENNY: Do you have a favorite one?

DR. JERRY: I recommend NutriBiotic's rice-based protein powder to start with. It's a very clean product. It may be crucial to give the digestive enzyme to help facilitate the digestion of the protein supplement. If not, undigested protein will be broken down by bacteria and through a process called putrefaction. And that's where we get the word "putrid," and the stools will smell as such. The bacteria in the colon will continue to break down the stool and liberate ammonia. Elevated ammonia levels in our children can cause a lot of behavior issues, social disconnect, and generalized fogginess (go to www.nutribiotic.herbsmd.com). One more thing: For children who absolutely shun proteins, it is important to supplement with zinc as well. It appears that low body-zinc conditions alter the taste of protein so much that children will avoid it.

JENNY: Wow! That's good to know. I really like your Kartner Health enzymes. They have not only been a great enzyme for Evan, but have helped me so much! How many enzymes do we give our kids?

DR. JERRY: I recommend $^1/_2$ to 2 capsules with each meal and snack. They do not work an hour or more later! They cannot be given after school due to an "infraction" hours earlier.

Probiotics

JENNY: Let's talk about additional important supplements like probiotics. It's amazing to me how many people don't know what a probiotic is. I tell them it's the opposite of an antibiotic. So many people forget how important it is to supplement good bacteria, and that's what a probiotic is: good bacteria. This is why people get infections in their gut or yeast overgrowth: because there are no good guys on the team. The only odd thing I wasn't able to figure out was why Evan would get a swollen belly or sick until we found the right probiotic.

DR. JERRY: Probiotics are healthy living bacteria that promote bowel health and restoration of the normal microorganisms that are supposed to be in the bowel. They are able to accomplish this by INHIBITING the growth of potentially harmful bacteria, yeast, and parasites. For many reasons (such as the heavy use of antibiotics), beneficial bacteria are no longer present and offering their protection to the bowels (as easily documented by stool analysis). There are many types of probiotics (the healthy bacteria) available, and each company insists that their product is the "best" for you and your child. There are two significant factors: the number of healthy bacteria given per serving, and the number of different types of healthy bacteria. Look for products that offer two to ten billion per serving. The second significant factor would be the type of healthy bacteria offered in the probiotic. There are many types of bacteria thought to be healthy for the bowel, and so there are many combinations available, each promising the best results. I recommend using a probiotic developed by leading companies such as Kartner

Health, Klaire, and Kirkman, to name a few. Keep in mind, just like any supplement, probiotics can cause some very bizarre behaviors. (I have seen increased stimming, hyperactivity, stomach cramps, and even self-injurious behaviors.) If this happens, cut the dose in half. If the child is still acting up, the probiotic will have to be switched out with another brand. (Order probiotics at www.kartnerhealth.com or at www.klaire.com.) Watch for results. Positive results will be seen in the stool color, size, and smell. Behaviors may improve dramatically as well.

When a probiotic is working, the stools normalize (reduction of diarrhea; normalization of stool size, smell, and consistency). It is also important to repeat the stool analysis to check not only on restoration of good, healthy bacteria, but that the abnormal bacteria, if previously noted in an earlier sample, is no longer present.

JENNY: Evan was on the ThreeLac probiotic for six months after being diagnosed with autism and he lost his freaking marbles, but I stuck with it and it killed so much yeast that he started talking in conversations.

DR. JERRY: And the next kid who tries it might have the same success as Evan did or it could be a complete disaster with no success. It is important to keep in mind that a probiotic that works well for one child could be a disaster for another.

JENNY: What about making your own good bacteria with coconut kefir? I know many moms who love it. I think they talk about it in *The Body Ecology Diet*. You can find more information on www.bodyecologydiet.com, along with books that have recipes for kefir.

DR. JERRY: Coconut kefir is an excellent source of probiotics and minerals. Many children have greatly benefited from it.

JENNY: It's hard to eat, I must say. I used to give Evan kefir, but then he came up allergic to coconuts!

DR. JERRY: These children can become allergic to anything given frequently to them. My son became allergic to nuts while on the Specific Carbohydrate Diet, in which the carbohydrates are nut-based. In Evan's case, too much coconut exposure sensitized him.

Sadly, any food that is sensitizing will need to be removed from the diet. We have to be diligent and try other avenues of healing for the gut. In the meantime, unhealthy bacteria and yeast will continue to survive and even thrive in the gut.

JENNY: Scary! There are so many more supplements that we can get into, but it would take up the entire book. So I'm just going to include your list, which does a really good job of going through each supplement and giving recommended doses.

SUPPLEMENTS FOR HEALING UNDERLYING AUTISM TRIGGERS

The following can be purchased from:

Kartner Health (Dr. Jerry's supplements)	kartnerhealth.com 866960-9251
Kirkman Labs	kirkmanlabs.com 800-245-8282
Klaire Labs	klaire.com 888-488-2488

Zinc: We feel it is safe to supplement just about everyone with ASD with 10–20 mg of zinc daily. Serum zinc levels or packed red blood cell element evaluations may reveal higher levels of supplementation are necessary.

Selenium: Many of our children with ASD require additional selenium. We will start with 50–100 mcg daily. Packed red blood cell element evaluations (a blood test) may reveal higher levels of supplementation are necessary.

Calcium/Magnesium: Since most of our children need to be dairy-free, alternative sources for calcium are necessary for proper growth and development. We typically recommend 500–1,000 mg of calcium citrate (not Tums) daily. Magnesium should be given with calcium to enhance absorption. Calcium and magnesium blood levels should be checked regularly. Remember, we need to be on a vitamin D supplement as well.

Chromium: If this is revealed to be low on blood level tests, we recommend 50–100 mcg daily.

Protein: Many children do not consume protein, or if they do, it's in very small amounts. We recommend supplementation with a rice-protein powder put directly into their drink. NutriBiotics makes a very clean product; 1 tablespoon typically is equal to 14 g of protein. The amount of protein our children require usually depends on age: If under three years, supplement with 1 g of protein per two pounds of body weight. Ages four to six years, 1 tablespoon daily; seven to ten years of age, supplement with 1 3/4 tablespoons daily. Older boys and girls require 2 tablespoons daily. This protein powder can easily mix into any fluid since it contributes only a very bland flavor. It does have "texture" that some of our kids can detect. This can be minimized if mixed into juice, rice milk, etc., with a blender.

Cod liver oil/EFA: Just about all children will require omega-3 fatty acids. When using cod liver oil, we recommend starting with the recommended daily allowance of vitamin A. Usually this is 1/2 teaspoon of cod liver oil for children ages two to five years; 1 teaspoon for children who are older. A blood test, called an Essential Fatty Acid Profile, will reveal other possible fatty acid deficits that can be supplemented. Some children react poorly to cod liver oil and can get very hyper and aggressive. This will resolve one to two days after discontinuing.

Iron: This can be easily evaluated by simple blood tests that need to include a Complete Blood Count (CBC), ferritin level, reticulocyte count, and total iron binding capacity. If iron deficiency is noted, your family doctor can prescribe iron and give a close follow-up.

Vitamin Supplementation

Vitamins: Given their extreme food selectivity, our children become measurably deficient in many of the vitamins. These vitamins must be replenished in order to ensure normal physiologic functioning. We also have to keep in mind that even though we may be giving them these vitamins, they may not be absorbing them well (see below). It is beyond the scope of this book to discuss each vitamin in detail (that could be a book in itself!), but here is a much abbreviated presentation of what each vitamin does:

Vitamin A: There are two forms of this vitamin: a "trans" form and a "cis" form. The "trans" form is found in most manufactured sources called vitamin A palmitate. This may not be as effective in many of our children. The "cis" form is found in natural sources such as oils from cod and salmon. Briefly, vitamin A is important to vision, cell membrane function, and the immune system.

Vitamin B group: Thiamin, riboflavin, niacin, pyridoxine, and methylcobalamin are the names they commonly go by. Each one must be supplemented. Vitamin B_6 (pyridoxine) and its activated form, called P_5P, and vitamin B_{12} (methylcobalamin) seem to be very important to the autistic child and can minimize many autistic behaviors. Vitamins B_6 and B_{12} have a major impact on the methylation pathway.

Vitamin C: Also known as ascorbic acid. We generally use 500–1,000 mg (or more!) in our kids. This is a potent antioxidant and important in many physiological operations of the body. With higher doses of vitamin C, be sure your source is buffered.

Vitamin D_3: Also known as cholecalciferol, it regulates absorption and deposition of calcium and phosphorus. It can be found in some fish oils (think omega!), and our body can generate vitamin D with exposure to sunlight. We recommend supplementing from 600 IU to 2,000 IU of vitamin D_3 daily, depending on the child's weight and measured 25-hydroxy vitamin D levels (blood test).

Vitamin E: This is another potent antioxidant. The recommended dosage for children is in the range of 100–400 IU daily, depending on their weight.

Vitamin K: This is important to the formation of blood-clotting factors. Bacteria in our gut produce this for us—another good reason to return the bowels to normal function as soon as possible. This generally does not need to be supplemented except in extreme cases of gut maldigestion, malabsorption, and inflammation. Vitamin K_2 is easily supplemented if thought to be deficient.

Treating Maldigestion and Malabsorption

It has been demonstrated repeatedly that many of our children lack the digestive enzymes needed for breaking down foods. This can be demonstrated in comprehensive stool studies offered at Genova Diagnostics or Doctor's Data Laboratory. It is advisable to start slowly with digestive enzymes, giving one with each meal AND snack.

Improving Function of the Immune System

Many children with autism have a dysfunctional immune system (that can be a Th1/Th2 imbalance). Critical nutrients to rebuild the immune system and balance the Th1/Th2 back toward normal will require:

Zinc: This mineral is almost always deficient in children with autism.

Selenium: This can raise immunoglobulin G-2 and G-4, which will decrease the number of infectious diseases and may also help those children with intractable seizures. Selenium also helps protect the body from mercury. We dose 10 mcg of selenium per two pounds of body weight up to a maximum of 100 mcg daily.

Chromium: This can aid in shifting Th2 to Th1 by promoting the formation of DHEA (which antagonizes cortisol). We recommend starting with 50–100 mcg for children we see in our clinic.

Vitamins A, C, E, and B_6: These vitamins are known to be quite necessary for normal immune system function.

Fatty acids: Omega-3, along with omega-6 and omega-9, are usually needed. The omega-3 fatty acids are supplied by cod liver oil, DHA Junior, and flax oil. Omega-3s are also supplied by using high oleic safflower oil as cooking oil. Omega-6s are also needed in some children.

Probiotics: These are friendly bacteria that live in our gut. They help to create an environment that is hostile for yeast and unfriendly bacteria.

Colostrum: Cow's-milk can also be considered a transfer factor. It appears to be toxic to many viruses and fungi (yeast) and promotes repair of intestinal cells.

Essential Detoxification

Improved Methylation: Genetic testing can determine if there are problems in this pathway. Specific supplements can raise the products of this pathway (Jill James, Ph.D.). We typically recommend:

- TMG or DMG taken orally.
- Start with 125 mg twice daily. Some children do better with TMG, others with DMG. Side effects, if seen, are hyperactivity and more emotional behaviors.
- Methyl B_{12} usually injected by parents every other night; we start dosing at 1,250 mcg of methyl B_{12} per injection. We tend to start the trio methyl B_{12}, folinic acid, and N-acetyl-cysteine all in one injection.
- Here is the formula we have compounded at the pharmacy: Methyl B_{12} 12.5 mg/folinic acid 50 mg/NAC 50 mg per ml.
- We then start with 0.1 ml subcutaneously every other day.
- Folinic acid is usually placed in the methyl B_{12} injections but can be taken orally. It, too, can cause some hyperactivity. If taken orally, 400 mcg daily is a good starting dose. This is a really safe vitamin, and toxicity is rare.
- Cysteine can be taken orally but, in some children, can cause yeast to grow. Cysteine can be applied transdermally (as a cream that allows the cysteine to enter the body) and if given this way (not in an injection), we recommend starting with 100–200 mg twice daily.
- Glutathione, transdermally or IV: This is so crucial for many children. This is one of the end products of the methylation pathway. When given orally it, too, like N-acetyl-cysteine, can cause yeast to bloom. Children do very well with IV infusions of glutathione (where we stick a small catheter in the arm and infuse the glutathione directly into the vein) but they rarely like the procedure/needle stick. We can give anywhere from 300 mg to 1,000 mg of glutathione IV once or twice monthly. Glutathione can also come in a transdermal preparation, and we recommend 200 mg twice daily. One other route to administer glutathione would be to inhale it. Using a special "nebulizing" machine (about $50–$70), glutathione can be aerosolized and breathed in by the child. We recommend 100 mg–200 mg once or twice daily if given by this route.

Enhancing Cognitive Abilities

- B vitamins: Many children really respond to the B vitamins, especially B_6, B_{12}, and magnesium.
- Essential fatty acids: Children usually have such a poor dietary intake, and the "good" fats are no exception. We will often get a blood test, a "Fatty Acid Profile," and will supplement according to the results. It is safe to assume the children will need omega-3 fatty acids. That is why we start with cod liver oil.
- Minerals: Because of dietary limitations, many minerals are lacking.
    1. CoQ10
    2. NADH
    3. TMG/DMG
    4. EFA
    5. Grape seed extract (GSE)
    6. Antioxidants in general: Vitamins C and E (to name just a few)
    7. Chelation in selected cases
- Removal of nitrites (cured meats)

Reducing Autistic Behaviors

- Normalize neurotransmitter levels. Supplement with:

    —Tyrosine, TMG, GABA, NADH, Cerefolin, Deptin

- Improve receptor site activity. Supplement with:

    —TMG
    —NADH (maybe)

- Remove substances that can interfere with normal function.

    —Digestive enzymes: one capsule with each meal
    —Remove MSG, NutraSweet, aspartame, hydrolyzed vegetable proteins, excitotoxins, soda

—Food dyes
—Reduce high-phenol-containing foods (blueberries, strawberries, etc.)

- Protect from excitotoxins. Supplement with:

—Vitamin C 500–1,000 mg daily
—Vitamin E 100–200 IU daily
—Magnesium 2 mg per pound daily
—Grape seed extract (50–100 mg/day—PhytoPharmica)

- Increase the seizure threshold (stabilization of neuronal cell membrane potentials). Supplement with:

—EFA
—Taurine 250–500 mg daily
—Vitamin B_6

- Improve gastrointestinal function.
- Improve motility.
- Secretin: This hormone is normally released by specialized cells in the duodenum (the channel that directly follows the stomach outlet) that tells the pancreas to secrete bicarbonate (neutralizes the acidic stomach content). Given through IV or transdermally, this has had profound positive effects on many of the children we see. It can normalize bowel function with respect to the child having formed one- to twice-daily brown stools that smell like regular bowel movements. Secretin can also have profound effects on autistic behaviors, with some of the children responding remarkably. The children who tend to benefit most from secretin have loose stools and have very limited to no language. Unfortunately, secretin needs a physician's involvement and prescription.
- Fiber: Fiber has always been helpful for developing regular stooling behavior. We currently are using Miracle Fiber and Fibersure.

- Calcium: As previously discussed, calcium HAS to be supplemented in our dairy-free kids. We follow general RDA guidelines, 500–1,000 mg daily, given with magnesium.
- Magnesium (avoid magnesium oxide)
- Probiotics

Nutritional Pharmacology for Specific Issues

- Hyperactivity

—Suspect gluten/casein leaks, consider specific carbohydrate diet
—GABA (500–1,000 mg three times daily)
—Taurine (500–1,000 mg three times daily)
—EFA (1,000–2,000 mg once daily)
—Calcium/magnesium (doses vary)
—TMG (125 mg twice daily and work the dose up slowly to 500 mg twice daily)
—DMSA (chelation by protocol in selected cases only)
—No refined sugars
—Elimination of artificial colors
—Magnesium glycinate (200–400 mg twice daily)
—Glycine: We start with 250 mg twice daily.

- Inattention

—Suspect gluten/casein leaks
—Tyrosine (500 mg twice daily)
—EFA (up to 2,000 mg once daily)
—CoQ10 (25–50 mg twice daily)
—NADH (2.5–5 mg twice daily)
—TMG (125–250 mg twice daily)
—DMAE
—Theanine

—DMSA (by protocol)
—Ginkgo biloba

- Self-Abusive behaviors and rage, impulsivity, disinhibition: This is often linked to disturbances in serotonin metabolism.

  —Suspect gluten/casein leaks
  —Inositol (1–6 g three times daily)
  —Chromium (100–200 mcg daily)
  —Taurine (up to 10,000 mg total daily)
  —GABA (up to 10,000 mg total daily)
  —Low-carbohydrate diet (no refined sugars)
  —Elimination of artificial colors
  —Often improve with chelation (DMSA)
  —Naltrexone (by prescription)
  —Consider Risperdal (Rx)

- Poor Sleep

  —Melatonin (1–3 mg at bed), Taurine (1,000–4,000 mg at bed)
  —GABA (1,000–5,000 mg at bed)
  —DMSA (by protocol)
  —TMG (250–500 mg once or twice daily)
  —Magnesium (400–800 mg at bed)
  —5HTP (50–100 mg at bedtime)
  —Naltrexone transdermal (1–4 mg at bedtime)

- Diarrhea: We often obtain an X-ray of the abdomen, because sometimes diarrhea is a sign of constipation.

  —Colostrum (variable dosing)
  —Probiotics (as discussed)
  —Digestive enzymes (food sensitivity—malabsorption—osmotic)

—Lauricidin (1/4 tsp three times daily and increase as needed to get normal stool consistency)
—Echinacea
—Aloe extracts
—EFA
—Specific Rx meds:
  - antibiotics such as metronidazole benzoate and vancomycin
  - antifungals such as fluconazole, ketoconazole, and itraconazole
  - antiparasitics such as Alinia, Flagel, and Yodoxin (parasites can be picked up when our kids chew on nonfood items such as grass, twigs, or leaves, and may need an antiparasitic to restore bowel health)

- Constipation: Get an X-ray of the abdomen (called a "KUB" X-ray).

—Soluble fiber is easily mixed in a drink and has no flavor
—Xprep (prune concentrate)/Fruit Eze
—Senna: Smooth Move TEA!
—Mineral oil
—Aloe resin (leaf, not gel), can be harsh
—Pedi Fleets (daily if necessary, until the plug is out)
—MiraLAX (1/2 or 1 teaspoon daily as needed, up to a tablespoon)
—HIGH-dose vitamin C
—Magnesium
—Colon cleanser from oxypowder.com

NOTE: Many of these supplements will be repeated throughout the book for many ailments. **DO NOT DOUBLE THE DOSE.** Always refer to this chart only for dosage and, if not listed, please consult your doctor.

4
THE IMMUNE SYSTEM AND AUTISM

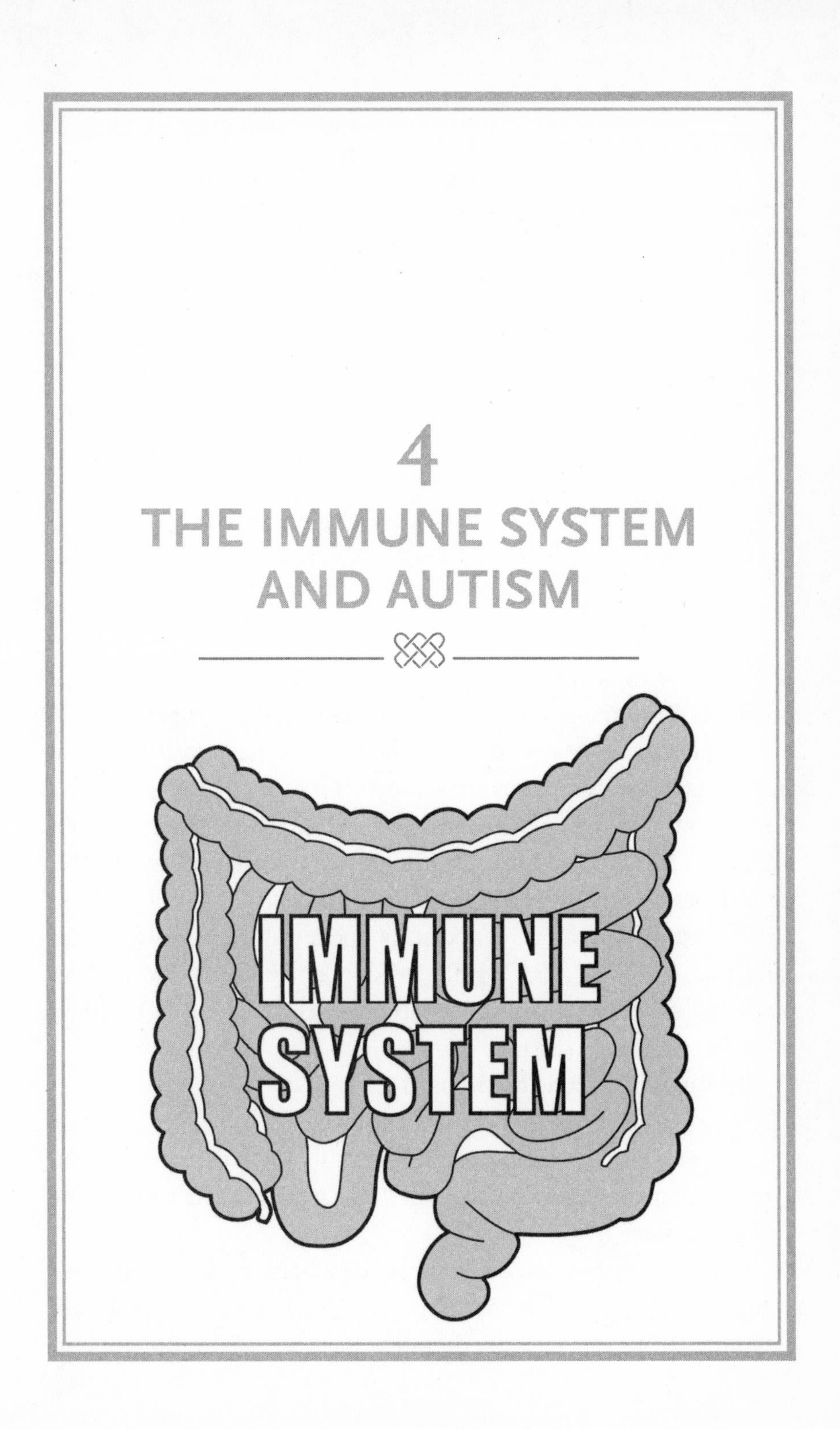

When I was a little girl, I was sick from school at least twenty to thirty times a year. I was also the most constipated kid in the neighborhood. My mom was giving me enemas until I was ten years old. It was so embarrassing when I would see her pull out a Fleet bottle, I would usually run and hide out by my friend's house until I was forced to go back. That being said, I firmly believe that because I was so constipated it led to many illnesses.

If most of our immune system is operating from our gut, how can it possibly do its job if it's filled with poop? It can't. Having clean pipes and excreting waste properly is truly the secret to a healthier immune system.

Not only in our kids but in us, too.

Jenny: It was hard for me to comprehend at first that the immune system is partly in our gut. I thought it was a gland or its own engine of some sort.

Dr. Jerry: Eighty percent of the immune system lines the digestive tube from the mouth to the anus and it's dedicated to keeping contaminants we put into the digestive tract (by way of our mouth) from the outer environment from entering into our internal environment as well as keeping the healthy organisms growing in our bowels in a delicate balance. If the immune system does not work properly, then infective agents can get into our body or set up "shop" along the gut lining.

JENNY: Like bad organisms?

DR. JERRY: Our body can normally keep many bad organisms at bay, but when the immune system isn't working properly they will actually increase in numbers, be prolific, and can potentially cause problems. Because they are living organisms, they are consuming their foods, whatever those foods might be, and they have waste materials and toxins that they liberate.

JENNY: Ew, so the bad organisms poop inside of us?

DR. JERRY: Yes, and we constantly absorb their waste. One of the major tasks of the large intestine is to reabsorb water and dehydrate the stool (so we don't have diarrhea, but rather, formed stools). Any toxins/waste materials that are dissolved in those fluids will be absorbed, too, and thus be delivered throughout the body.

WHAT ALTERS THE IMMUNE SYSTEM?

JENNY: Are vaccines the only things that can alter the immune system?

DR. JERRY: No. Exposures to a developing baby start at conception! Harmful agents may be derived from a mom's exposures to various toxins. These potential sources include a mother's amalgams (the "silver" fillings in her teeth), or the fish, for example, she consumed. We cannot even discount exposures at the worksite. Some of these exposures may even extend back one to two decades. Keep in mind that the placenta gets everything Mom gets and preferentially makes it available to the developing baby. So we have to look at the whole human being, the history of exposures, not just at a set of "shots."

SIGNS OF AN ALTERED IMMUNE SYSTEM

JENNY: Many moms talk about how their child was prone to recurring ear infections. Is this a sign that the immune system may not be in healthy shape?

DR. JERRY: Absolutely. The most common marker for immune system dysfunction is frequent ear infections in babies and very young children. This "red flag" may be letting you know that something is wrong with the immune system. If you get one ear infection, it's no big deal, as that does happen. But if you get an ear infection and three weeks later you have another one and four weeks later you have another one, that *is* a big deal! The next thing you know, your child has been on ten or fifteen different courses of antibiotics. The medical community, as a whole, should have been evaluating this child's immune system, probably after the third infection requiring an antibiotic, to see what was not working properly. But that's rarely, if ever, done. Rather, the next step after numerous ear infections (the most common antibiotic-related infection of childhood) is to see the ear, nose, and throat doctor. This will predictably result in the insertion of pressure equalization tubes (also known as PE tubes) in an attempt to drain a persistent abscess living behind the eardrum. With this procedure, one is opening a sterile environment (the space behind the eardrum) to a nonsterile environment, exposing the middle ear to non-sterility because of a tube placed there. So the tube does its one job (draining any potential abscess), but no one has ever looked for the CAUSE. No one is asking WHY! They're just going ahead and putting one more Band-Aid on.

JENNY: What about recurring fevers? Evan was one of those kids who had a fever a week and no one could figure out why.

DR. JERRY: Yes, some of these children can have recurring fevers. My son was one of those who would have a 102-degree temperature, and I would do my doctor thing from head to toe and say, "I don't know what's going on here. He's clean!" Then, four hours later, the fever was gone, and then three days later he would have a fever again. This recurring fever, without an obvious source (like an ear infection) led me to strongly consider that something infectious or inflammatory is recurring in these children. So, we have children with intermittent fevers and no physical findings. There were no findings in the ankles, knees, or hips. These children aren't limping. It's certainly not in their lungs or in the heart, or they would be gravely ill. The only other place that could be infected would be the GI system. With this in mind, one must really wonder about what might be going in there. Now, the GI tract is usually *not* without symptoms. Many of these children have problems with chronic constipation, chronic diarrhea, abnormally colored stools, foul-smelling stools, and even undigested material in stools. These medical findings, with or without fevers, justify a medical procedure called endoscopy. Endoscopy requires placing a small camera down the throat and into the stomach to see what is going on in there, as well as placing a camera up the bottom to look at what is going on in the bowels. Obviously this involves finding a GI physician who will look at autistic children with a mind to help. Some of the early GI docs who helped define what was going on in the bowels were Drs. Karoly Horvath, Arthur Krigsman, and Timothy Buie.

JENNY: What did the endoscopies show?

DR. JERRY: What was found in the large majority of these children is that they have inflammatory bowel disease, documented with biopsy specimens. Chronic inflammation, whether it is due to reflux, infection, or autoimmunity, is going to have a negative impact on the brain.

AUTOIMMUNE PROBLEMS RESULTING FROM ALTERED IMMUNE SYSTEMS AND BOWEL DISEASE

JENNY: Can you explain what "autoimmune" means?

DR. JERRY: Simply put, the immune system "knows" every cell in your body. If something foreign enters the body, the immune system quickly distinguishes "self" from "non-self" and removes it. But, in the case of autoimmunity, the body loses this ability (discerning self from non-self) and starts destroying specific tissue, such as the thyroid in autoimmune thyroiditis or, in this case, the bowel.

JENNY: Okay, to break it down even more, we could say that the mom or the child has a toxic overload from the environment or vaccines and this overload could damage the immune system and when that happens, the immune system can start to attack its own organs and tissues, which you call autoimmune.

DR. JERRY: Yes, and there are lots of other models for autoimmune disease. Rheumatoid arthritis is thought to be autoimmune; some thyroid disease is thought to be autoimmune. Diabetes is thought to be either autoimmune or triggered by a virus. In other words, in the case of diabetes, the immune system is going after the virus, and it thinks the islet cells of Langerhans (these are little cells in the pancreas that create insulin) are the virus and starts munching on them. We see that in rheumatic heart disease, where the body mistakes the mitral valve of the heart for streptococci and starts munching on it after a strep infection and we lose that valve. Keep in mind I am really oversimplifying this concept so it can be easily understood. Bottom line: We know that there are certain triggers that can initiate the immune system to do bad things against our own body.

JENNY: One of them being inflammatory bowel disease.

DR. JERRY: There are other causes of inflammation of the bowels, such as the overgrowth of what we call dysbiotic bacteria and fungus (yeast). These are organisms that shouldn't be there and they are just wreaking havoc.

JENNY: Yes, the yeast beast is at it again!

DR. JERRY: Yes, a fungal infection. Again, there are a lot of people in the medical community who will say there's no evidence that a fungal infection can cause problems in children's intestines. Where else can you culture a fungus in large quantities and it *doesn't* wreak havoc? Fungus can cause problems, whether it is in fingernails, in the mouth, in the sinuses, or in the bowels. Only recently have studies determined that there can also be a fungal component to sinus infections in children. If you have a fungal skin infection or a nail infection or a vaginal infection, we're going to treat it. But, when we talk about an intestinal fungal infection, the medical community will say, "Oh, no, that can't possibly be the source of problems for your child."

JENNY: It drives me crazy.

DR. JERRY: When we do treat these kids with an antifungal, they have remarkable changes in their behaviors and their disposition.

Hyperimmunity

JENNY: I've heard moms also talk about how their child never got sick. They went through flu seasons without their child catching one thing. Evan was this way before I knew he had autism. He was so healthy when all of his friends were sick and then all of a sudden, BOOM! He had a fever a week for a year.

DR. JERRY: This is what I call hyperimmunity. When the immune system gets stressed, it can go into a mode of hypervigilance. People who live out on the streets can be a good example of having a hyperimmune system. Many of them are heavy drinkers/drug users with very poor nutrition. They can remain in a "non-ill" status up to a point and then all of a sudden they crash and end up in the emergency room. For a long time their immune system went into a hyperdrive mode and was able to keep up despite significant stressors until it just collapsed on itself. So I think this hyperimmune system is similar to what develops in some of our children and they never get sick. Remember, I can see just the opposite of this in my clinic. These are the children who are sick all the time. They come to me having had sixty or seventy different courses of antibiotics through the past three years. Their immune systems are dysfunctional, too, just in a manner that makes them very susceptible to disease.

JENNY: When I took Evan to an immune specialist, the doctor told me that Evan had the immune system of a dying AIDS patient. Fortunately his immune system is now back to normal, but I was terrified that it wasn't going to get better.

How Does the Immune Deficiency Happen?

DR. JERRY: Immune systems can get better. We see that all the time. AIDS patients have a very specific virus that is altering the immune system in a potentially very deadly manner. AIDS is an acronym for acquired immune deficiency syndrome. Now, either you are born with an immune dysfunction, which you would call congenital immune deficiency syndrome, or you can acquire it, like from a virus such as the one that causes AIDS. This is how the malady was named: acquired immune deficiency syndrome. It was *acquired*.

But our kids have another type of acquired immune deficiency syndrome. I can say this because they were not born with it. Can I prove it? No. We do not do routine immune system evaluations on our children prior to vaccines. Thus, I cannot demonstrate, with laboratory documentation, that a normal immune system existed PRIOR to vaccines. So the medical community will surely default to "they were born with this defect." One has to wonder if a vaccine-induced immune dysfunction syndrome may exist? It does exist in animal studies.

JENNY: VIIDS?

DR. JERRY: Essentially, yes.

JENNY: And if the immune system was damaged from environmental toxins like from emissions liberated from a factory, you could call it EIIDS, for environmentally induced immune deficiency syndrome?

DR. JERRY: (Smiling) I'm glad you, and not me, are naming these, but you are getting the idea: that some external factor or factors (not inherited) caused the immune system to become dysfunctional.

REPAIRING THE DAMAGED IMMUNE SYSTEM

JENNY: What can we do to boost the immune system in our kids?

DR. JERRY: Well, it depends on what part of the immune system needs boosting. When you hear about companies selling products stating, "This will make mitochondria stronger" or, "This makes liver cells healthier" or, "This cleanses your blood," how do you know what they're saying is true? Show me weak mitochondria, show me your product, and show me strong mitochondria. If you tell me this cleans the liver, fine. What markers do you have for a dirty liver, and how do you know that after you take the product, your liver is better? Just because we're dealing with autism doesn't mean that we have to check our scientific brains at the door. For the children who do not have a doctor yet, the best way to get their immune system to improve is to DECREASE THEIR SUGAR INTAKE!

JENNY: AMEN!

DR. JERRY: Sugar compromises the white blood cells' ability to fight infection. A study out of Loma Linda University published in the *Journal of Clinical Nutrition* demonstrated that glucose (sugar/energy source in humans), fructose (fruit sugar), sucrose (table sugar), honey, and orange juice all significantly decreased the capacity of our immune system (specifically, the white blood cells) to engulf and destroy bacteria. Interestingly, a fast for thirty-six to forty-eight hours significantly improved the immune system's ability to engulf and destroy bacteria. So Grandma was right: "Starve a cold, feed a fever!"

Decrease Sugar to Boost the Immune System

DR. JERRY: We know that sugar, and it does not seem to matter from what source it is derived (for example, table sugar, fruit sugar, and honey), compromises white blood cell function. There are a lot of functions for the white blood cells, but we can think of them as cells that police our internal cities. They go around and fight disease. If they become compromised, the bad guys win. That's why I recommend the diet be as pure and as organic as possible.

JENNY: What about honey?

DR. JERRY: Honey, maple syrup—these are all sugars. My son was actually allergic to cane sugar, so we used beet sugar for a sweetening agent as well as maple syrup crystals.

JENNY: I thought you said no to maple syrup.

DR. JERRY: If you take maple syrup and boil it down completely, you get maple syrup crystals. You can buy it this way. It's a great alternative to cane sugar and is great in gluten-free coffee cake. So, table sugar substitutes are good, but keep in mind that the overall goal is to drastically decrease all sugar sources. If a recipe calls for a cup of sugar, you do half a cup, or a quarter cup, of sugar. To a child who's on a very low sugar diet, that is still really sweet and delicious because their taste buds are more sensitive to sweet (since we have scaled back on the overall daily sugar intake). Back in the old days, when my grandma was making apple pie, she would slice up the apples, and she would sprinkle just a little bit of sugar and cinnamon on top and that was it. She made pies this way out of habit from the sugar rationing during World War II. The pies were always sweet and delicious. That's how they made things then. Over time, sugar has popped up in all kinds of foods that historically were sugar-free. The amount of sugar consumed by Americans has increased tremendously over the past few years. So much so that now, when you order a slice of apple pie, there is a gooey gelatinous super-sweet glaze incorporated throughout.

JENNY: It's the sugar generation!

DR. JERRY: Yes, and it's weakening the immune system. Different studies from the USDA all correlate that there has been a marked increase in the consumption of sugar and sweeteners over the past two decades.

IVIG for Boosting the Immune System

JENNY: Let's talk now about IVIG. This is another treatment that parents talk about and I don't think they even know what it stands for.

DR. JERRY: IVIG is intravenous immunoglobulin. IVIG is more of an immune system therapeutic intervention. IV just means intravenous; it's put in by the vein. IG stands for immunoglobulins, which are antibodies. But before we talk about replacing them, which is what IVIG does, we have to know what they are, and there are generally four types that we talk about.

WHAT THE IMMUNE SYSTEM IS, THE FOUR TYPES OF IMMUNOGLOBULINS, AND HOW TO TEST THE SYSTEM'S FUNCTIONING

JENNY: I guess now would be the time to expand on the different types of immunoglobulins.

IgG

DR. JERRY: Yes, and do you remember what those are?

JENNY: Hmmm . . . let's start with IgG. I know it has to do with food sensitivity because I see the little IgG on the top of Evan's food sensitivity test.

DR. JERRY: Yes, but it also does something else.

JENNY: I'm getting to it! I'm blond and it takes me a minute to recall past the bleach damage.

DR. JERRY: (Laughs) Okay, okay.

JENNY: It's also supposed to remember what disease or whatever you got in the past and not let you get it again.

DR. JERRY: Very good! In the allergy chapter we described immunoglobulins as protein substances that have the ability to tag cells, viruses, fungi, for destruction. Immunoglobulin G gives you long-term protection from a disease. So, for example, if you were to measure my IgG to chicken pox that I had forty-two years ago, you would see that mine would come back on the lab report as elevated. It doesn't mean that chicken pox is bothering me right now; it just means that I have these little Patriot missiles specifically designed to blow up chicken pox virus should I get exposed to it when, say, I am visiting a second-grade classroom. The virus enters my nose or mouth, and then these IgGs that are primed and ready to immobilize and "tag" the chicken pox virus before the virus can replicate. I won't ever get clinically ill with chicken pox because of these very specific IgGs.

JENNY: I used to get so confused when I saw Evan's IgG viral panel come back and it said he had human herpes virus 6 (HHV-6).

DR. JERRY: And that's why you asked me to start him on Valtrex (an antiviral prescription medication that can kill some of the herpes viruses). I had to explain to you that the panel just tells us he was indeed exposed to human herpes virus type 6 and that there are many types of herpes viruses, not just the "one" we learn about in school (HHV-2). HHV-6 is another one of these types that is "caught," like a cold, out in the community. Evan was just exposed to HHV-6 in the past (like my chicken pox IgG). It does NOT mean that this virus is CURRENTLY acting mischievously in Evan's body. Almost all of us (95 percent of the world's population have IgG antibodies to HHV-6) have had exposure to human herpes virus 6, but it doesn't mean that it's actually a problem today. With that said, HHV-6 can reactivate and has been associated with autoimmune disorders, mononucleosis syndrome, and neurological complications.

JENNY: So Evan's IgG just means that he is making Patriot missiles to human herpes virus 6.

DR. JERRY: Chicken pox is a herpes virus, too, and is also known as HHV-3. The IgG test can show us that the disease has been there in the past, but it doesn't mean that it's actually a problem today.

Bottom line: We really like the IgGs because they give us long-term protection from certain diseases.

IgA

JENNY: Okay, so I really understand IgG and its job in the immune system. What about IgA?

DR. JERRY: The next group, IgA or the A class, are the immunoglobulins that float on body parts that are generally wet, like the eyes, the nose, the mouth, and down all the way to the anus (because that whole small intestine and large intestine tube is "wet"). The vaginal area and the urethra are included, too.

JENNY: So these IgA dudes will protect you from colds?

DR. JERRY: Yes, these will protect you from bacteria and viruses that enter the nose, the mouth, and the eyes. That's how you catch disease. If somebody coughs, the droplets will get into the eyes, the nose, or the mouth, and we inhale them and that's how we get disease.

JENNY: That kind of grosses me out to picture these bacteria bugs coming out of someone's sneeze and entering my eyeballs.

DR. JERRY: And many of our kids have deficient levels of IgAs and will experience multiple respiratory infections, sinus infections, or ear infections. These children may have chronic gut infections as well because they have too little IgA to start the process of "invader destruction." A child can get two or three ear infections during the first year of life. This is very common following a cold. They will often be put on amoxicillin and will improve rapidly. The scenario I am concerned about is the recurrent ear infections and multiple antibiotic usages. Where is the immune panel? Why didn't the pediatrician or the family practice doc who was taking care of this child look and evaluate the child and say, "We have an immune system problem. There is something really wrong with this immune system's ability to fight disease. Let's see what it is."

JENNY: What would it have shown on that panel?

DR. JERRY: IgA deficiency. Perhaps IgG deficiency, or even both.

JENNY: So now moms can tell their doctor, "Hey, Doc, this is the sixth ear infection in eight months. It's time to check his IgA, and since we are drawing blood, let's check his whole immune system while we are at it!"

So something is causing the IgA to drop because these kids are getting sick suddenly. They aren't born like this, so what happened?

DR. JERRY: I believe that they were not born like this, but something has come along and modified the way the immune system behaves.

JENNY: Wow, so if vaccines can cause the lower IgA levels and our kids become sick all the time, how are they supposed to detox or handle the viruses we are injecting into them when they can't even fight off an ear infection?

DR. JERRY: Now you bring up a very good point here. If infections are not handled well, such as a chronic sinus infection or chronically recurring ear infections, the immune system will sustain a state of chronic inflammation. In this particular state, small signaling proteins (cytokines and interleukins, for example) that help with the immune function also seem to impact behaviors of the child in a very negative way. This can contribute the "fog" or "disconnect" that these children seem to exhibit. IgA can help protect mucous membranes from infection, which in turn protects the child from a chronic inflammatory state and its behavioral impact.

IgM

JENNY: So let's move on to the next type, which is called IgM.

DR. JERRY: These guys are the first responders. Early in the course of an infection, it's the IgM's job to start the immune response to remove the offending agent.

JENNY: Do these guys actually go in and destroy, or do they just kind of say, "Hey, everybody, check out this stuff we found?"

DR. JERRY: They generally tag and let the immune system know that there's a real problem going on here. If you have too low a level of IgM, you are more prone to disease.

JENNY: So basically what I'm learning thus far is that we are going to ask our pediatricians not only for an IgA test, but we want to ask for the entire immune panel to be done. IgG, IgA, IgM . . .

IgE

DR. JERRY: And IgE! We will mention more about IgE in the allergies chapter. Do you remember what they do?

JENNY: Hold on, gimme a second, it's coming to me. I can hear the *Jeopardy* music playing in my head, waiting for me to answer. One more second.

DR. JERRY: Ha, ha!

JENNY: IgEs have something to do with severe food allergy or pollen allergy.

DR. JERRY: Yes, these are the ones that give you problems with allergies, and very often they are sky high in our kids. Their role in the human body, besides making us miserable with allergies, is still being worked out. Current thinking is that they do have a role in protecting us from parasitic and protozoan infection. The allergist is concerned with IgEs and allergic symptoms, and will perform scratch tests to environmental and food sources. IgE levels are commonly found to be elevated in autism. What this translates to in our children is significant multiple allergies to everything from house dust mites to timothy grass pollen to mold spores to foods. Children's allergic behaviors are often very difficult to manage as they can appear to be "dull," "checked out," or they can head bang or perform other self-injurious behaviors, and can also be prone to temper tantrums, loss of focus and concentration, to name just a few findings.

IG Deficiency

DR. JERRY: Now, if you're deficient in the G class, the M class, or the A class, we call that an immunoglobulin deficiency, and is technically termed hypogammaglobulinemia. This is not autism. This is an immune system deficiency and it's recognized by insurance companies along with the accepted therapeutic intervention: intravenous immunoglobulins (IVIG). That is, we are replacing the low immunoglobulins measured with a preparation derived from human blood. Now, this is not to be trifled with, this is a human blood product. It generally comes from fifty thousand donors or more, so the child will have a huge exposure to potential illness-causing components (though very rare). We know scientifically how to clean up this preparation so it will not be a source of infection itself, but risks remain.

JENNY: So in a nutshell, IVIG is taking roughly fifty thousand people's blood donations and it's pulling out antibodies (immunoglobulins) so that it can fight bad guys that our kids can't fight.

DR. JERRY: Yes, it's pulling out their immunoglobulins that they have made against a whole host of diseases (not *the* diseases, but rather the infection-fighting immunoglobulins). Typically, these donors have "seen" and made antibodies to chicken pox, human herpes virus 6, rhinovirus, adenovirus, and many, many other diseases. We are giving the children these donor-derived antibodies to circulate through their bloodstream so when they get exposed to a disease entity, or have some disease festering, they will now have the antibodies to go after it.

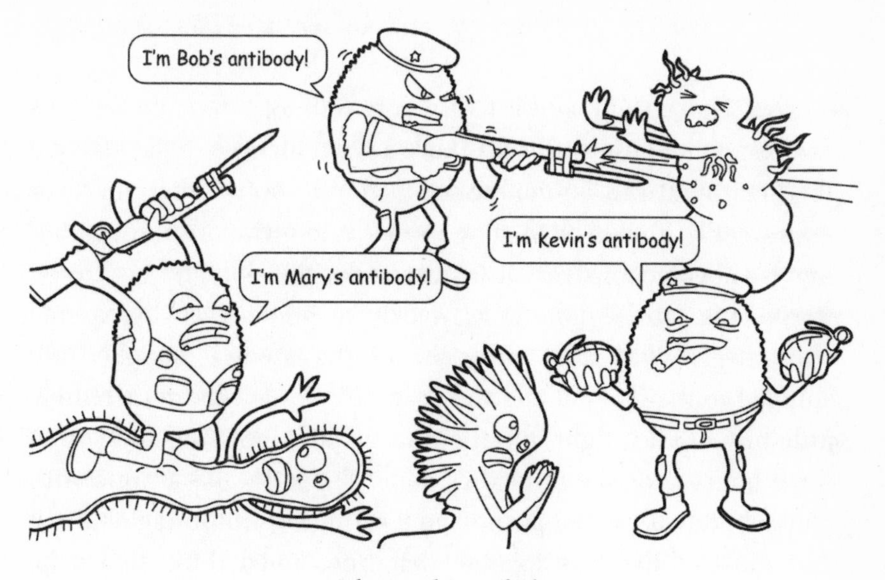

Other people's antibodies

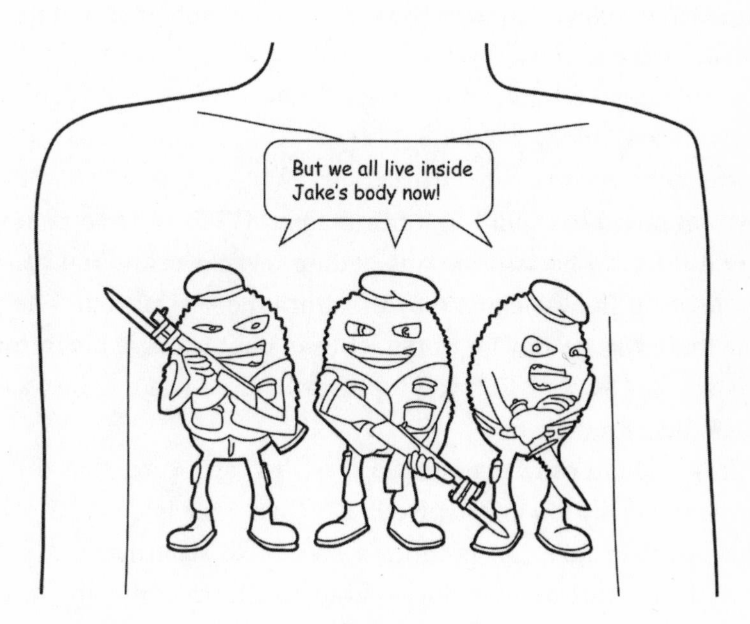

After IVIG

JENNY: Wow, I had no idea that you can transfer these IGs to someone else!

DR. JERRY: That's right, and it's very, very well tolerated and the kids can respond. These antibodies have a short lifetime in the body, so this treatment can be done once a month, every other week, or even weekly, if need be. A new approach to giving immunoglobulins is subcutaneously (that is, just under the skin and not in the vein). This can be done once weekly, at home, even by parents themselves. With this approach, all the medical supplies are shipped to the parents and they can actually put these incredibly little tiny needles right into the tummy fat, tape it up, and two to three hours later, the infusion's done. The kid walks around with a little buddy pack (the pump and a syringe of immunoglobulins) and most of the kids tolerate that fine. You'd think they'd be pulling them out, screaming and yelling the whole time, but they do just fine. Insurance companies like this approach because it is less expensive to administer. The subcutaneous approach also has fewer side effects—patients treated this way usually avoid the headaches and vomiting associated with the more traditional intravenous approach.

When IVIG Is Dangerous

JENNY: I remember when I first heard about IVIG. I was so excited to get it for Evan because he was getting fevers weekly. You had me go to see if he was eligible by this immune specialist and he told me there was no way he would let Evan do it because his immune system was SO bad. Can you explain why Evan was told he was not a candidate for it?

DR. JERRY: There can be a situation, as in Evan's case, that the IgA level is actually too low to give IVIG. Giving the body IVIG, which does contain IgA, can produce a shock-like state that can potentially be life-threatening. So, for Evan, this form of therapy was not an option.

JENNY: And because of that, Evan never received IVIG, but I would like to say that since we have "cleaned him out," his last IG panel came back normal. It happened without IVIG.

DR. JERRY: That's exactly right. This is what we are trying to do. The interventions discussed in this book are shutting down vicious cycles that perpetuate abnormal physiologic functions. Reversal is brought about by removing toxins and quenching inflammatory reactions. Yes, the good news is, once we removed the disease process, restored the pristine cycles, the body can reset not only the immune system but also other bodily functions back to the way that God designed it.

JENNY: That just happened to be Evan's case, but I do want to say that the moms I talked to who did IVIG had seen amazing results, including some recoveries. Have you seen that?

DR. JERRY: Yes, and it is very exciting. Think of it this way. Children with autism, or any of us, for that matter, will have much more success in learning if we are feeling great as opposed to sick. If I were a teacher, therapist, etc., give me a healthy, non-hurting child any day of the week to teach, for I will have much better results, as opposed to the sick, hurting, and angry child. So, these children will make dramatic progress in a short time. One of the downsides is expense. That is why we have to be so careful to document what we are treating so as to garner the insurance company's willingness to participate in the therapy (isn't that a nice way of saying it?).

IVIG Cost and Procedure

JENNY: How expensive is the treatment?

DR. JERRY: It is very, very expensive and the cost varies according to the child's weight. On average, though, it runs $1,500 a dose. So, if you're doing twelve doses a year or twenty-four doses a year, depending on how you're breaking it down, it can be prohibitively expensive if not approved by insurance. I have had some very determined parents go to their churches or their synagogues, asking for support. Some raise the money in very exciting ways. One mom had some "bad boy" bikers raise thousands of dollars (all legal!) for her son Jared. He received all the IVIG he needed.

JENNY: So IVIG is not a treatment for autism at all; it's a therapeutic treatment for immune deficiency.

DR. JERRY: Absolutely, ESPECIALLY where the insurance company is involved, and if, by chance, the patient's autism dramatically improves, *oh, well!*

Interpreting Immune System Tests

JENNY: When parents go into their pediatrician's office and demand they get these tests done, whether it's the immune system testing or any other type of testing, a lot of the lab work comes back telling us that it's high or low only in an adult range. There is no kid range, most of the time, so how do we know if it really is high or low?

DR. JERRY: You're right. "Normal" is usually reported as high or low according to ADULT ranges. We have to be very careful when we look at it and pronounce, for example, "The thyroid is normal." We have to ask ourselves several questions. Is that normal for an adult? Is it normal for our kids? In addition, there is a wide range of what's normal for each child. So, despite falling in a normal range, it may be abnormally low for the one child we are seeing in the office. In other words, using our example of the thyroid study, if a child presents with a low body temperature, constipation, decreased energy, and irritability (common symptoms of low thyroid function), I am going to treat him regardless of how normal his thyroid studies are. I treat the child, not a piece of laboratory paper. Laboratory values give us some good ideas where to start, but the clinical and historical findings trump the computer printout on the laboratory report. That's just how I was trained.

JENNY: So you're saying, besides looking at the lab work, you also always look at the child's behaviors to treat because the lab might not be telling the whole story.

DR. JERRY: Yes. I was clinically trained in medicine, and all the laboratory provided was support and additional clues. These clues can be very helpful indeed, but not the last word. You still have to look at the child. That's what I do.

JENNY: That's why I want to marry you.

DR. JERRY: Ha, ha! I don't think my wife would give me up.

JENNY: I'm completely into sharing you. I will live in the attic.

DR. JERRY: I don't think so, but I'll ask Donna. (I actually did, and she said we can adopt you!)

JENNY: How do parents trust that the pediatrician even knows how to read these tests correctly since he's looking at "adult" normal ranges and not "children's" normal ranges?

DR. JERRY: There are so many different ranges for the laboratory testing; the doctor will have to refer to textbooks that have the normal ranges. Every value can be researched in these texts. These texts break down the different findings to age brackets. It just takes time to look them up, which is not so easy if the doctor is running from one patient to the next every ten minutes. This is inconvenient. But, hey, one could easily argue that autism is inconvenient.

IMPROVEMENTS TO AUTISM SYMPTOMS DURING ILLNESS

JENNY: Continuing on with the immune system . . .

Can you explain why some of the kids' autism symptoms seem to disappear when they're sick? I've called you in the past, saying, "Evan has lost his diagnosis during a fever."

DR. JERRY: This is actually common. Some children can be so "with it" when they are sick with fever or on antibiotics. Another consideration, too, is when they are ill, they usually are not eating very much as well. There are many theories here. One thought is that the foods the child consumes are significantly affecting the behaviors. These kids typically do best when they do not eat, or if they are getting a major bowel clean-out for endoscopy (they usually are placed on a clear liquid diet, and given lots of laxatives to remove ALL the stool in their colon). This is a big clue. Another thought is that while the child is ill, the immune system is focusing its attention on the disease process and is basically not acting "mischievously," if you will. There is a lot of work going on looking at the autoimmune nature of the immune system and the diseases caused by this harmful process. In a nutshell, autoimmunity results in tissue destruction and inflammation.

JENNY: You said earlier that "autoimmune" is when your immune system attacks your own tissues, right?

DR. JERRY: Yes, and when the child gets sick, the immune system goes to work on the illness and forgets its mischievousness and takes off to go do its job of preventing a bacterial infection from spreading or a viral infection from worsening. The disease process (a vicious cycle) that goes on while the child is well stops when the child is ill and the child becomes very coherent. They can all of a sudden have terrific use of language, heightened awareness, and increased calmness. The parents comment, "You know, when he has a fever or is sick, he is his very best."

JENNY: That makes so much sense! I just got a big lightbulb moment. My dad, who had rheumatoid arthritis, which is autoimmune—

DR. JERRY: I know.

JENNY: I know you know; I'm telling everyone else. Well, when my dad caught a fever for four days, he was sicker than a dog, but he suddenly could move freely and walk. Before his fever, his arthritis made him frozen stiff like a zombie. That's a perfect example of his immune system being mischievous by attacking his joints with arthritis, but when a virus came in, it left it alone and went and fought the infection. That's why his arthritis went away temporarily. Once the fever went away, his arthritis came back! The immune system became mischievous again.

DR. JERRY: That's right. This could be a very big clue for his management. He has a chronic inflammatory autoimmune condition. When he was sick, his immune system was sidetracked for a time and he felt great. What we do in the management of autism may have significant implications in the management of other inflammatory and autoimmune conditions.

T-HELPER CELLS

JENNY: Okay, moving on. I'm so excited to talk about the Th1 cells and the Th2 cells!

DR. JERRY: Wow, does Jim know you get that excited about Th1 and Th2 cells?

JENNY: Actually, yes. All I talk about are new medical words I've learned. I think he might daydream half the time when I explain what they mean, but I don't really mind. I have a ball!!

DR. JERRY: Okay, so let's hear you explain, then, what the Th1 and Th2 cells do?

JENNY: "Th" just means T-helper cells, and I need a pen so I can draw on paper what they do.

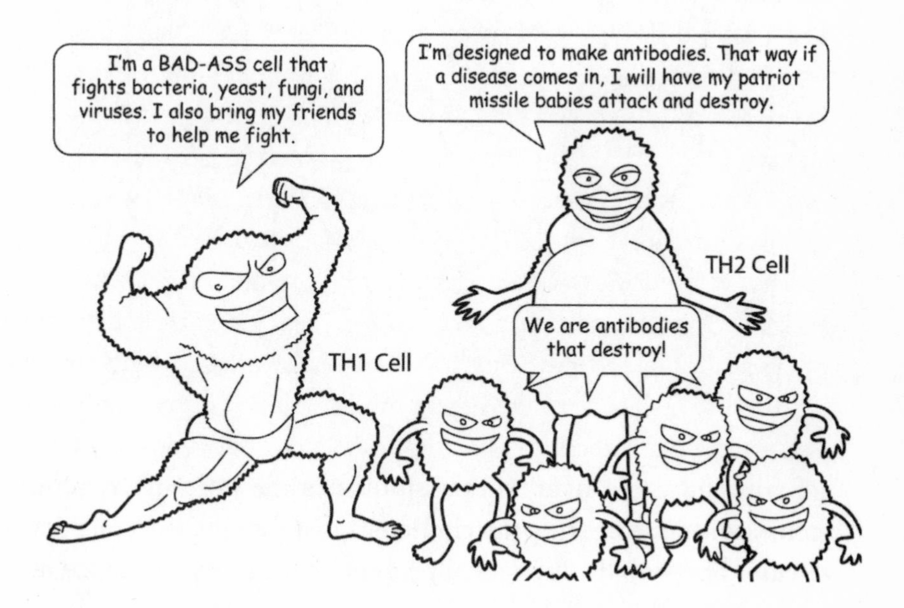

DR. JERRY: That's right, and the Th2 side of the immune system is really responsible for making the antibodies for the vaccines that we're exposed to. Thus, if you are ever exposed to that disease again, such as chicken pox or roseola (human herpes type 6), you have antibodies for it.

JENNY: And the vaccine makers really count on those Th2 cells to make tons of antibodies to ensure long-lasting protection from diseases. However, this is not always the case. For example, in the original formulation of the tetanus shot, it didn't cause that much of an immune response, so it didn't give long-lasting protection.

DR. JERRY: To ensure a vigorous response to vaccines, the vaccine makers discovered a way to further stimulate the immune system. By adding a substance called an adjuvant, the response to the vaccine was better than when giving the vaccine alone. This ensured that there would be antibodies made to the vaccine and the immune memory would be robust . . . that is, the protection would be for many years.

PHARMACORP
How will we make our vaccines last longer in humans?
I know! Let's add aluminum!

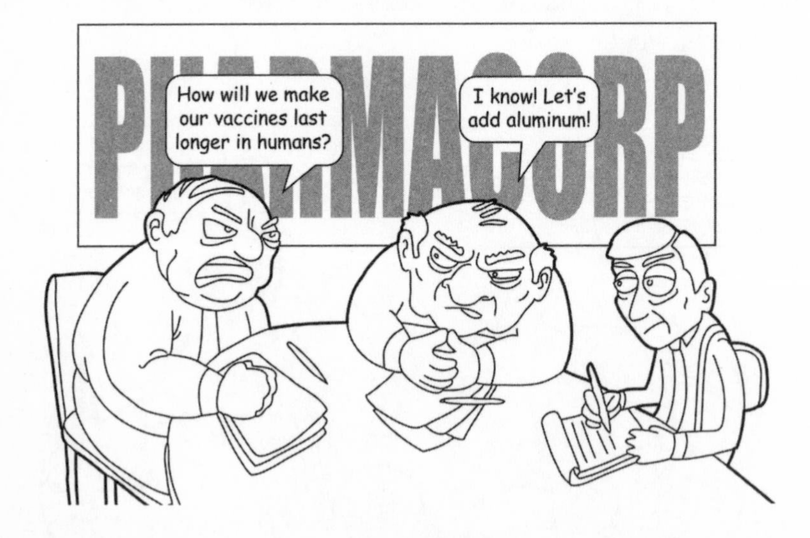

Adjuvants are anything that stimulates the immune system, such as aluminum. The problem here is that they did not consider whether this would stimulate anything else or if this substance itself could be toxic to the body. There is a long list of other ingredients aside from adjuvants that can be readily found in vaccines.

JENNY: I don't know how anyone could think aluminum wouldn't be toxic.

DR. JERRY: The problem is that all this foreign matter is being injected into our very young children without sufficient testing, except for the demonstration of antibody response by the human body. So that when a pharmaceutical company wants to demonstrate to the FDA that these vaccines work, they say, "Look, we've looked at a large number of kids, we gave them a shot of tetanus, and three months later, we drew antibody titers to tetanus and they all converted!" And they said, "Shazam, it works." But they don't look any farther down the road to see the consequences of their actions.

JENNY: There is a downside to increasing the role of the Th2 cells that no one talks about and I'm going to draw it.

This is after using adjuvants like aluminum and/or many other different adjuvants.

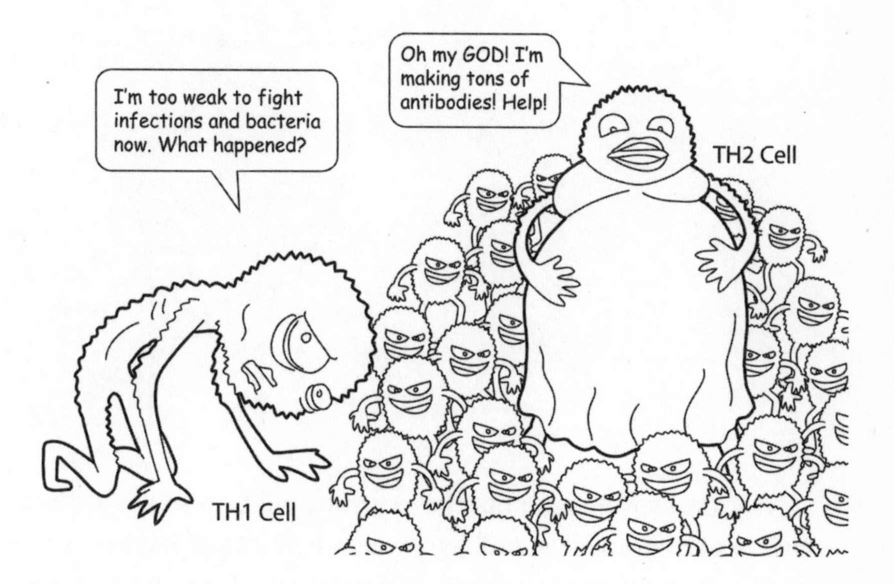

That's when parents start to notice a change in their child's health and the scene usually looks like this.

Doctor, I don't understand why my son gets so many ear infections now...
Twelve ear infections is nothing! Don't worry!
It's almost like his TH1 cells became weak and he can't fight anything.
What's a TH1 cell?

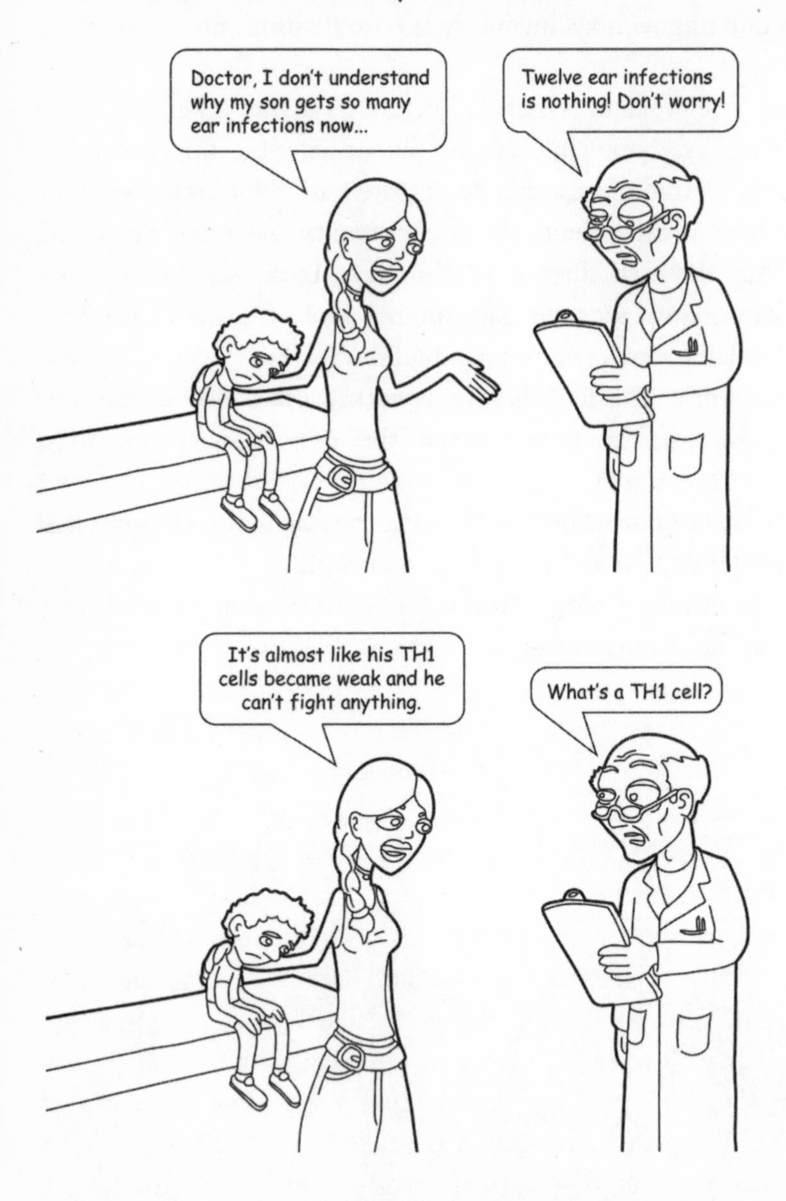

DR. JERRY: That's right, and they keep getting colds. Doctors will say, "You have to get him out of day care," trying to put the blame on Mom when what really happened was the Th1 cells are not able to fight anything and the Th2 has become a superpower. Due to the Th2 hyper response, these children develop allergies, asthma, and eczema, along with a whole host of behavioral changes.

IMMUNE REPAIR AND THE GI TRACT

Depending on the damage, many immune systems can recover, or at least improve greatly. There are many different protocols one could follow. Let's just discuss a few of them. I would like to start with the gastrointestinal tract. This is a great place to start, since the vast majority of the immune system lines the GI tract.

First of all, it is important to ensure daily bowel movements. You know, just having a huge amount of stool in the bowels can be the source of a lot of bad behaviors. So, we will clean out the children first (see the stool section for further instructions on how this is accomplished, page 217).

Next, we have to add a lot of good, healthy bacteria, which are called probiotics. These should be given twice daily. It is important to find good-quality probiotics that are dairy-free (www.kartnerhealth.com and www.klaire.com). If you have a physician who is willing to do stool and urine tests, it can be determined if your child has an overgrowth of yeast or pathologic bacteria in the GI tract. If so, most often, prescription drugs are needed to rid the colon of these invaders. If a physician is not willing to help and you are on your own, adding supplements like caprylic acid and monolaurin can really help. In addition, one must decrease the "nutritive" materials reaching the colon (so we don't keep feeding the bacteria/yeast), so we should drastically reduce the daily sugar consumption (juices, fruits, and carbohydrates) and consider adding a digestive enzyme with each meal. There are many options out there for cleaning the gut, but most of these preparations are herbal and have a very strong smell and taste that most children who do not yet swallow capsules will just not take. But you can try my recommendations for laxatives in the poop chapter on page 217.

The next step to improving the immune system will include removing as many toxins and stressors as possible. This includes cleaning up the child's environment, starting with the bedroom. Many synthetic carpets give off gas toxins that are not tolerated well by children. I removed the carpet in my son's room right down to the concrete slab! Both the carpet and the pad underneath it were off-gassing. One must thoroughly consider all allergic sources and remove them as well. More strategies will be discussed later in the allergy section of the book.

In the meantime, here are some clinical nutrients that can assist in rebuilding the immune system and bringing the brain back into balance in the Th1/Th2 equation. Please see the supplement chapter (page 53) for dosage:

Zinc
Selenium
Chromium
Vitamins A, B_6, C, and E
Cod liver oil

The transfer factor is a collection of disease-fighting elements taken from another species (such as cows) and given to humans. This can be very helpful, too, by identifying foreign invaders and triggering your immune response. One transfer factor we like to use is the colostrum in cow's milk. Colostrum is the "first" milk of the mammal that is rich in immunoglobulins. Hence, we are "transferring" the immunoglobulins from one source (usually the cow—after breastfeeding, that is) to the child. Even the antibodies (IgG, IgA, IgM, IgE) from a cow can be very helpful when ingested by our children as it really helps the GI tract. Depending on the product, one to two teaspoons one to three times daily can be a real help. It is interesting to note that even though this is a cow's-milk-derived product, the casein has been removed and is usually well-tolerated by children who are strictly dairy-free. A brand that I like is Kirkman's Colostrum (www.kirkmanlabs.com).

5
ALLERGIES AND FOOD SENSITIVITIES

I don't feel so good.
That's because they're feeding us antibiotics and hor-mones now.
No wonder our farts are destroying the atmosphere.

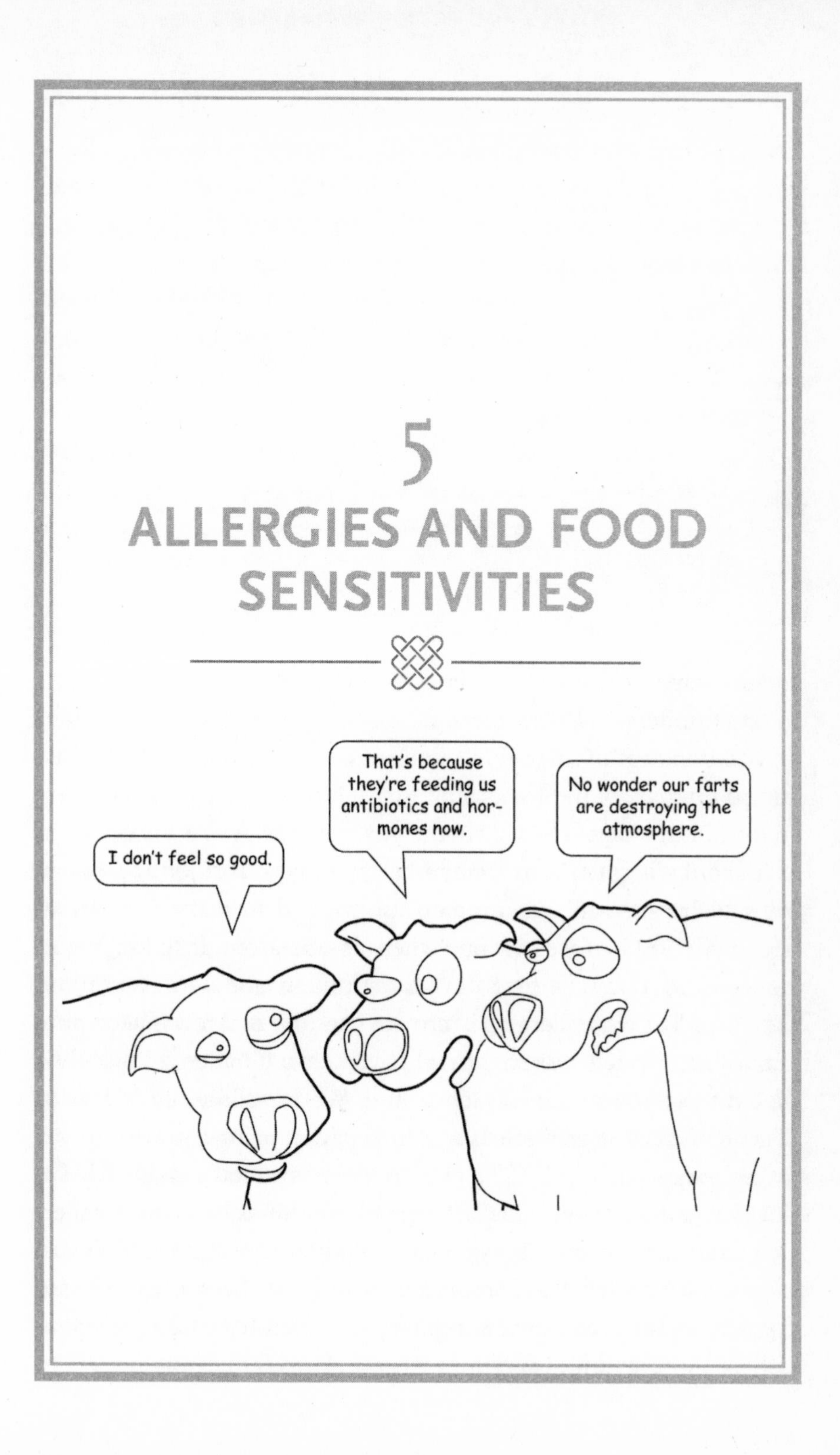

WHEN I USED TO GIVE EVAN his scrambled eggs in the morning, I couldn't understand why he would lose his mind five minutes after he was done eating. I couldn't understand why Evan would get red bumps on his face moments after I gave him pineapple. Growing up on the South Side of Chicago in the 70s, we didn't experience or even hear about allergies. I only remember that my cousin Johnny was allergic to bees, so in the summertime we had to make sure we all screamed "BEE!" if we saw one when he was around. Today, one in three children has allergies and I don't understand why every mom who has a kid with allergies is not questioning it. Are we becoming numb to it because our friends all have kids with allergies also? We shouldn't accept this. It's absolute bull. We are filling our kids with Claritin and acting as if this is a normal part of being a human in our society today. When I finally took Evan in for his food allergy and sensitivity test, I was amazed to find out all the things he came up allergic to and how many things he came up sensitive to. And that was just for food. Aside from common food allergies, he was also allergic to grass, certain trees, pollen, dogs, cats, dust mites, and I can go on and on. I lost my mind and immediately started educating myself on what happens to the body when you have an allergic reaction. I learned that the body creates histamine, which then causes a neurological reaction. Evan would tantrum and itch or scream for hours till it settled down. I immediately removed everything that he had an issue with. If my ex-husband would have let me rip out all the grass and put cement down so Evan wouldn't suffer anymore, I would have done it. I eventually learned that by killing Evan's yeast and strengthening his immune system, his allergies went from severe to minimal. I beg EVERY parent to get their child an IgG test. It made such an incredible difference in Evan's life and I know it will in your child's, too.

JENNY: Seriously, it's gotten out of control. I don't know one mom who has a child who is free from allergies. Everybody got hit. It's the allergy generation. Can you explain what the hell happened?

ALLERGIES AND THE IMMUNE SYSTEM

DR. JERRY: There will be a common thread throughout this book about the immune system being responsible for many issues. Virtually all allergies are the result of an improperly regulated immune system. Now, there are different types of allergic responses that the immune system can make. We will keep it simple. IgE is responsible for the "classic" response to allergens. This causes the runny, itchy nose, itchy eyes, cough, eczema, asthma, and more seriously, anaphylactic shock. IgE allergies are what the allergist will test for with the skin "prick" test. Many children have markedly elevated levels of IgE. My second son, John, runs levels between 900 and 1,200 with a normal being less than 150. He would develop hives if he played in the grass. He had "allergic" croup quite often growing up. Having elevated levels of IgE will make one more sensitive to environmental exposures such as house dust mites, mold, pollens, and foods.

As you know, Jenny, since the mid to late 1980s, the large

increase of allergic symptoms in children also corresponds to the increase in asthma, attention deficit disorder, and autism. There are many published medical journal articles that show that the MMR vaccine could be "switching on" the overproduction of IgE.

"Infection of Human B Lymphocytes with MMR Vaccine Induces IgE Class Switching" by Farhad Imani and Kelley E. Kehoe (2001, *Clinical Immunology*) is just one article illustrating that we really do have evidence that vaccines, along with environmental toxins, may be ushering the epidemic of dysfunction we are currently seeing in our children. Have we merely substituted one potential epidemic (say, a measles epidemic) for another very real and current epidemic (autism)?

WHAT TO TEST FOR, HOW TO TEST, AND WHAT TO TREAT

JENNY: Can you explain the food allergy tests that our kids should have?

DR. JERRY: We certainly can look for the IgE responses to foods. Fortunately, they are not very common. We are very aware of the potential of peanuts to cause anaphylactic shock in some children with an IgE allergy to peanuts. The "skin prick" test can be a very difficult test for children with autism because they are already sensitive to touch, let alone to a prick from a needle. Another method to find out if a child is IgE allergic to foods AND environmental substances is what is called provocation/neutralization/desensitization (aka PND). In this testing, the allergist will determine the very smallest amount of an allergen that does NOT cause a skin reaction. It is this a minute concentration that is placed in sublingual drops, nasal spray, or weekly shots and given to the child daily. The end result of this therapeutic intervention is actually desensitization of allergies and, over time, actually a cure.

JENNY: Is it true, then, that when the IgEs are elevated in our kids, like in Evan's case, that they then become allergic to everything, and I mean everything, from dust mites to mold to forty different foods?

DR. JERRY: Yes, that's what happens when the IgE becomes elevated.

JENNY: What happened that caused this?

DR. JERRY: When we get vaccinated, there are things that are purposefully put into vaccines to wake up the immune system to make antibodies. Remember, antibodies are like specifically "crafted" Patriot missiles, and in the case of vaccines, they are specific for a particular disease, for example, tetanus. One method to get the body to make a large amount of specific antibodies is to put into the vaccine a substance that will stimulate this production. This substance is called an adjuvant. Aluminum is a very common adjuvant. Bottom line here: The stimulated immune system is responsible for causing the child to become allergic to many environmental and food exposures.

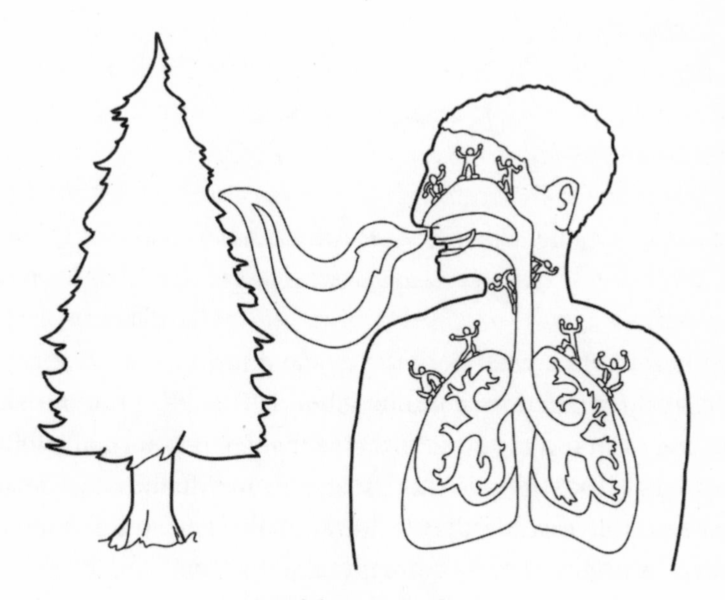

IgEs fighting tree pollen

IgG

Dr. Jerry: Another type of allergy can be triggered by the immunoglobulin IgG. The medical community generally does not officially recognize this type of reaction as "allergic." These reactions can occur shortly after eating, but can even happen two to three days later, making it difficult to figure out which food is causing the behaviors seen in the child (something just eaten, or something eaten two to three days ago).

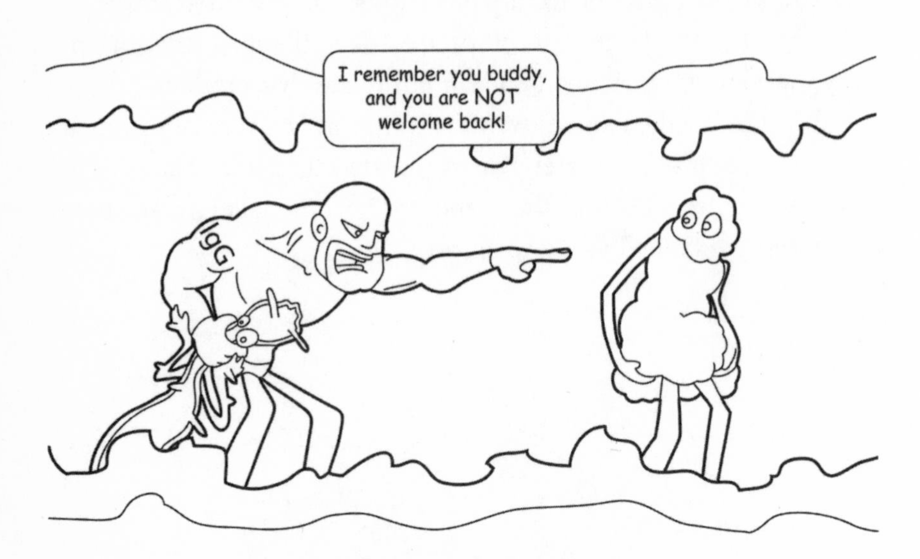

IgG remembers old diseases you once had or diseases it was vaccinated for and destroys them!

Jenny: Remind me, what does the Ig stand for?

Dr. Jerry: Ig stands for immunoglobulin. This is a protein made by the body that can tag other proteins that are not normally found in the body. This "tagging" is a first step in an inflammatory response and immune cascade that will eventually remove this foreign invader from the body. Generally, the IgG will tag bacteria and viruses and protect you from illnesses. When it starts tagging food, we can have a real problem. It is believed that the constant inflammatory response going on in the body (by repeatedly eating the foods that we are "allergic" to) will significantly contribute to the brain fog and "disconnect" our children have. The IgG reaction is different from the IgE reaction we just mentioned. Keep in mind, though, we have two other types of Ig, IgA and IgM, which are also involved in keeping us healthy. (Note: We also have IgD, but it is not yet well understood.)

You are going to die, foreign invader!
But I'm just broccoli. How can I be bad?
IgG

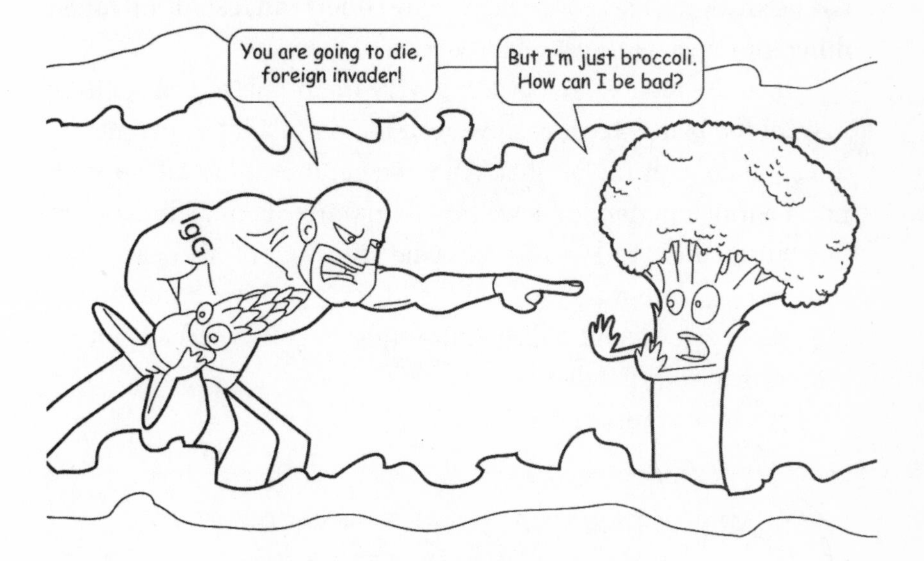

IgG also attacks food like it's a foreign invader.

As we discussed before, most of the foods we eat contain protein. After the food is swallowed, the digestive juices are supposed to chop this protein into smaller and smaller pieces, which we call amino acids. The amino acids will be absorbed into the bloodstream and later, into cells, will be reassembled into another protein that our body needs. BUT, if some of the proteins in the food we eat are NOT broken down, and *leak* into the bloodstream, the IgG part of the immune system will take great notice of this and attack them as if they were bacteria or viruses. Okay, so we have problem number one with the digestive tract allowing food proteins into the bloodstream instead of being properly digested and sent to the colon. Problem number two is the immune system makes IgG antibodies to some of these foods, IgG to dairy foods, IgG to apples, to wheat, etc. Now, for example, every time the child eats an apple, he goes foggy!

There is a wonderful blood test, called an IgG Food Sensitivity Panel, that will inform a parent of which foods need to be avoided in order to help remove the cloudy "funk" the child may continually be stuck in. These food sensitivity panels can test for up to 184 different foods with just one teaspoon of blood.

Once the results are back, it is very important to totally eliminate all foods that have positive results. I have a lot of parents try to negotiate with me on that. After we get the child really operating at a much higher level, we may then think about adding one or two things back. I have a patient who stims out of his head when he eats rice . . . but he received the lowest "positive" value on the IgG panel. He would still be stimming today if we had not removed rice from the diet.

Let's look at just one article below:

ALUMINIUM AS AN ADJUVANT IN VACCINES AND POST-VACCINE REACTIONS

Fiejka M, Aleksandrowicz J. Zakladu Badania Surowic, Warszawie. Rocz Panstw Zakl Hig. 1993;44(1):73-80. PMID: 8235346 [PubMed—indexed for MEDLINE]

Aluminium compounds have been widely used as adjuvants in prophylactic and therapeutic vaccines. Adjuvants are able to stimulate the immune system in a nonspecific manner, i.e. high antibody level can be obtained with minimal dose of the antigen and with reduced number of inoculations. Adjuvants use has been mostly empirically determined by such factors as efficacy and safety. The mechanism of action of the aluminium adjuvants is not completely understood and is very complex. The basic factors of the mode of action: 1) the com-

> plex of antigen and aluminium gel is more immunogenic in structure than free antigen, 2) effect "depot"—The antigen stimulus lasts longer, 3) the production of local granulomas. Vaccines absorbed onto aluminium salts are a more frequent cause of local post-vaccinal reactions than plain vaccines. 5–10% of those vaccinated can develop a nodule lasting several weeks at the injection site. In some rare cases the nodules may become inflammatory and even turn into an aseptic abscess. The nodules persisting more than 6 weeks may indicate development of aluminium hypersensitivity. Finally aluminium adjuvant immunogens induce the production of IgE antibodies.

As thimerosal was removed from vaccines, aluminum continues to be one of the many ingredients commonly found in vaccines, and in greater concentrations per vaccine. A quick search on PubMed or even Google can reveal some potentially worrisome findings. In this case, the above article illustrates the potential effects of aluminum on the immune system with respect to IgE production. We have not discussed other effects, such as diminished response to viral, bacterial, or fungal infections, nor have we considered the induction of autoimmune diseases. Keep in mind there are twenty-plus different ingredients used in the formation of vaccines, under three main listings: adjuvants, preservatives, and stabilizers. There can also be an "acceptable" amount of contaminants as well. I am very concerned that as the number of vaccines given to each child has grown substantially over the past twenty years, we are finding very quickly the children who are not able to detoxify these ingredients. This poisoning manifests as the diseases discussed in this book.

JENNY: I cover that whole nightmare about adjuvants in the immune system chapter, but what I've learned from you is that the adjuvants cause the body to make TONS of antibodies and can cause the IgEs to go bonkers. So you're saying when they go bonkers, that's when they elevate and cause crazy allergies.

DR. JERRY: Yes. I am also very concerned to see the increased rates of children being diagnosed with autism, ADHD, asthma, allergies, and autoimmune diseases over the past twenty years. I am thrilled to see the attention given lately in the media, and yet I am very sad that it has taken such large numbers of sick children with their parents to finally be recognized as an "epidemic."

JENNY: Do parents need to go to an allergist for the IgG test or can they have their pediatrician do it?

DR. JERRY: Any physician can order an IgG "RAST" food allergy panel.

YEAST AND THE IMMUNE RESPONSE

JENNY: In Evan's case, many allergies went away after we killed his yeast. Can you explain why that happened?

DR. JERRY: Dr. William Crook, in his book, *The Yeast Connection,* put forth a possible explanation. Yeast can grow along the lining of the bowel wall much like ivy can "creep" along a wall. As the ivy attaches itself to the walls, yeast can also attach itself to the bowel wall. Each attachment site is inflamed and is a possible point for leakage from the gut to the bloodstream for partially digested proteins. Remember, we discussed the concept of food proteins (perceived as foreign by the body) sensitizing the immune system. Let me make this a little clearer. Your immune system "knows" every cell in your body, from brain tissue, to colon tissue, to the kidneys. It is able to do this by recognizing the proteins imbedded in the membranes of cells that make up each organ. Thus, foreign proteins, such as found on viruses and bacteria, are quickly distinguished as NOT belonging to the body and are quickly destroyed by specific missiles generated by the immune system. We call these missiles antibodies. Now, if food proteins are allowed to enter the bloodstream, these "foreign bodies" will be recognized by the immune system as NOT belonging to the body and will generate antibodies to these foods (called IgG antibodies). This is how food sensitivities come about.

JENNY: What exactly does a mom say to her doctor to order a test like this? Does she just say she wants to run an IgG test?

DR. JERRY: I would recommend that the parent actually go to the lab Web site and order the kit. Bring the kit to the physician so he can sign the order. Then, the parent can take the child to a laboratory to have the blood drawn and sent. Many labs can do IgE, IgG to foods and there may be some environmental testing available as well. I would prefer the simplest, though: IgG to foods without any wellness program/rotation recommendations (they usually charge for that).

GETTING YOUR CHILD TESTED FOR YEAST

Your doctor may not be fluent in getting this done, and he or she may give you some resistance, but you as a parent can take charge.

- Go to the lab Web site (Urine Organic Acid: The Great Plains Lab, www.greatplainslaboratory, 913-341-8949; Stool Cultures: Genova Diagnostics, www.genovadiagnostics.com, 800-522-4762; or Doctors Data, www.doctorsdata.com, 800-323-2784 for U.S.A. and Canada) and order the test.
- Take the test to the doctor so that he can sign the order.
- Take your child to your local lab to have the blood drawn and have the lab return the kit.

JENNY: Now, let's try to explain what exactly happens after an IgG antibody finds its target—say, orange juice—and tags it for its "ultimate demise." This inflammatory response will lead to the formation and release of cytokines, interleukins, as well as many other modulators of immune function.

I listened to Dr. Jerry explain to me about why it's not good when cytokines and interleukins are generated continuously, so I'm going to break it down in a Jenny version what I learned from him. Here it goes.

When our kids become allergic to everything, their bodies are constantly releasing these cytokines and interleukins. Let's pretend those are FedEx and UPS and they sound an alarm once in the bloodstream, which causes the glial cell (which I like to call "chef cells" because they deliver nourishment to the brain's neurons) to become secret double agents and morph into the macrophages, which I like to call Rambo cells. Unfortunately, the Rambo cells won't turn back into chef cells (glial cells) until FedEx and UPS go away. But they won't go away if the body is constantly dealing with an allergic reaction. So these poor neurons in the brain are starving for nourishment because the chef cell (glial cell) has been turned into Rambo, and Rambo doesn't deliver food. Rambo attacks enemies and often thinks a friend is an enemy in an allergic reaction. We have felt this happen to us when we have a head cold. We can't think correctly and just want everyone to shut up and stop talking to us because we have a foggy brain. That's because Rambo is busy being a bodyguard at a nightclub, leaving no chef to nourish our brain. That's what our kids feel like if you don't minimize their allergies. It's what they feel like if you feed them something they are allergic to.

DR. JERRY: Allergies play a huge role in behavior. Not only can you see the dark circles under the eyes, nasal congestion, scratchy throat, and possibly reflux, you can witness brain fog and the disconnect in the children. Allergies also do play a major role in chronic inflammation. Remember what an allergy is: Something enters into the body that the immune system is going to perceive as a foreign protein. Our own military force, the immunoglobulin system, is going to have it removed, and in the process, causes an inflammatory response. If you have enough inflammatory responses, you're going to send signals to the brain that cause the children to have a lack of focus, concentration, loss of short-term memory, difficulty with verbal expression, and difficulty with fine motor skills, such as writing. Furthermore, they can become irritable, hyperactive, and inconsolable. Emotions can become deregulated as well, and one may find a child just sitting and weeping. I remember asking my son Josh why he was crying, and he would say, "I don't know, Daddy. I am just sad."

So the allergens, for many of our children, are out there. It may not be food, or pollen, but could be in the home as well.

CHEMICAL SENSITIVITIES, INDOOR TOXINS, AND VOCS

JENNY: What are some of the things that can cause allergies in the home?

DR. JERRY: Now, some of the following may be allergies, or may be chemical sensitivities, or both. Where one crosses the line of "allergic reaction" to "chemically sensitive" is a real gray zone. Let's get down to the nuts and bolts here. The allergist will generally consider an "allergic reaction" to manifest with symptoms that include itchy eyes, sneezing, and runny nose. These symptoms are usually treated with allergy medications and, if severe enough, with allergy shots. These reactions are typically mediated by antibodies of the E class, termed IgE. Food sensitivities are not as obvious. They can manifest with symptoms that include red ears, red cheeks, headaches, nausea, diarrhea, constipation, sleep-cycle irregularities, personality changes, cognitive changes, reflux (GERD: gastroesophageal reflux disease), asthma, and recurrent infections. These reactions are typically mediated by antibodies of the G class, termed IgG. There is another group of sensitivities, termed chemical sensitivities. How these come about is not well-understood. These patients exhibit allergy-like reactions to chemicals such as perfumes, cleaning agents, carpet smells (off-gassing), and pollutants. The best treatment for this group of sensitivities is avoidance.

A major contributor to what is now being referred to as "indoor air pollution" is carpeting. Carpet can off-gas toxic compounds for years. Underneath the carpet is a foam cushion, which will also contribute volatile compounds (a fancy term for giving off toxic gases) that can be dangerous. Some of these compounds are referred to as volatile organic compounds, or VOCs, which are harsh chemical compounds that could cause long-term health problems, including cancer and kidney and liver disease. One must do a lot of research when replacing flooring.

JENNY: What kind of floor would be the best with these kids?

DR. JERRY: Tile is probably the best flooring. Using no VOC glues to tack it down, it is one of the cleanest of the floorings. Cork is also a nontoxic, environmentally friendly material. Some cork flooring is "floating" and not glued down. Next are the hardwood floors, but a lot of research has to be done here on the finish—again, we really want to avoid the volatile organic compounds. The glue must be no VOC as well. Finally, if carpeting is a must, it appears that wool is the lowest of "offenders" and, if worsted (no glue on the back side), with natural dyes, and installed over environmentally safe padding would be an acceptable choice (though very pricey!).

WEB SITES FOR HEALTHY PAINT

www.ecofriendlyflooring.com
www.ecospaints.com
www.freshairechoicepaint.com
www.greenplanetpaints.com

Organic Recommendations and Nontoxic Household Products	
Location	**Web site**
Whole Foods Market	www.wholefoodsmarket.com
Wild Harvest Organic Found in many major grocery stores	www.wildharvestorganic.com Listings (by state)
Food co-ops, health food stores, and natural food stores	Green People www.greenpeople.org/healthfood.htm Organic Consumers Association www.organicconsumers.org/foodcoops.htm
Seventh Generation	www.seventhgeneration.com
Earth Friendly Products	www.ecos.com
Organic Valley Family of Farms	www.organicvalley.coop

MOLD

JENNY: What about molds?

DR. JERRY: Mold and mold spores are part of the environment. They come into the house anytime a door or window is opened, and also on children, pets, husbands, and guests coming in from outside. Molds can produce allergens (things we are allergic to), irritants, and in some cases, toxic substances called mycotoxins.

They can be responsible for common allergic symptoms: itchy eyes, sneezing, congestion, and asthma. They also have been implicated in more complicated and serious disorders that are so vast they cannot be discussed here. Mold needs some moisture in order to grow and usually gets started with a water leak from a pipe, a roof leak, improperly sealed windows, and condensation. It is very important to remove the damaged material and fix the water source.

JENNY: Any tests for house dust mites?

DR. JERRY: You can test for house dust mites, but basically you know you've got them. Everybody has house dust mites. They eat the little flakes of skin that fall off of your body. Protected mattresses and pillows make it difficult for them to accumulate. Likewise, a solid surface (i.e., no carpet) for the flooring also aids in keeping their numbers down. The problem with the house dust mite is that we can be very allergic to them. This can easily be demonstrated with a skin test at your local allergy specialist.

JENNY: I had read somewhere about stuffed animals. They are actually apartments and condos for dust mites, isn't that true?

DR. JERRY: Absolutely. I would recommend removing all "nonessential" stuffed friends from the child's room. Those remaining can be placed in the dryer under low heat and cleaned that way. It will scratch the eyes of the stuffed friends, but they will be mite- and dust-free!

JENNY: What about bedding?

DR. JERRY: Old mattresses should be replaced. A prescription from your physician is mandatory if you want to get a mattress free of a chemical fire retardant. Encase the mattress with a mattress protector that is mite-resistant.

JENNY: Flame retardants. They show up in our kids' blood!! I had no idea most kids' pajamas are filled with it, along with mattresses and bedding. That stuff is toxic.

DR. JERRY: The current flame retardants are boric acid and antimony. Antimony is a toxic material and can act very much like arsenic in the body. Again, you have to have a doctor's prescription to get mattresses and bedding that are flame-retardant-free. Finding sleepwear that is chemical-free is a chore, but can be done.

JENNY: I'm coming out with a line called Too Good; that's a toxic-free line of food, bedding, cups—you name it. But in the meantime, www.hannaandersson.com sells nontoxic clothing.

DR. JERRY: Of course you are. That doesn't surprise me at all!

JENNY: What else should people look out for in their homes to help minimize allergies?

DR. JERRY: You have to change your furnace air filters every month. It appears the HEPAs are better, according to allergists. When the heating and air-conditioning units are not in use (in spring and fall, for example), small, portable HEPA filters may be of great help. The most important room to put this filter (please, do not buy an expensive one!) would be where the child spends a lot of her time—for example, the bedroom.

JENNY: Now that we have convinced people to go get allergy testing done, do you suggest a particular kind of lab for IgG?

DR. JERRY: There are many good and reputable labs that are performing IgG RAST tests for food allergies. There is a lot of competition, and like politicians, they all claim that they are the best while the others are severely lacking in one technique or another. For those on a real budget, use what you can through your HMO such as LabCorp and Quest Diagnostics. They can run some of the IgG and IgE food allergy panels. If you want to go out of the "system," both Alletess and Immuno laboratories do a fine job.

GETTING AN IgG RAST TEST

Within Your HMO:

LabCorp (www.labcorp.com or call 504-838-8250)
Quest Diagnostics (www.questdiagnostics.com or call 610-454-4158)

Out of Network:

Alletess Medical Laboratory (www.foodallergy.com or call 800-225-5404)
Immunolabs (www.immunolabs.com or call 800-231-9197 or 954-691-2500)

PETS

JENNY: What about buying a dog?

DR. JERRY: Please do not go out and purchase a dog or a cat as a "therapy" animal until your child (and siblings) have been tested by an allergist. Again, remove carpeting, if possible. If not, purchase a good-quality sealed HEPA vacuum cleaner (check *Consumer Reports* for some reputable brands, and please do not buy one of those expensive $800 vacs!). You may also want to purchase one or two portable HEPA air cleaners.

Nirvana Safe Haven (www.nontoxic.com)

Think LOW VOC in whatever you do: paint, glue, cabinets (pressboard off-gasses—so that is a BIG no!). Consider new bedding that is free of chemicals and flame retardants. Clothing should also be as "organic" as possible.

Perfumes, house "fresheners," and even candles with fragrances all contribute to an environmental load that needs to be detoxified. Cleaning agents should be as natural and nontoxic as possible.

JENNY: What about allergy suppression?

DR. JERRY: Though some natural allergy medications can work fairly well, such as Quercetin, many of the children we manage need something much stronger. We will use a combination of oral antihistamines, such as Claritin RediTabs, or Zyrtec, along with nasal steroid sprays, such as Nasonex. In addition, Singulair has been very helpful in combination with the above. Nasonex and Singulair are prescription medications. Some children, like my Joshua, are unable to tolerate allergy medications. We therefore took him to an allergist, Dr. Marvin Boris, in New York, who was able to determine his exact allergies. He then prepared a nasal spray that Josh receives once daily to desensitize him to our world of molds, dusts, and pollens. No more dark circles, swollen eyes, or "bad days" at school.

ADVICE

Ask for an IgG food allergy panel test and an IgE test from your doctor.

- Within Your HMO:

  —LabCorp (www.labcorp.com or call 504-838-8250)

  —Quest Diagnostics (www.questdiagnostics.com or call 610-454-4158)

- Out of Network:

  —Alletess Medical Laboratory (www.foodallergy.com or call 800-225-5404)

  —Immunolabs (www.immunolabs.com or call 800-231-9197 or 954-691-2500)

Make the home environment as allergy-free as possible:

—Stay away from VOC paint.
—Use organic cleaning products that do not contain ammonia or chlorine.
—Do not install new carpeting or padding; if you have it, remove it.
—Use laundry detergent, dishwashing detergent, and cleaners from brands such as Planet, Ecover, Seventh Generation, and EcoFriendly.

Give an antihistamine to relieve symptoms, such as Claritin RediTabs: Break in half (for small children) and put directly into the mouth (it melts like cotton candy) or in a drink.

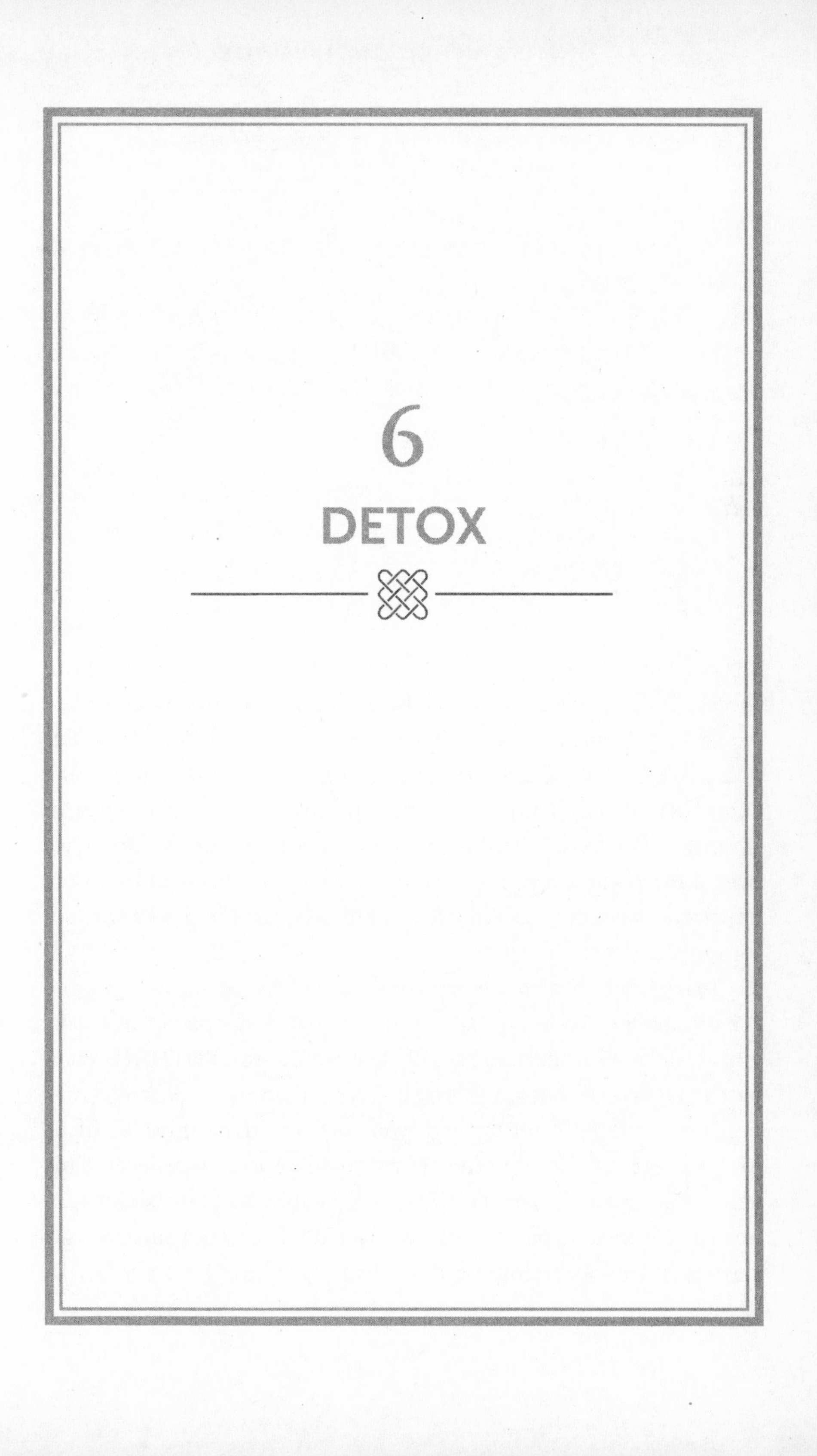

6
DETOX

I DON'T KNOW HOW MANY PEOPLE remember the Skylab falling from the sky back in the late 70s or early 80s, but I sure as hell do. I wouldn't play outside the entire summer because I thought it was going to fall on my head. My mom thought I was crazy, but I didn't care. There was a chance that something could harm me in the environment. The Skylab finally fell into an ocean, and I couldn't have been a more ecstatic eight-year-old. Nothing outside could harm me anymore—well, maybe Micky Bearbend, who used to punch me, but for the most part, I felt safe.

Today when I watch the news and I see oil barges leaking into the ocean, mercury polluting fish, poor air quality, chemicals in foods, global warming, I think to myself, **The Skylab was NOTHING compared to today.** Of course I'm much more acutely aware of things now because of what I went through with my son, but I think all of us would agree our environment is much more toxic than ever. This generation of kids is constantly teaching adults that our bodies cannot handle these types of assaults and it's becoming increasingly clear that kids suffering from Autism Spectrum Disorder, ADD,

ADHD, OCD, and other difficulties are the canaries in the coal mine. They're much more sensitive to toxins such as chemicals and heavy metals and have a harder time getting rid of them. But when they do begin to shed the poisons, the changes can be miraculous. Detox is absolutely necessary for EVERYONE to maintain a healthy lifestyle. People outside the autism community might view detox only as a means to get rid of drugs or alcohol. This is not the case anymore. Witnessing the detox of metals and chemicals out of thousands of children who have then improved or recovered from autism has proven to me that detox will be an essential part of everyone's health in the future.

JENNY: Why are these kids such sponges? Why do they absorb metals and toxins so easily?

DR. JERRY: We're all exposed to metals, but some of our kids have a hard time getting rid of them. They actually accumulate metals through life, and life starts in the mother's womb. So whatever the mom has is going to be preferentially accumulated by the infant. Toxins can be checked in the umbilical cord blood at the time of delivery.

The table below is courtesy of Environmental Working Group's study "Body Burden: The Pollution in Newborns" (July 14, 2005). The entire study and results can be found at www.ewg.org.

Chemicals and Pollutants Detected in Human Umbilical Cord Blood

Mercury (Hg)—tested for 1, found 1 pollutant from coal-fired power plants, mercury-containing products, and certain industrial processes. Accumulates in seafood. Harms brain development and function.

Polyaromatic hydrocarbons (PAHs)—tested for 18, found 9 pollutants from burning gasoline and garbage. Linked to cancer. Accumulate in food chain.

Polybrominated dibenzodioxins and furans (PBDD/F)—tested for 12, found 7 contaminants in brominated flame-retardants. Pollutants and by-products from plastic production and incineration. Accumulate in food chain. Toxic to developing endocrine (hormone) system.

Perfluorinated chemicals (PFCs)—tested for 12, found 9 active ingredients or breakdown products of Teflon, Scotchgard, fabric and carpet protectors, food wrap coatings. Global contaminants. Accumulate in the environment and the food chain. Linked to cancer, birth defects, and more.

Polychlorinated dibenzodioxins and furans (PBCD/F)—tested for 17, found 11 pollutants, by-products of PVC production, industrial bleaching, and incineration. Cause cancer in humans. Persist for decades in the environment. Very toxic to developing endocrine (hormone) system.

Organochlorine pesticides (OCs)—tested for 28, found 21 DDT, chlordane, and other pesticides. Largely banned in the U.S. Persist for decades in the environment. Accumulate up the food chain, to man. Cause cancer and numerous reproductive effects.

Polybrominated diphenyl ethers (PBDEs)—tested for 46, found 32 flame-retardants in furniture foam, computers, and televisions. Accumulates in the food chain and human tissues. Adversely affect brain development and the thyroid.

Polychlorinated naphthalenes (PCNs)—tested for 70, found 50 wood preservatives, varnishes, machine lubricating oils, waste incineration. Common PCB contaminant. Contaminate the food chain. Cause liver and kidney damage.

Polychlorinated biphenyls (PCBs)—tested for 209, found 147 industrial insulators and lubricants. Banned in the U.S. in 1976. Persist for decades in the environment. Accumulate up the food chain, to man. Cause cancer and nervous system problems.

WHY SOME KIDS CAN'T DETOX

JENNY: What's different in some of the kids that doesn't allow them to chelate (detox metals) on their own?

DR. JERRY: We have natural pathways that are designed to clear toxic metals from our body. We are all born with different capacities to accomplish this. Some of our population is more easily poisoned than others. We know the very young and the very old are especially sensitive to poisonings and heavy metal. Now this brings us to the methylation pathway. If the major detoxification pathway is genetically functioning at 60 percent, and then gets poisoned by mercury, the body becomes compromised in a major way. Toxins will continue to accumulate and exert their effects on growth and development. Specifically, toxins will compromise the production of cysteine, glutathione, and metalothionine (which binds to heavy metals and removes them from the bloodstream).

JENNY: Why are they deficient in cysteine or metalothionine?

DR. JERRY: That's just the way they were genetically made. And again, if they were never exposed to toxins in the womb, they might never have had a problem. If they were exposed to just "regular" toxins of day-to-day living, they would be fine. You see, if they never were exposed to heavy metals from vaccines, heavy metals in the fish that the mom ate while she was pregnant, then they wouldn't have had to push so hard on their detox pathway. Remember, we are speaking of a total body burden of heavy metals and toxins. This burden starts just after conception. By the time these babies take their first breath, their ability to mitigate the damage of toxic exposures is already taxed. Some children are barely taxed. Some children are almost maximally taxed. Those children born with a robust ability to detoxify sail right through childhood immunizations and everything else this world throws at them. For others, though, clinical signs and symptoms start becoming evident at a very young age. So when we hear, "Well, my kids get these vaccines and they're fine. They don't have ADD or autism. They're valedictorian scholars in schools. What about them?" My answer to that is that they were blessed with a detoxification pathway that works.

JENNY: Why are the kids metal-toxic?

DR. JERRY: Because they can't get rid of it (through the process of detoxification and elimination) and thus accumulate the toxic substance.

METAL EXPOSURE

JENNY: And where exactly are the metals coming from?

DR. JERRY: Well, the first exposure you have is in utero (the womb). If the mom has silver amalgam fillings, they are 50 percent by weight mercury. Every time she brushes her teeth, every time she has her teeth cleaned, every time that she consumes something warm or hot, it's going to accelerate the off-gassing of this mercury in its vaporous state. It's going to end up in her blood (by inhalation or mucous membrane absorption). It's going to be stored in her body.

The problem lies with the delivery system of nutrients to the developing baby. Everything gets preferentially delivered to the placenta. The minerals, vitamins, amino acids, and sadly, even the toxins. So the baby gets the very best of the minerals, the vitamins, and the amino acids to help that baby grow. If there are toxins present, they, too, as the cord blood study on pages 129–30 has demonstrated, will end up in the child as well. Now, if the mom happens to get a flu shot for her baby at six months (many flu shots still contain thimerosal as a preservative), we're going to have a problem.

JENNY: It doesn't make any sense!

DR. JERRY: No, it doesn't make any sense. The media doesn't pick up on it. And we've all just not being trained to discern. We're not able to think by ourselves and grasp what's going on here. And that's why there's not a huge uproar. Why do we have mercury in the seas? What's going on? Why are all of these fish polluted? What's going to happen to us twenty years from now if the rates of pollution continue? Each generation, despite some pretty impressive medical advances, is sicker at younger and younger ages.

JENNY: If the fish are so toxic with mercury, why don't we have autistic fish?

DR. JERRY: The predator fish eat the plant-eating fish. The plants the fish eat are rich in selenium. Selenium binds to mercury and renders it markedly less toxic. So both the plant-eating fish and the predator fish have a great source of selenium to protect them from the mercury in their environment.

JENNY: God, that's fascinating.

DR. JERRY: Kind of cool. Okay, so, anyway, now we have exposures in utero. Then the baby is born.

JENNY: Has anyone ever looked at what toxins might be in breast milk?

DR. JERRY: We have had moms who would express their breast milk and send it off to Doctor's Data Laboratory. The results of the breast milk would surprise a lot of us. So we have contamination that could possibly be coming in through the breast milk, through the air that we breathe, and obviously through vaccines.

HOW DO METALS POISON YOU?

JENNY: How do metals poison us?

DR. JERRY: To keep it simple, they disrupt metabolic pathways that generate components needed by the cells. Dr. Boyd Haley, one of the most knowledgeable researchers on the effects of mercury, has said, "I have never found an enzyme that can't be poisoned by mercury."

It's obviously not lethal poisonings, except in a few, but rather, major alterations that manifest as disease. Dr. Haley is especially concerned with mercury. You just can't get rid of it. It binds almost irreversibly to their proteins. So once it's clamped on, it is constantly poisoning that system. We all survive because, thank God, we have a lot of redundant pathways. If all the pathways were blocked, then the affected individual would die. The body really operates in harmony. One note off and it will affect the chord, which will mess up the tune. In "system talk," this translates into this: The immune system is no longer functioning the way it should because it's depending on enzyme systems that are working suboptimally, yeast then grows, mucosal membranes begin to inflame, stool removal is hampered, anaerobic bacteria flourish, and toxins are liberated. The body shifts into an oxidized state, a chronic inflammatory state sets in, and on and on. We have a very, very sad song.

JENNY: I learned that with Evan. I killed his yeast and I said, "Oh, great. He's recovered." And then he started to grow yeast again and I said, "I have to go back and clean his metals out, otherwise he will just keep growing yeast and get sick."

DR. JERRY: Right. Exactly.

JENNY: When did all this mercury start?

DR. JERRY: We've been working with heavy metals for a long time. The hatters used to use mercury in the tanning of skins. That's where the term "mad as a hatter" came from, because eventually they would go crazy. Dentists have the highest suicide and divorce rate as a professional organization. You have to wonder if working with amalgams for many years has caused these problems.

JENNY: And they also seem a little antisocial.

DR. JERRY: Yes, they're kind of odd (except for my dentist, of course!).

JENNY: Well, I guess we're not going to be invited to The Dentist Association Ball this year!

CHELATION: DETOXING METALS

This should ONLY be done with a qualified doctor.

Chelation is always doctor-supervised. If it's not doctor supervised and you're using over-the-counter preps, then you don't know if you're chelating. You don't know what you're chelating. And you don't know if you're moving metals from point A to point B, with point B being the brain. Blood tests need to be followed. This just cannot be done with hair analysis.

DR. JERRY: Some medications that have been tested and studied to remove heavy metals:

The Chelators and How They Work

Disodium EDTA

- This is an amino acid that bonds onto heavy metals in the bloodstream.
- This chelator removes calcium from the bloodstream, posing a huge risk; this form of EDTA is not recommended for children. If too much calcium is removed, the heart stops beating and this could, and has in recent years, resulted in death. If given very slowly by a knowledgeable M.D., over the course of hours, it is very safe.

Calcium Disodium EDTA

- Works to remove excess lead from the body, but is not specific to mercury and methylmercury like DMSA or DMPS.
- Can be taken orally, can be administered through an IV drip, or can be given as a suppository.
- This is an amino acid that attracts lead, other heavy metals, and some minerals from the bloodstream and expels the toxic elements via urination.
- This particular form of EDTA does not remove the calcium from the bloodstream and is, therefore, a safer option.

DMSA

- Has been approved by the U.S. FDA as a means of removing lead from people (primarily children) with lead poisoning.
- This can remove heavy metals, including lead, arsenic, and mercury as well.

- Available in capsule form.
- This agent is rich in sulfur and removes the lead, or other heavy metals, by attracting them (like a magnet) to leave the body by way of the digestive tract.

DMPS

- Is intended to remove mercury from the body as well as other heavy metals via the kidneys, liver, and gastrointestinal tract.
- This agent can be administered either intravenously (IV), intramuscularly (IM), or by subcutaneous injection (SQ).

JENNY: But removing them can sometimes make the metals wander around the body instead of coming out in the poop, right?

DR. JERRY: That's right. We don't want to get into the metal-moving business. We do not want to move metals just to move them. I would hate to move metal from one part of the body into the brain.

JENNY: Don't some chelators escort metals out to the poop shoot?

DR. JERRY: Chelated metals may be removed through the stool. Constipation is certainly not going to help here. If mercury is in the stool and just sits for days in the colon, there is a very real risk it could be absorbed back into the bloodstream and redistributed. Another concept is that some toxic metals have certain target tissues they gravitate toward. For example, lead preferentially deposits in bone tissue, and mercury preferentially deposits in metabolically active tissue. The brain, which is very metabolically active, happens to be a great target for mercury. Mercury in newborns will most likely deposit in the brain.

JENNY: What about the little boy and girl who died from chelation? Everyone on the other side always talks about that, using death as a warning to parents to not do biomedical.

DR. JERRY: That's a common tactic used to cast dispersion. In those two cases, the children did die tragically. But they did not die from IV chelation but rather from a medication error. The wrong medication was injected in both cases and the end results were tragic. Anytime, anywhere, if the wrong medication is infused, it can be fatal. This is an ongoing issue in hospitals. Large numbers of hospitalized patients receive the wrong medications and die every year. But that doesn't mean we don't go to the hospital and get infusions if we need them. They can be life-saving. Medication errors happen in hospitals with FDA-controlled drugs and with regular mainstream doctors.

In the case of the wrong chelator, the medication that the doctor selected was supposed to be infused over hours, but it was infused over minutes. This caused both the children's calcium levels to drop and the heart does not beat without calcium. The heart, in both cases, ceased to beat.

This article was published on January 18, 2006, at 12:00 a.m., and can be viewed at: www.post-gazette.com/pg/06018/639721.stm

DRUG ERROR, NOT CHELATION THERAPY, KILLED BOY, EXPERT SAYS

By Karen Kane, *Pittsburgh Post-Gazette.*

One of the nation's foremost experts in chelation therapy said she has determined "without a doubt" that it was medical error, and not the therapy itself, that led to the death of a 5-year-old boy who was receiving it as a treatment for autism.

Dr. Mary Jean Brown, chief of the Lead Poisoning Prevention Branch of the Atlanta-based Centers for Disease Control and Prevention, said yesterday that Abubakar Tariq Nadama died Aug. 23 in his Butler County doctor's office because he was given the wrong chelation agent.

"It's a case of look-alike/sound-alike medications," she said yesterday. "The child was given Disodium EDTA instead of Calcium Disodium EDTA. The generic names are Versinate and Endrate. They sound alike. They're clear and colorless and odorless. They were mixed up."

Both types of EDTA are synthetic amino acids that latch onto heavy metals in the bloodstream.

Dr. Brown said she obtained the child's autopsy report on behalf of the CDC after reading an article about the death in the *Pittsburgh Post-Gazette*. She said it didn't take long to figure out what had happened.

Essentially, Tariq died from low blood calcium. Without enough calcium—a metal—in the blood, the heart stops beating. Dr. Brown said the Disodium EDTA the child was given as a chelation agent "acted as a claw that pulled too much calcium" from his blood.

"The blood calcium level was below 5 [milligrams]. That's an emergency event," she said.

Officials from the state police, the district attorney's office and the coroner's office will meet soon to decide whether to hold an inquest into the child's death and whether it should remain listed as accidental.

Dr. Brown said the same mix-up happened in two other recent cases: a 2-year-old girl in Texas who died in May during chelation for lead poisoning and a woman from Oregon who died three years ago while receiving chelation for clogged arteries.

Dr. Brown said that in each case, the blood calcium level was below 5 milligrams. Normal is between 7 and 9.

The correct chelation agent—Calcium Disodium EDTA—would not have pulled the calcium from the bloodstream, she said.

The Butler County coroner's office confirmed last week that

Tariq had died as a result of his chelation treatment, but the findings that were released didn't indicate whether the treatment had been improperly administered.

Dr. Brown said chelation was once a common and necessary therapy that was used on children and adults alike for lead poisoning. Chelation means administering an agent into the bloodstream that causes heavy metals in the body to cling to it and then be excreted in urine.

Though its only approved use, according to the U.S. Food and Drug Administration, is for lead poisoning, Dr. Brown said she is aware that it is used by some people for other medical problems, ranging from clogged arteries to autism.

She said there have been no reputable medical trials demonstrating the effectiveness of chelation as a therapy for anything but lead poisoning. But if it were administered accurately, the procedure would be harmless.

She said it is well known within the medical community that Disodium EDTA should never be used as a chelation agent. She quoted from a 1985 CDC statement: "Only Calcium Disodium EDTA should be used. Disodium EDTA should never be used . . . because it may induce fatal hypocalcemia, low calcium and tetany."

"There is no doubt that this was an unintended use of Disodium EDTA. No medical professional would ever have intended to give the child Disodium EDTA," Dr. Brown said.

Tariq was brought to the United States from England last spring by his mother, Marwa, for the chelation therapy. He was in the Portersville, Butler County, office of Dr. Roy Eugene Kerry when he went into cardiac arrest.

In recent months, chelation treatments of a wide variety ranging from IV to oral to topical have been gaining popularity for autistic children due to anecdotal information from parents indicating a reduction in symptoms. The underlying belief is that autism is caused by a sensitivity to heavy metals in the bloodstream.

Howard Carpenter, executive director of the Advisory Board on Autism and Related Disorders—the largest autism advocacy group in the region—said the determination by Dr. Brown clears up the mystery surrounding Tariq's death but not the uncertainty over chelation itself.

"Since this child died, there have been parents who are pro-chelation who have been very angry that there's talk against it. On the other side, they say the death was a natural consequence of a dangerous activity. Maybe what happened to [Tariq] is explained, but we still don't have a conclusion about whether chelation is an effective treatment for autism," he said.

Tariq's father is a medical doctor who practices in England.

Dr. Kerry could not be reached for comment. A board-certified physician and surgeon, he advertises himself as an ear, nose and throat doctor who also specializes in allergies and environmental medicine.

Karen Kane can be reached at kkane@post-gazette.com

JENNY: A lot of parents talk about the regression that happens during chelation, which is another reason parents are scared to chelate.

DR. JERRY: After doing this for ten years, I've realize that it's very important to go slowly and steadily when you pull heavy metals from a child, rather than give them a wallop of stuff. Fortunately, by doing this, we don't see that regression you are talking about. We may see some little bumps and a little less sleep at night—a little more irritability, appetite down a little bit—but overall, parents are thrilled with what's going on. So I think it's very important that when I'm doing any kind of new therapeutic intervention, even antifungals, I always start with a half dose to make sure that it's the right drug for that particular child, and that what we're doing isn't going to cause the child to regress or have some difficult times—though it can be expected. Once again, during the treatments, we give Motrin if they're getting headaches or are really irritable. Epsom salt baths given along with minerals really help the kids out. It gives an extra boost of magnesium sulfate, which they need for calming and detoxifying. We use a lot of glutathione, either via:

- IV (intravenous)—administering a liquid substance directly into a vein
- transdermal—a cream that administers a specific dose of medicine via the skin
- nebulized—medicine administered through a mist form, as seen with inhalers

JENNY: How do you choose the correct chelator?

DR. JERRY: I usually let my children choose the chelator. First, I do a pre-chelation urine test to have the lab give me a report on what metals are in it. This represents what the child is effectively able to remove from his body on any given day. This is called the pre-chelation study. We may find this urine to have a little bit of lead and arsenic, and maybe a little bit of mercury. Now it is time to select the first chelator. For this example, let's just pick EDTA. I give the child EDTA and we grab another urine sample. I send it to the laboratory and it tells me that under the influence of EDTA, here's how much lead, mercury, or arsenic is coming out. It better have higher concentrations than what came out in the pre-chelation urine. Then I'll select DMSA. Under the influence of DMSA, this is how much lead, mercury, and arsenic comes out. So I let the child, depending upon the urine excretion of heavy metals, determine which chelator is best for him. This is important to consider, as there are a lot of products that claim they chelate heavy metals.

We need to have some kind of laboratory test to determine if the product is living up to its claims.

JENNY: I've heard that some chelators cause the yeast beast to come. Which ones do that?

DR. JERRY: The sulfur chelators like DMSA and DMPS, if given orally, have a pretty good track record of inducing yeast flare-ups. These chelators can be administered transdermally. In some children, they work very well, again, as determined by urinary excretion of heavy metals.

JENNY: Explain the transdermal route to me again.

DR. JERRY: The compounding pharmacy can put DMSA into a cream that's absorbed through the skin. Once again, we've seen some very, very good results just with that. You put the cream right on the wrist and they rub it in just like a woman putting on perfume.

JENNY: You can also give it as a suppository, right?

DR. JERRY: Yes, this is a suppository that has a chelator and is placed into the child's bottom. In older kids it may not even be a negotiable consideration. For our younger kids it is usually not a problem. So that's a good route. Suppositories tend not to induce the growth of yeast.

JENNY: Why a suppository in the first place? Does it really work that well up the bum?

DR. JERRY: The vasculature around the colon is very rich and is constantly drawing water out of the colon and will just absorb whatever is put into it. We can put in medications in suppository form, such as Tylenol and seizure medications. We know that the rectum is a great way for delivering medicine if it's still tolerable for the patient. Urine for toxic metals is once again obtained to evaluate the medication's effectiveness. You look as if you have a question.

JENNY: Yes, I do.

DR. JERRY: I could tell. You have that "I have a question" look.

JENNY: You've said to me, "Oh, Evan is high in lead. I'd like to use EDTA." Do you have a specific chelator that goes with certain metals?

DR. JERRY: The children I was seeing five to ten years ago had much higher mercury exposures. So I was going to really go after that mercury with DMPS and DMSA since they have a greater affinity for mercury. Affinity just means a strong attraction. The different chelators seem to have a pecking order with respect to which metal they have the strongest attraction to. They will pick up different metals, but if they see the metal they have a strong affinity for, they may dump what is in their "arms" and go after their metal of choice. Let me use the orchard analogy. If you're walking in an orchard, the best fruit is at the top of the tree. But since you're kind of lazy, you'll pick the one on the lower branches and on the ground first. When DMSA, which has a really nice affinity for mercury, is introduced into the body of a child who has mercury toxicity, the first things that you may see coming out are lead and maybe arsenic. And everybody gets depressed and says, "Oh, I thought my kid was one of those mercury kids. All I see coming out is lead and arsenic." Yes, for now, because it's going after the easiest "to reach" stuff first. The harder stuff will come later.

Another consideration is the location of the heavy metals. Many of the chelators will not travel into fat tissue. There is very little data to support the notion that any chelator can cross the blood-brain barrier. Though we are working hard to decrease the total body burden of heavy metals, we may not be making much of an impact in the brain. With that said, how does one account for the marked improvements we see in the children while chelating? Something is working and it is hard to argue with success.

JENNY: Will it ever come out of the brain?

DR. JERRY: Well, I hope as chelators are developed, the newer ones will cross the blood-brain barrier.

JENNY: It doesn't now?

DR. JERRY: No. That's why chelation can be so frustrating. Those molecules that are responsible for binding heavy metals can't get through the blood-brain barrier. The next generation of chelators will be able to cross the blood-brain barrier, go into the brain cell, find the heavy metal, pull the heavy metal off of where it's bound, take it out of the brain cell, and back out of the kidneys or the colon to be excreted. And that's how we are really going to be able to clean up the human body.

Intravenous Chelation

JENNY: Let's talk about intravenous chelation.

DR. JERRY: IV chelation is just one other route. We talked about an oral route. We talked about a transdermal route. We even talked about a rectal route. This is just one more route. It's been done safely for many, many years for all different types of applications.

JENNY: Why wouldn't everybody off the street want to just come in and get IV chelation?

DR. JERRY: Well, like I said in the beginning, because of the fact that some people are detoxifying themselves daily. They're doing okay. But what about the others?

Let's formulate this into a simple model. If genetically you are not able to keep up with detoxification, then the toxins will accumulate in your body. This will result in oxidative stress and inflammation. So now we present to your specific "genetic box" this triad: toxins, oxidative stress, and indirectly, inflammation. You have just activated your genetic box, and you are going to get ill—genetically determined, but ONLY after toxic exposures, the ensuing oxidative stress, and inflammation. For some, this illness may look like Alzheimer's disease, Parkinson's disease, rheumatoid arthritis, attention deficit disorder, and autism, just to name a few. Another word picture: You are genetically born to be allergic to cats. But, you are just fine if you are never exposed to cats. If a cat jumps in your lap, introducing "toxins" to your nose, the inflammation quickly follows with swelling of the nasal passages, itching, sneezing, and before you know it, you are "ill." Remove the toxins, treat the inflammation, and you are better. What if we do the same thing with these other diseases? If we remove the toxins, put water on the fire of inflammation, and reverse oxidative stress, might we reverse a lot of disease processes? What a novel approach.

JENNY: That explained it perfectly.

DR. JERRY: So what we're doing, then, is asking the question, "Is whatever disease process we're trying to deal with—chronic fatigue, fibromyalgia, Parkinson's, autism, attention deficit disorder—reversible if we can alter those vicious cycles that are hurting us, remove the toxins that trigger them, and remove the inflammation that seems to perpetuate them? Can we turn these cycles back to their pristine condition? Will we see an abatement of disease?" And the answer looks like yes.

JENNY: So by removing the toxins, cleaning up the diet, removing heavy metals, giving supplements, and draining that bucket, our kids' symptoms will dissipate or disappear completely. Symptoms like jumping, spinning, not speaking, poor eye contact, irritability, and crankiness will disappear. It also improves focus and concentration. We remove the toxins that are triggering these symptoms.

DR. JERRY: Yes.

JENNY: What is the percentage of patients you see improve from chelation?

DR. JERRY: Oh, I'd definitely say there's a good 20 to 25 percent who clinically improve. Now, sometimes you can't tell. I'll tell parents, "Look, when we go to chelate, you may be one of the twenty percent who see immediate benefit right away." We all get excited about that. But for the others, if they have a large toxic metal load—it may be a process of years to reverse.

JENNY: Do you think every child with autism needs to chelate?

DR. JERRY: If a child is totally mainstreamed in school and doing great but just a little quirky and Mom says, "I want IV chelation," I'm not going to do an IV chelation. The better a child is doing, the less invasive I want to be. Every time you do a medical procedure, you run the risk of it backfiring. If I have a kid who's doing well, I don't want to run the risk of chelating him only to find out he's got a sensitivity to one of the chelators. But the story changes when the child is still rocking in the corner, biting his wrists, and smearing his poop on the wall. If the benefits outweigh the risks, I'll do it. So IV chelation is really important for our severely affected individuals, and less so for the children who are doing really well.

JENNY: I so badly want to chelate Evan, but he's doing so well that I think, what if I make him worse when to me he's perfect?

DR. JERRY: Every intervention can give you quite a backlash and sometimes the hardest thing to do in pediatrics is "nothing." If they are doing extremely well, maybe IV chelation is not the answer.

JENNY: Did you chelate your son Josh?

DR. JERRY: Yes, we've chelated Joshua. We were never really able to capture the metals from Joshua. So, either the metals have been beyond the reach of the chelators (i.e., the brain-fat tissue) or they have since been removed by all the nutritional support given to him through the years.

Nutritional Support During Chelation

JENNY: Please talk about how imperative it is to get your child nutritional support during chelation.

DR. JERRY: You constantly need to be on vitamins, minerals, and oils. I would refer people back to the supplements chapter (on page 53) to find dosages. During chelation, it is important to be monitored by your doctor and be checked regularly for mineral deficiencies and blood work to ensure the liver is tolerating the intervention. Chelators have a nasty habit of grabbing some good minerals as well, such as zinc or selenium. Also, while chelating, it is important to monitor liver, kidney, and bone marrow function. The physician involved with chelation is quite aware of how to do this type of monitoring.

JENNY: Because I think people don't realize that it does strip minerals in the body. That's a big, important thing.

DR. JERRY: Yes, I remember one of the children I saw back in 2000.

He was given oral DMSA for thirty days straight. When I saw him in my clinic, he had sores around his mouth, nose, and anus. This was classic for zinc deficiency. He healed just fine after stopping the chelation and rebuilding his zinc levels.

JENNY: What about homeopathic-type chelators, like the foot soak or zeolyte or even giving cilantro? Any of these work?

DR. JERRY: There are a lot of therapeutic interventions available for chelation. It is good to have a healthy skepticism about everything offered for your child, including what we do in our clinic. It is very important to have some kind of measurements to validate that what you are doing is working. If the particular intervention is based only on testimonials, walk away!

ADVICE

Chelate *only* with a doctor!

Chelators can have some interesting side effects. The most common would be mineral depletion. This happens when the chelator inadvertently binds to a mineral (such as zinc or selenium) and removes it from the body. While chelating, it is advisable to have mineral levels checked frequently. Other common side effects include headache, fatigue, cramps, irritability, changes in sleep, diarrhea, and skin rashes. Some chelators have some potentially serious side effects that include problems developing in the bone marrow, liver, or kidneys.

The routes of administration depend on the type of chelator used. Some are applied transdermally (skin cream), in the rectum (suppository), orally, and intravenously (IV).

7
FIGHTING YEAST/CANDIDA

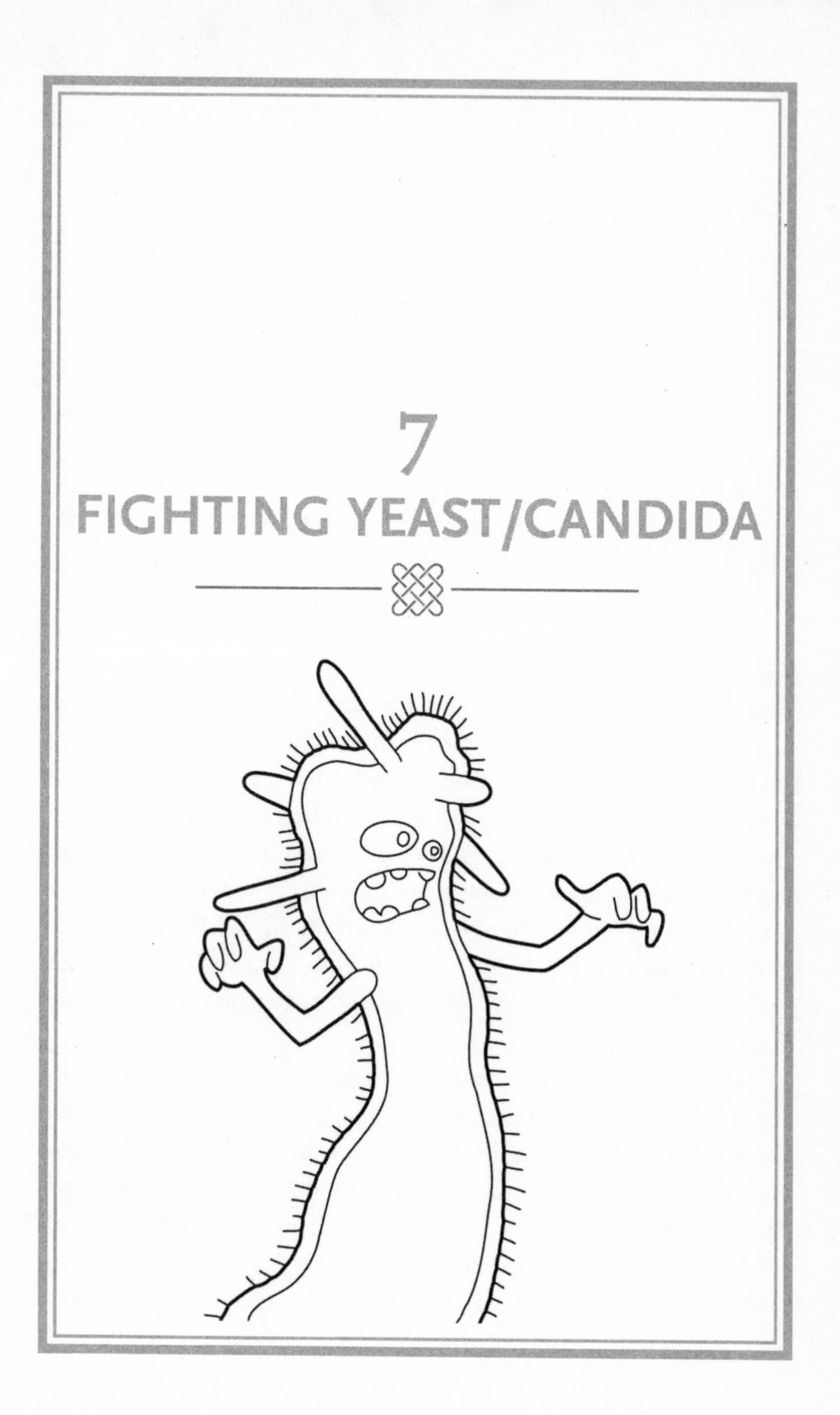

I THINK IF I BRING UP the words "candida," "yeast," or "antifungal," which is a yeast killer, around any of my friends again, they are going to disown me. Candida is one of the most fascinating topics for me and I know someday I'm going to write a book called *Yeast Sucks* because, well, it does! I was in a little bit of denial when Dr. Jerry first told me about candida. I had no idea the full scope of damage that could be done from it. I am now a firm believer that yeast is one of the causes of many diseases, even for adults! I am a firm believer that many of our kids, including those who don't have autism, are LOADED with yeast and this is one of the reasons so many childhood allergies exist.

When I started Evan on an antifungal, he went almost catatonic. Truth be told, I was excited. I was glad he started vomiting and went psycho. I knew this was a die-off reaction and I prayed that the other side of it would be rainbows. It turned out to be more than rainbows. After killing candida, Evan began to fully converse in back-and-forth conversations. This doesn't happen for every child, but it does help many, many children's OCD behaviors. Also, their allergies minimize, and in some cases, their eczema is totally resolved. I couldn't wait for this day to talk to Dr. Jerry about it. Like I said, I've become obsessed with killing yeast.

WHAT IS CANDIDA/YEAST?

JENNY: First, what is candida?

DR. JERRY: Candida is a type of yeast. We all have it. It is in all of our bodies, but in very small amounts. The problem with candida is that if the immune system becomes dysfunctional or compromised in any way, candida can get out of control and grow. This is certainly NOT discussed in medical textbooks. Most of the information contained in textbooks is ten to twenty years old, and since these children were not around in the numbers we now see, there is relative silence on this subject. We know that there are certain chemicals liberated when they grow in the gastrointestinal tract and if they are present in the urine, that can be a laboratory clue that yeast is, indeed, growing (these chemicals are arabinose and tartaric acid and can be detected in a test called the urine organic acid test).

What I commonly see as yeast "issues," that is, the complaints that children present with, are: Up in the middle of the night laughing, intermittent laughing during the day, and itching (the itching and redness can be perianal, genital, or generalized); climbing all the time; "standing" on the head; bloating of the abdominal region; marked increase in "gas" production (flatulence), constipation, or diarrhea; change of smell in stool—it could smell "yeasty/bready," foul, or even "sweet"; giddy/super-silly behaviors, brain "fog," or they are just "out of it"; a loss of energy; infections.

SIGNS OF YEAST ISSUES

Behaviors

- Demanding
- Noncompliant
- Aggressive
- Stimming
- Hands over ears
- Chewing (on everything and anything) and teeth grinding
- Laughing for no reason, in the middle of the night or spontaneously during the day
- Climbing all the time
- Standing on head or hanging upside down all the time
- Brain fog: giddy super-silly behaviors
- Loss of energy
- Seeming out of it
- Cravings for bread, pasta, and sweets

Clinical signs

- Rashes
- Eczema
- Funky-smelling scalp (the "wet dog" smell)
- Itching: perianal, genital, and/or generalized
- Redness: perianal, perivaginal
- Abdominal bloating
- Increase in flatulence
- Constipation or diarrhea
- Change in smell of stool (yeasty, bready, foul, or sweet)

CONSEQUENCES OF YEAST: LEAKY GUT SYNDROME

JENNY: Sometimes leaky gut syndrome can happen due to overgrowth of yeast. Can you explain leaky gut syndrome?

DR. JERRY: "Leaky gut" is another new term that will not be found in the medical textbooks. We use this term to illustrate the concept of substances that usually do not have access to the bloodstream actually passing through the GI tract into the bloodstream. This is a term we use to describe the condition where the lining of the gut wall becomes MORE permeable. Let's put it another way: After digestion, only simple sugars, fatty acids (breakdown products of fats), and amino acids (breakdown products of proteins) are allowed to "permeate" (pass through) the gut lining and into the blood, along with other small molecules. On the other hand, when a gut is "leaky," it allows larger and larger molecules to pass, and this may include partial proteins that children can't break down. It appears that when yeast overgrows in the bowel walls, they, too, may contribute to the gut becoming more permeable and the toxins and byproducts of the yeast growth will be allowed to enter the bloodstream and thus be distributed throughout the body.

JENNY: But give me a play-by-play of how it happens.

DR. JERRY: When we talk about leaky gut, we are talking about a complex set of circumstances that allow "foreign" proteins (partially digested food) and substances to gain access to the bloodstream. Proteins are made up of amino acids (the amino acids are linked together, much like pearls on a strand . . . the whole strand is a protein), and when we eat food, our digestive enzymes are meant to break down each one of those proteins to their components—the amino acids (individual pearls). We are not supposed to put protein into our bloodstream, just amino acids. Our body recognizes friend or foe by its protein. In other words, the immune system knows every protein in your body; whether it would be heart protein or brain protein or colon protein, it knows every protein. And it also knows if something foreign comes in, like a virus or bacteria, because they, too, are made of proteins (in this case, foreign proteins). And when it sees this foreign protein, it mounts an immune response to it. It makes antibodies to it. Think of "antibodies" as little Patriot missiles designed to destroy very specific targets. So, we are not supposed to put proteins from the foods that we eat into our bloodstream because it will make us allergic or sensitive to the food. We're supposed to break down those proteins to amino acids. Our body's digestive enzymes are normal in most of us, but in our autistic kids they can be lacking digestive enzymes (or they are just blocked from being able to work) and thus the foods that the kids are eating are not breaking down properly. That's okay until you get to the point where you have a leaky gut, because if you have a leaky gut, then those small bits of proteins will enter the bloodstream. Like with foods containing gluten and dairy, our kids cannot break these proteins down, so they enter the bloodstream and exert an opiate-like effect on the brain, making these children appear to be stoned.

Causes of Leaky Gut

JENNY: What are the causes of a leaky gut?

DR. JERRY: There are many causes that can ultimately wound the gut, that is, make it more permeable to substances that should NOT enter the bloodstream. One widely publicized theory is the measles virus from the MMR vaccine. This theory was put forth by Dr. Andrew Wakefield ("Ileal-lymphpoid-nodular hyperplasia, nonspecific colitis, and pervasive developmental disorder in children," *Lancet*, 1998) and basically describes a situation where measles virus promotes a chronic inflammatory bowel disease. Anytime you have an inflammatory condition in the bowels, you tend to have more of an issue of leaky gut as well. Environmental toxins, too, can play a role in contributing to the formation of a leaky gut. On the top of the list here are the inorganic mercurial compounds, and that is why we hear so much about thimerosal, a mercury-containing preservative that is still used in many of the childhood vaccines at the time of this writing. Contributing to the total body burden of mercury would be the mercury contained in fish, as well as other sources from the environment.

JENNY: I know this is an ongoing question, but why doesn't the medical community believe in the leaky gut syndrome?

DR. JERRY: You are so right. The medical community still doesn't believe in this whole thing called leaky gut syndrome. They don't get the diets, such as gluten-free, dairy-free diets. They say it hasn't been proven, but if they come to look at our science within the autism community, we have plenty of proof.

HOW YEAST GROWS UNCHECKED IN SOME KIDS

JENNY: Why doesn't the immune system recognize yeast as a pathogen (a germ) and go kick its ass?

DR. JERRY: Let's talk about some very possible mechanisms that seem to interfere with the immune system's ability to detect and destroy yeast. Some of the children are sick right after delivery and require antibiotics very early in life. These antibiotics may create an environment just right for children to develop yeast growth on mucosal membranes. At this young age, the body's immune system is still learning about itself and may consider yeast as "self." Thus, the immune system won't attack "self" and allows it to grow. In another group of children, those who start off well but later in life lose their ability to regulate yeast growth, apparently the "pathogen recognition" button has been switched off and an immune response is not generated, and there is the same result: unfettered growth of yeast.

JENNY: I finally got myself tested for yeast overgrowth, thanks to you, and I'm in the middle of killing the tons of yeast I have in my body. Many moms don't realize that if a kid has tons of yeast and metals, the kid's mom probably does, too.

DR. JERRY: I have taken care of many mothers of autistic children who complain of chronic fatigue, mental clouding, aches and pains, and unexplained skin rashes. Many times when they see their physician, they are "reassured" that their issues are "to be expected" or due to an especially "difficult" child, or some other lame excuse. The approach to removing yeast from parents parallels the approach to our children: limit sugars, use antifungals and probiotics, and make sure of daily bowel movements. Adding digestive enzymes with each meal can really help, too.

FOOD CRAVINGS, SYMPTOMS, AND ALLERGIES CAUSED BY YEAST

JENNY: One of the main issues I'm having right now as I experience the yeast die-off is my incredible craving for sugar. I usually crave sugar during PMS, but while I'm killing the yeast it has taken on a life of its own. I want to gorge on chocolate bars and buy cases of Hostess Cupcakes. Why is the craving for sugar so strong during this die-off period?

DR. JERRY: Food craving is a topic unto itself! Your craving for Hostess Cupcakes is not too far off from what many of our kids crave, too. They are what I call "carbo junkies." Very often it is the foods you crave that are the foods you should avoid. This is definitely true in our kids. Sugar seems to be at the top of the list of food craving for many people. In fact, it has been said that sugar can be downright addicting! So what do sugar craving and yeast have in common? Well, one of the by-products of yeast growth is the formation of alcohol. (The process of fermentation: Just add yeast to a sugar solution, such as grape juice, and you get wine.) So it may be the reason you're addicted to sugar is to feed your yeast, so then your yeast can make alcohol (you have this "microbrewery" going on inside of you). Now, you just can't go to your local doc with this idea. . . . You will be laughed out of the office. But I have to tell you that after treating many parents and their children with antifungals, many of the sugar cravings, mental cloudiness, and overall behaviors markedly improve.

JENNY: And that's why our kids seem drunk sometimes?

DR. JERRY: YES, and this can manifest as the giddy behavior you see, or just the plain meanness (like the "mean" drunk) they can exhibit. They are laughing for no reason (or at least no reason we can discern!), they have a drunken-sailor walk, and they can be irritable and crave sugar. These kids look stoned because they are. They can be very detached, have poor eye contact, very poor speech, etc. When they are treated, these behaviors improve dramatically.

JENNY: Can you name a few more behaviors you have seen due to yeast overgrowth?

DR. JERRY: Being demanding, noncompliant, aggressive, stimming, hands-over-ears, passing gas, and teeth grinding. Sometimes there can be a lot of chewing going on. They can chew on their shirt or they can be found chewing everything in sight because they're just uncomfortable. It is interesting to note that one of the ways we pacify pain when we're young is by chewing. In fact, that's why babies have pacifiers. Just that sucking motion helps them calm down. Some other signs include painful bloated bellies, diarrhea alternating with constipation, and rashes. One can find eczema on the skin and scaly stuff on the scalp. Even a funky-smelling scalp (my wife called it the "wet dog" smell when Josh's scalp became odiferous) can emanate from a child with yeast overgrowth.

JENNY: Is the yeast we have in our bodies that is causing havoc the same as the yeast that's in bread?

DR. JERRY: Not exactly. They are indeed different, but they ferment sugar in the same way. In the process of making bread dough, we put live yeast organisms into the recipe. Bread has sugar in the dough and when you let it sit at room temperature, the yeast munches on the sugar and makes alcohol and carbon dioxide gas. Carbon dioxide gas lifts the bread up and makes all those air pockets. Then we put it in the oven and bake it and it bakes off all the alcohol and KILLS the yeast. And out comes this beautiful bread.

So these kids can come to me, if you will, bloated, passing a tremendous amount of gas, and they are tooting all the time. The living yeast is thriving on the sugar and warmth producing the products of fermentation: some alcohol, carbon dioxide gas, and some toxins.

JENNY: Many moms have said to me that their child would wake up with a flat belly and by the end of the day it would be bloated like a Buddha belly.

DR. JERRY: Yes, and when you push on their bellies or tap on their bellies, it feels like air. If you take an X-ray of the abdomen (called a KUB X-ray), it just shows dilated bowel loops, that is, it's full of air. If you've ever had gas pains and cramps, it's miserable. It hurts. And you wonder why these kids are banging their heads or pushing on their bellies.

JENNY: Here's the million-dollar question, Doc: How does a parent get a pediatrician to test for yeast in their kid's gut when doctors don't even believe in it?

DR. JERRY: The first thing I would ask your physician to do is to ask for a stool sample to be done at your local hospital or lab. Ask for fecal leukocytes, occult blood, a culture and sensitivity, ova and parasites and fungal elements (this is "yeast"). The physician will give them the order, and then you will go to your local laboratory—whether it be Quest (www.questdiagnostics.com) or LabCorp (www.labcorp.com) or whatever hospital you live nearby—and that lab will give you the proper collecting kits that they use. You'll have your prescription in hand and they will handle everything and explain to you how to collect the stool and how much stool to collect.

JENNY: What do you do if the doctor refuses?

DR. JERRY: Get a new doctor, or keep demanding it if you feel your child really has this problem.

JENNY: I don't have a problem demanding it, but many moms are scared to.

DR. JERRY: Moms need to keep pressuring their doctors. Moms have to get their "Black Belt" in the art of persuasive communication.

This may include pulling articles off the Internet for the doctor to read or something as primitive as bringing into the exam room one of "those" loaded, foul-smelling diapers and allow the fragrance to permeate the office. You know, I don't really think the doctors grasp just how bad the bowel issues are until, how should we say it, they have the opportunity to come face-to-face with Mom's daily reality.

JENNY: Okay, so now the test comes back and the child has yeast—then what?

WHAT FOODS TO AVOID

DR. JERRY: So the tests come back and we've got yeast. Now the doctor is going to be more apt to write a prescription for an antifungal. Remember, there are some things that the parents can do, such as limit the sugar/starches/juices and anything that is "sweet," no matter how natural the product is. Yeast is an organism that feeds on sugar. It ferments it and the products are alcohol and toxins in the colon. The colon is the water reclamation plant. It dries stool so you don't have diarrhea. Anything in the water—such as the alcohol and toxins produced by yeast living in the colon—is entering the bloodstream. In this case it causes the giddy stoned behaviors.

Yeast is an equal employment opportunist, that is, it doesn't care if the sugar is derived from organic honey, pure maple syrup, or another carton of juice. Sugar is sugar, and it's hard, but you have to get them off it. The consumption of sugar feeds yeast, and it is addicting.

JENNY: Yeah, right. Get a kid off sugar. How?

DR. JERRY: If a child's sugar source is fluid, start weaning them by slowly, slowly diluting their drinks. If a child is consuming six ounces of juice, then begin by giving them five ounces of juice, with one ounce of water the first week, and gradually increase the water while reducing the juice. You can take months to wean them. If your child is truly an addict, there will be withdrawals. Make a progress sheet and back off if your child has trouble. Slow the weaning down. Some kids are so dependent, if you don't give them their sugar, they won't drink. They will go to their graves without drinking because they won't feel thirst the way we do. So you have to be careful not to dehydrate them in the process.

A trick you can use is putting stevia in the water. Stevia doesn't react like sugar.

And if candy or cookies is your child's problem, switch them to Stevia-based candies from health food stores or online—this might be a long wean. Also, you can start by switching them from candy to dried fruit, especially organic dried apricot and organic dried raisins. Cut the fruit into small pieces. Then slowly move from the fruit to Stevia candy.

JENNY: Is there an antifungal you prefer over another one?

THE BEST ANTIFUNGALS AND COURSE

DR. JERRY: The first drug of choice is going to be Diflucan and the generic form is called fluconazole. I like this because it can come in the form of suspension, a liquid that has solid particles dispersed throughout a liquid. Like sand in water . . . you can shake it well, and the sand will be "suspended" in the water for a time. It is available everywhere, but for a dye-free, sugar-free product, you will have to get it specially made by a pharmacy that "compounds" (that is, makes their own medications to your specifications). This is covered 90 percent of the time by the insurance company (and cheap enough, when compounded, to buy if insurance does NOT cover it). The pediatrician may want to use an antifungal called Nystatin, but I have found that it is usually very ineffective with yeast overgrowth.

JENNY: How long should these kids be on it?

DR. JERRY: Diflucan is best given once a day, and somewhere between fourteen and twenty-one days. It's not a five-day course and it's definitely not a one-day dose. Some of these kids actually need thirty days of treatment.

JENNY: Evan was on it for three months.

DR. JERRY: Some children are on an antifungal treatment for a year! Again, two things are happening: You can never totally eradicate yeast from the human being, and it takes a normally functioning immune system to keep the yeast population small.

JENNY: Why so long?

DR. JERRY: Remember you asked why the immune system does not see yeast as a pathogen (germ) and will not effectively mount an immune response to it? We really need the immune system's help at keeping yeast colonies small and negligible. Until that happens, we will have to keep pressure on the yeast growth with an antifungal.

Our hope is to create an internal environment that does not favor the growth of yeast and reestablish an immune system that can keep them from surging in population.

HOW TO GET THE BODY TO LIMIT YEAST GROWTH

JENNY: Yeast is in all of us, isn't it?

DR. JERRY: Yes, you cannot eradicate yeast from the human being; it prefers dark, moist, wet (mucous) areas. It goes by different names, depending on its location. If we get it on the feet, we call it athlete's foot; if it's in the crotch, we call it jock itch, or we call it vaginitis. But because our immune system keeps it under control, it doesn't manifest itself unless certain conditions are met, even in healthy individuals. The key to minimizing yeast growth is to make conditions unfavorable for yeast to grow! This is accomplished by decreasing sugar and complex carbohydrate consumption, decreasing the number of fruit servings per day, and adding probiotics and digestive enzymes to the diet.

JENNY: Once the yeast is under control, how does one switch their child off those medications to something that is less hard on the system?

DR. JERRY: After treatment with what I call a systemic antifungal, like Diflucan, I will switch to Nystatin or oral Amphotericin, which are nonsystemic. "Nonsystemic" is a term used to mean that it does not leave the digestive tube. In addition to lowering sugar, I always recommend probiotics (see the supplement recommendations on page 53). These are healthy bacteria that help make the gut less favorable for fungal growth. There are some wonderful natural antifungals like caprylic acid, monolaurin, oregano, and olive leaf extract (see the chapter on supplements for more information). The problem with the natural antifungal agents is that they generally don't have a taste that our kids can appreciate!

JENNY: I had to have Evan's Diflucan compounded. Why do some meds need to be compounded?

DR. JERRY: Compounding refers to the process where a pharmacist actually takes a medicine, usually in its purest form, and puts it into a suspension that is made just for our kids: gluten-free, dairy-free, dye-free, sugar-free, corn-free, etc. He can also make encapsulations or transdermals (medications that are put into a cream that is rubbed on the skin and absorbed into the bloodstream). This type of pharmacist is called a compounding pharmacist. Basically this is done in order to minimize allergic exposures that may be in the "off the shelf" brand.

JENNY: Are there any side effects from the pharmaceutical antifungals?

DR. JERRY: Everything that we do can have side effects. These children have the most metabolically fragile systems! I have had kids come completely unglued with cod liver oil or vitamin C! So now, you ask about an antifungal. Keep in mind that any drug can cause an allergic reaction, which has a tremendous range: from dark circles under the eyes, itchy skin, raised rashes (hives), coughing, and irritability, even to life-threatening rashes (Stevens-Johnson syndrome) and complete airway compromise (anaphylactic shock). In addition, each medication may have its own "niche" that it can cause problems in. The antifungals, for example, can cause liver problems, and thus, need to be monitored. So, anything we do in medicine has to be weighed carefully: benefits versus risks.

Another yeast killer I like to use is Amphotericin B because it works great and doesn't do any harm to the liver or kidneys. It goes in the mouth and out the anus. It kills the yeast. It can be taken for long, long periods of time. It does have to be compounded and has a very, very high safety threshold.

JENNY: What about over-the-counter antifungals?

DR. JERRY: There are many, many antifungal preparations available. I am so right about the taste, though. Unless the child is able to swallow capsules, it may be very challenging to get these preparations in. But some children will take anything (which is amazing to me), and we can make a lot of progress in controlling yeast. Some of my top choices for yeast control, in addition to the dietary changes, probiotics, and the addition of digestive enzymes, include:

Olive leaf extract
Caprylic acid
Candex

JENNY: I've heard that yeast can't grow if you do the Specific Carbohydrate Diet—is this true?

DR. JERRY: For some people, that's very true. I think one of the best ways that we can limit the growth of yeast is by removing its food supply. Yeast typically grows at the end of the digestive tube, called the large intestine (or colon), and is dependent on nutritive material to come to it. Thus, we need to aid digestion so that much of the food ingested is actually absorbed by the small intestine, way before it gets dumped into the colon. This way, whatever ends up in the colon has a very low nutritive value. The idea, then, is yeast isn't going to be able to thrive. There are many diets for "yeast," and the Specific Carbohydrate Diet is one of them. In a nutshell, all the grains are removed from the diet. Carbohydrates for these kids are made from flours derived primarily from nuts. When grains are removed from the diet, some children respond terrifically—but, like with any other diet, some children do not. Yeast is a terrific survivor, and our kids can have some very peculiar immune deficiencies that allow it to grow. In some cases, I have had to place some kids on a fruit-free diet, which I hate to do, but the sugar in the fruit (which is not being absorbed in a fructase deficiency) was feeding the yeast.

JENNY: And moms need to know that just because something is gluten-free doesn't mean it's okay. GFCF pancakes and waffles are still carbs, and carbs turn into sugar.

DR. JERRY: That's right. Keep in mind that carbohydrates and starches (include French fries here!) are broken down in the digestive process to sugars. It is wonderful that there are many GFCF ready-to-bake, ready-to-eat treats for our kids. They might taste delicious, but if you have a yeasty kid, he's going to crave those carbohydrates because that's how he is going to get his sugar fix. Moms and dads are going to have to limit these. Now, keep in mind that there are some kids who will eat only the carbohydrate-dense foods. That is a real problem for menu planning.

BOWEL MOVEMENTS AND YEAST

DR. JERRY: Okay, let's look at one of my "grandmother-isms." Grandma says: "If you don't take out the garbage daily, the rats will grow."

So no matter how we stress digestive enzymes and the right foods, if the children aren't having daily bowel movements, then they are not taking out the garbage. That is, they need to clean out their bowels! The material that we call poo is a very fertile nutrient source for things to grow. Some of the worst bowel infections I've seen have occurred in constipated kids. The stool stagnates and decays. This type of stool has a really putrid odor because the digested materials are undergoing a bacterial process called putrefication.

JENNY: I will completely second that, Doc! When Evan didn't poop during the time we were yeast killing, he went crazy and all of his language would disappear. When I finally got him to poop, he was so happy and talked more than he had ever done.

YEAST AND DIE-OFF REACTIONS

DR. JERRY: You have spoken a few times now about killing yeast and Evan going crazy. Maybe we should talk about the yeast die-off reaction these kids go through.

JENNY: Hey, buddy, I'm doing the interview. We'll get to that when I'm ready. . . . So, let's move right into the die-offs that these kids go through.

DR. JERRY: (Smiling) I like to think of yeast as little water balloons that are ruptured when killed. The problem is that their contents can be pretty toxic. How do these toxins get access to the bloodstream? Picture this: The job of the colon, besides being the garbage container, is to extract water from the stool. When the stool enters the large colon, it enters like water (very loose from the whole digestive process). The work of the colon now is to reabsorb the water and dehydrate the stool (thus, we don't lose water). Any toxins (like from the yeast we just managed to "pop") in the water will be reabsorbed, too. These toxins tend to cause behavioral issues.

Now, if we discuss this with the GI doctor, he will say, "It can't possibly happen, because all of these fluids and toxins from the large intestines and small intestines are then filtered by the liver and will never get to the brain."

JENNY: You're right. They would say that because they have said it to me. How do you respond to it?

DR. JERRY: By wholeheartedly agreeing and then reminding him or her about the effects of alcohol as it, too, goes to the liver, and then it goes right to the brain. We also give drugs by the rectum. There are medications that we give intentionally in the rectum. So we do have toxins that we've created by killing off yeast that can actually be filtered and still be bothersome. The children experience a die-off reaction because toxins are being released in large amounts and are absorbed by the colon in the process of dehydrating the poo. These toxins are then delivered to the rest of the body, the target organ being the brain.

JENNY: What are the behaviors some moms might see their child go through during these yeast die-off episodes?

DR. JERRY: The signs are irritability, lethargy, hyperactivity, and stimming. In other words, whatever your child does for autism, he will do ten times worse. He'll bite, scream, slap himself, and can head-bang. If it is so out of control, what I tell parents in that particular situation is to cut in half whatever it is we're using to kill the yeast. We will approach this slower. If I'm using Diflucan, and I said a teaspoon a day, I'll say, "Let's go to half a teaspoon." Remember, even the natural antifungals can cause a die-off reaction.

JENNY: What are some other things outside of cutting back on the meds to help those die-off episodes?

DR. JERRY: Epsom salt baths. One cup of Epsom salts in a tub of water. If we can, I also recommend taking activated charcoal two or three times a day, orally. Charcoal absorbs everything in the digestive tract. It'll absorb our zinc supplements. It'll absorb our selenium supplements. It'll absorb seizure medication, if the kids are on these things. So be careful not to give the charcoal with something. It should be given by itself, but at least an hour or two before or after something that we needed to get in there is in there. Keep in mind that charcoal will turn the stools black. So don't be shocked if you see that. But it'll absorb the toxins, too, and that's what we want, and they'll poo that out. During this period, which we call "die-off," the children may be experiencing headaches or bowel cramps. It may be a good idea to add some ibuprofen (Motrin or

Advil). Look for dye-free or obtain some compounded dye-free, sugar-free ibuprofen. Bottom line: When your child is in distress, think charcoal, Epsom salt baths, and ibuprofen.

JENNY: Activated charcoal is available at Whole Foods and doesn't taste like anything, so you don't have to force it down.

DR. JERRY: That sounded like a commercial.

JENNY: I used to be a performer, you know.

DR. JERRY: You're not anymore?

JENNY: No. Trying to help the world is much more fun.

DR. JERRY: I agree.

JENNY: I also want parents to know that if they see a die-off reaction, it's actually a good sign, right?

DR. JERRY: Yes. It's a good sign. It tells us we are on the right track. But where you have to be a little bit careful is that sometimes the child can actually have a bad reaction to the drug itself. It is important to run negative reactions by the doctor, just to make sure the child is okay.

If the child is having a rash or hives or when behaviors are so extreme, stop the drug and call the doc.

JENNY: I know you said that you don't know if you can actually see the yeast coming out of the butt of our kids, but I did with Evan. It looked like slimy, shiny, booger membranes that I think you could stretch a mile long.

DR. JERRY: Did you actually try to stretch it?

JENNY: (Laughing) You're darn right, I did. I was fascinated by it. Yeast awareness is something that is one of the many gifts these children are giving society today. I firmly believe once people take it seriously, many lives will be saved because of it.

DR. JERRY: I couldn't agree more!

ADVICE

If positive for yeast:

- Fluconazole: 4–6 mg per 2 pounds of body weight once daily.
- Ketoconazole: 4–6 mg per 2 pounds of body weight once daily.
- Itraconazole: 4–6 mg per 2 pounds of body weight once daily.
- Amphotericin B: For ages 2–5, 100 mg given 3–4 times a day (4 times per day is better, but for some parents it is very difficult to get in that fourth dose).

  —For 5-year-olds and older, 250 mg given 3–4 times per day.

- Nystatin

  —Infants: 200,000 units 4 times daily.
  —1–4-year-olds: 500,000 units 4 times daily.
  —5-year-olds and older: 1,000,000 units 4 times daily.

Natural antifungals can be very effective as well. Their use can be limited in children who are not able to swallow capsules due to the very pungent aromas and flavors. A short list follows that has been very helpful to some of the children I treat. Dosing depends on concentration, which varies from one manufacturer to another, so just follow the package's instructions.

Oregano
Garlic
Caprylic acid
Grapefruit seed extract
Probiotics
Olive leaf extract

CHOOSE A PROBIOTIC!	
Name of probiotic	**Where to get information and/or purchase the probiotic**
Kartner Health	www.kartnerhealth.com Phone: 866-960-9251
Kirkman Labs	Pro-Bio Gold www.kirkmanlabs.com 800-245-8282
MindLinx	NRG Solutions www.nrgsolutions.net Phone: 630-853-8383 Nature's Choice www.natureschoicetn.com Phone: 417-889—4184 Rockwell Nutrition (United Kingdom) www.rockwellnutrition.com Phone: +44 207 742 6700
Therbiotic	Klaire Labs www.klaire.com Phone: 888-488-2488
Primal Defense	Garden of Life www.gardenoflifeusa.com Phone: 800-819-6742 or 810-281-5507
Healthy Trinity	Organic Pharmacy www.organicpharmacy.org Phone: 800-819-6742 or 828-232-2842 Natren (United Kingdom) www.natren.com Phone: +44 134 231 2811 The Vitamin Store (contact via Web site only) www.shopthevitaminstore.com

DIGESTIVE ENZYMES: MANY TO CHOOSE FROM	
Kartner Health	www.kartnerhealth.com Phone: 866-960-9251
Kirkman Labs	Peptidase Complete www.kirkmanlabs.com 800-245-8282
Creon 10	A prescription enzyme that is very good and can save you some money (if you have pharmacy coverage) Informational Web site (contact via Web site only): www.revolutionhealth.com/drugs-treatments/creon-10 Purchasing Web site: www.drugstore.com Phone: 800-378-4786
TriEnza	Houston Enzymes www.houstonenzymes.com Phone: 866-757-8626
Enzyme Complete with DPPIV (DPP4)	Kirkman Labs www.kirkmanlabs.com Phone: 503-694-1600 or if outside Oregon 800-245-8282

- Be sure the child is not constipated. A laxative may be required during the yeast killing. (See the "poop" chapter on page 217.)
- Get activated charcoal, Epsom salt (for baths), and dye-free ibuprofen (e.g., Motrin) to lessen behavior problems.
- Stay away from sugar, and lower the carbohydrate intake.
- Yeast thrives on sugar! That's it, plain and simple. In fact, yeast does not care about the source of sugar—be it organic honey from California or pure maple syrup from Vermont. Pure fruit juice is loaded with sugar. Remember, sugar is sugar. In fact, carbohydrates

and starches (complex forms of sugar) are rapidly metabolized to sugar, and feed yeast as well. So we have children who crave sweets and we have children who are carbo junkies! One way to decrease the number of yeast colonies thriving is to limit their food availability. This means decreasing the source of sugars in a child's diet and replacing them with vegetables and proteins.

8
VIRUSES/BACTERIA

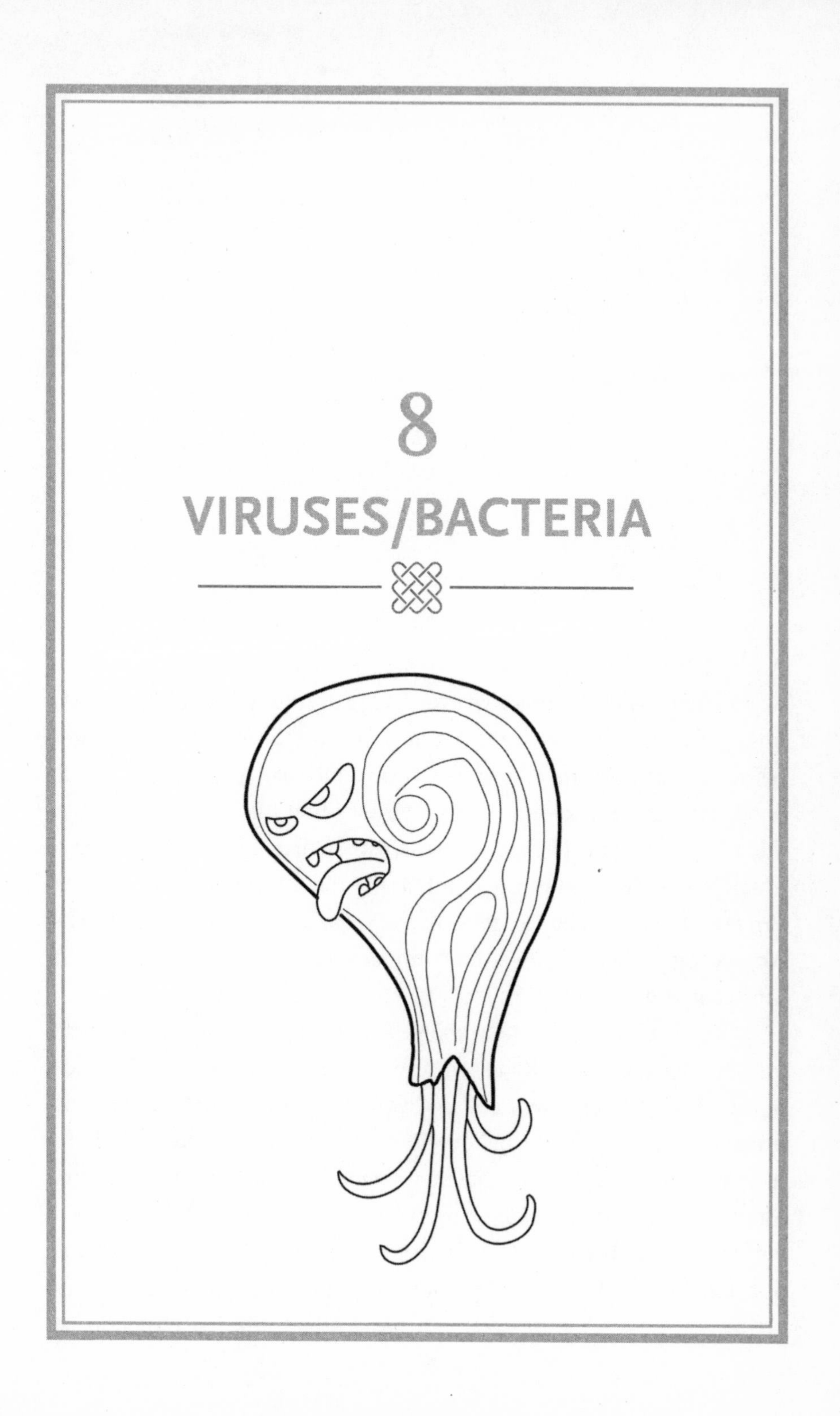

As I'm writing this chapter, I'm sick in bed with one of the worst bacterial infections I've ever had. I used to get strep throat as a little girl at least three times a year. I became used to this feeling of being invaded by an enemy we commonly call bacteria. The only good thing about bacteria versus a virus is that I get to take an antibiotic to help me get rid of it, whereas with a virus I would be forced to tough it out. The bad thing about taking the antibiotic though is that I'm going to be forced to deal with the yeast beast, which really sucks. And being a celebrity, it's a little embarrassing going to the store for Monistat and Vagisil.

After learning so much about the immune system from writing this book I'm a little pissed off that I allowed myself to get sick. Some of you might say, "It's not your fault you caught a bacterial infection," but I firmly believe it could have been prevented if I hadn't stayed up all night having a good ol' time the night before. Sleep is essential in keeping the immune system healthy, and I'm suffering now because of it. I can't even imagine how miserable our kids must be who are constantly fighting bacteria, viruses, or fungi. These kids are so much more susceptible to infection because of their dysregulated immune systems, which makes their behaviors heighten to the extreme. Having our kids get sick after already being sick makes living with a child who has autism almost unbearable.

GERMS	
TYPES OF GERMS	**HOW THEY ARE COMMONLY TREATED**
Viruses: chronic, low-grade infections from Herpes I, II, and VI; Epstein-Barr and Lyme	Antivirals, both natural and pharmaceutical: Lauricidin (monolaurin, coconut derivative); acyclover, valcyclovir, L-Lysine
Bacteria: Streptococcus, Clastrydia, and bacterial overgrowth in the bowel	Antibiotics, both natural and pharmaceutical; probiotics to be taken indefinitely
Parasites (diagnosed by stool test)	Antiparasitic agents, Alinia (Dr. Jerry's preference), Yodoxin and Flagyl
Fungus (yeast is part of the fungus family—it's in our bodies waiting for an opportunity to grow)	Antifungal agents, both natural and pharmaceutical (Diflucan), and dietary changes, i.e., cutting out all sources of sugar

DR. JERRY: Let's talk about all the different germs here, because people get confused. We have viruses, bacteria, parasites, and fungi. Yeast is part of the fungus family. These are all different entities. We don't treat viruses with antibiotics. Antibiotics go after bacteria. We treat yeast with antifungals but not antibiotics.

JENNY: Isn't it true that most of our kids need an antifungal when they are given antibiotics when they are sick?

DR. JERRY: Yes. Generally, antibiotics have an ability to kill bacteria that is harmful for us, but may incidentally kill bacteria that is beneficial to us. Some of these beneficial bacteria keep yeast from flaring up. Thus, if these bacteria are killed by the antibiotic, yeast can flare. This is where the antifungal (a yeast killer) comes in and keeps the yeast growth at a minimum.

JENNY: People also get confused about a virus in a vaccine and a bacteria that we're trying to protect. It all gets a little confusing.

DR. JERRY: Most viruses, like cold viruses, can be eradicated from the body. They come in, they set up shop, and our immune system recognizes that they're a pathogen (germ) and figures out how to break them and destroy them. Finally, they're removed.

THE HERPES VIRUS AND AUTISM

JENNY: But some viruses are forever, like herpes.

DR. JERRY: Yes, some viruses are forever. Herpes is notably one of the viruses that, once you contract the illness, the virus does not go away. In high school we were taught that the difference between love and herpes is that herpes is forever. The word "herpes" is derived from the Greek word meaning "to creep," referring to this group of viruses' ability to alternate between latency and reactivation.

JENNY: I went to Catholic school. They only taught me about burning in a pit of flames with Satan. No mention of herpes whatsoever!

DR. JERRY: There are currently eight distinct herpetic viruses in this family. Type 1 typically is responsible for canker sores and fever blisters, type 2 is usually associated with the genitalia, and type 3 is associated with chicken pox and shingles.

JENNY: Why do so many of the kids on the autism spectrum come up positive for herpes?

DR. JERRY: Remember, there are different herpes viruses out there. We are not talking about sexually derived herpes here. Herpes is generally spread by either droplets (sneeze, cough) or direct contact, depending on which of the eight herpes viruses we are discussing.

JENNY: Okay. Why are they having problems with them?

Dr. Jerry: Herpes has always been around. Other herpetic viruses include cytomegalovirus and Epstein-Barr virus. These manifest with cold and flu-like symptoms. We may take no special notice of them during the illness. These viruses have also been associated with mononucleosis or "mono." When severe, they can give you about six weeks of fatigue and maybe the spleen will enlarge, or your tonsils may become big and uncomfortable. Some children may actually have to be hospitalized. As with any infection, antibodies will be made against the virus in order to destroy it and to prevent its return, called immunity. The physician can actually test the blood and determine that the child is still making antibodies to protect him from future infections of that type of virus.

The question is, if your immune system is NOT acting properly, can these herpetic viruses be mischievous? By mischievous, I refer to an immune chronic inflammatory response to the virus that has reactivated. It is the inflammation that's going to affect the brain in a negative way and make the brain dull in thinking and dull in focus. Some people will describe a brain in that state as feeling like the first day when you have a head cold and you're just dull, and you don't really want to talk to anybody. You certainly don't want to be going to a calculus class. You actually want to be left alone. But remember after a couple of days of having an upper respiratory tract infection how marvelous you feel—just really wonderful because the inflammatory response is gone. In our group of children with autism, their immune system is dysregulated. There is also a medical theory that considers that certain families with an autoimmune history (for example multiple sclerosis, rheumatoid arthritis, Hashimoto's thyroiditis) may have a child who will also develop a form of autoimmunity when faced with chronic viral activation. When the child is induced to make antibodies to certain viruses, he will actually make antibodies to the protective "insulating" covering of nerves, called the myelin sheath. Thus, his own immune system is gnawing away at the insulation of nerves (much like the insulation of electrical wires). We see this in our clinic all the time. We routinely check titers (presence of) of antibodies against herpes type 1, type, 2, type 6, Epstein-Barr, and cytomegalovirus. We also check for autoimmune titers such as those directed toward myelin basic protein (the protective nerve sheath). Equally important is the evaluation of the entire immune system.

JENNY: All the parents I know talk about how herpes 6 comes up positive.

DR. JERRY: Herpes 6 comes up very often. Again, please note that having positive titers does not necessarily mean that there is a current problem with the virus. If I find that there are high titers (titer is a measurement of antibodies to a particular entity) and, in the immune system I find that there are a low number of natural killer cells (specialized immune system cells that play a major role in the destruction of cells infected with viruses), I know that this is a disease I can consider treating.

TESTING FOR VIRUSES THAT CAN CAUSE LOW-GRADE CHRONIC INFECTIONS:

Herpes I, II, and VI: Ask for the IgG antibody to these viruses
Epstein-Barr: EBV panel
Cytomegalo Virus: CMV panel

ANTIVIRAL THERAPY

JENNY: When you have a child with autism, do viruses play a role in those autistic behaviors? And if you're able to suppress or eradicate the viruses, does the child improve?

DR. JERRY: A lot of children do improve markedly with antiviral therapy. We are reducing the viral load of the body and decreasing inflammation, which in turn allows the brain to respond to stimuli in the environment in a much more natural way. We have several options to consider when prescribing antiviral medications.

JENNY: Okay gimme option one.

DR. JERRY: I like to start with an antiviral called Acyclovir. This is a prescription medication that is given three times per day. I also work with L-Lysine, which seems to have a viral inhibitory effect I can take advantage of. Some children may actually do better with another antiviral, called Valcyclovir.

JENNY: Okay, option two . . .

DR. JERRY: Intravenous immunoglobulins is another viable choice if there is enough immune system dysfunction (as per insurance company guidelines). This is a pooled blood product that has antibodies to most infections.

JENNY: Many parents who have children who've recovered from antiviral therapy actually have said their children developed a rash on their whole body. Why the rash?

DR. JERRY: Interesting. We always hear about rashes. If you're chelating and you get a rash, I've heard parents tell me, "Well, that's the mercury coming out." Well, how do you know that? Did anybody ever biopsy that and look for it? If you're treating any viruses, they develop a rash and all of a sudden it is supposed to be the "virus" coming out of the skin. We have never biopsied the skin to know for sure what is happening—but clearly something *is* happening and that cannot be argued with. It is important for rashes to be evaluated by a physician to be sure that it is not a dangerous type of rash (for example, hives).

JENNY: Like what?

DR. JERRY: The typical rash-like reaction I see is a slightly pink, slightly raised, non-itchy rash that loses its color when I push on it. It is typically present for about four to seven days, and then fades. It is most commonly seen on the back, chest, tummy, and upper arms. This is all we know about it, and it just does not raise any excitement in the medical community. Bottom line: We don't know exactly what is going on with the rash.

JENNY: Not yet.

DR. JERRY: Not yet.

JENNY: There are a lot of kids who will come up without any viruses in their blood work and recover with an antiviral. How can an antiviral work so well when there're no viruses showing up in the blood work? Explain that, Doc.

DR. JERRY: These antivirals may be working in different avenues that we have yet to describe. They may be working on other viral infections that we don't even know exist or even know how to test for. They may be working in the methylation pathway. So the bottom line is, we're not treating a piece of laboratory paper. We're treating a child. And if Mom tells you, "My kid's getting better," how do you argue with that? These autistic kids don't give you a placebo effect. What you see is what you get. If parents say, "When I give him Valtrex, the therapists are saying his language is blooming and he's being a lot more cooperative," then he's developing what I call the "F" word—Flexibility. Their obsessive-compulsive behaviors are down. The self-injurious behaviors are nonexistent now. He's sleeping through the whole night. And by the way, instead of going to bed at 11:00 P.M., he's going to bed at 8:30. The laboratory work just gives me an idea of where in the pond to go fishing. But I've got to get a fish on the line. So I'm ultimately always treating the child and the history that the parents give me.

JENNY: So what makes you, as the doctor, say, "Let's start antiviral therapy, even though I don't really see any viruses in the blood panel"? Is it that you've tried so many other therapies that hadn't worked on a child, so you're going to give it a try? What's the philosophy?

DR. JERRY: The stepwise approach that I take is that I really first focus on the bowels because the majority of children with autism have bowel disease. The bowel problems should be taken care of first, so when viral issues are addressed, the subtle improvements (or not so subtle) will not be masked.

Once we've managed the bowel issues, a new "inventory" of behaviors can be obtained. If the labs or history support the use of antivirals, then they are begun.

JENNY: Good answer. So it really wouldn't benefit a parent to go to their pediatrician to say test for herpes, would it?

DR. JERRY: Yes, it will if you will get the darn doctor to do some work. Again, ask for titers for human herpes virus 1, 2, and 6, cytomegalovirus, Epstein-Barr virus, along with immunoglobulin levels (IgG, IgA, IgM, and IgE), and include what is called a lymphocyte enumeration. He should also order a CBC with differential (looking for increased monocytes, indicating a viral infection).

These tests will look for evidence of chronic herpetic viral infections (there are currently eight known types of herpes infections), and the lymphocyte enumeration will give the doctor information on how well the immune system is working.

JENNY: You said damn! I can't believe it! I've been trying so hard not to say bad words and you said damn! I love it!

DR. JERRY: I said darn—it may have sounded very much like damn, but it was darn. Sometimes it comes out. Let me think of how I'm going to phrase this. Generally, a parent can convince a doctor to do a stool sample and look for fungal elements and bacteria. Understanding the laboratory investigations of the viral realm is a different matter altogether. The proper interpretation of the laboratory results coupled with state-of-the-art treatment is very intimidating for the general practice physician. It will take searches of the literature, conferring with colleagues, thoughtful consideration of the symptoms, and creating a treatment plan. Again, in all fairness, most doctors have had almost zero training in this arena. It is so much easier for the doctor to not do anything rather than take the opportunity to greatly improve a child's life.

I have a patient who was just incredibly stimmy, irritable, and aggressive. One of his biggest improvements in stimming behaviors came when we removed rice. The other huge improvement came when he was started on Valtrex. His changes were nothing short of remarkable! Rice was a huge problem, and his maternal exposure to herpes type 2 seemed to play a major role in his day-to-day behaviors. Children aren't supposed to have herpes type 2 problems, but some apparently do. They don't play by the rulebook. You just have to think outside the box. It's not written in textbooks, but you have to wonder especially when you see it. Valtrex and acyclovir are two of the drugs that I use for antivirals.

IF YOUR CHILD HAS HERPES, IT'S NOT YOUR FAULT

JENNY: Some moms say that they feel guilty that they passed down the herpes to their child.

DR. JERRY: Oh, I'm glad you brought that up. I have moms who feel guilty because they had an epidural or because they had sex in the third trimester. I have moms who feel guilty because they were cheerleaders and they were mean to other girls, and that this was God's punishment to them. I have moms who feel guilty for the ultrasound of the baby. Some mothers are concerned about receiving Pitocin to help with the contractions and now they think it's their fault their child developed autism. The way I answer this is that most of these interventions or behavior patterns were around well before autism rates soared. Pitocin was first synthesized in the 1950s and was commonly used for support of labor in the 1970s . . . well before autism was the problem it is today. We used epidurals before autism was a big problem. Women have been having sex in their third trimester for thousands of years, and again, we have never seen the rates of autism as we have now. So autism really is something new and not something that the moms could have caused. Women have had herpes or infections or dental work or whatever in their pregnancy and this isn't because of that. Things like flu shots, Rhogam shots, amalgams, and an aggressive vaccine schedule may be contributing, yes. But most of the things that women feel guilty about didn't cause the autism. It wasn't even contributory to the autism.

JENNY: Human papilloma virus, HPV—I'm interested in this because the majority of women these days have it. That's a virus that is down in the cervical area, so could that contribute to it in any way?

DR. JERRY: Well, again, prior to 1989, when we really saw an uptick in autism, was HPV still present? Yes, it was. So that's been around for a long time. So the question that you're asking is, do sexually transmitted diseases contribute to the escalation of autism? Sexually transmitted diseases have been around for a very long time. Since HPV is a viral disease, it may need to be considered in the overall contribution of toxic events the developing baby is exposed to, but no one knows for sure just what, if any, role the HPV has in autism. A point here: There are plenty of moms out there who don't have HPV or hepatitis B and their children develop autism and there are plenty of moms with HPV or hepatitis B who do not have children with autism. I feel strongly that the biggest contribution to the development of autism lies with the aggressive vaccine schedule and the contents of the vaccines.

OTHER VIRUSES: HOW THEY GET IN AND WHAT THEY DO TO THE BOWEL

JENNY: Well, you know I'm not going to argue with that! Let's continue with another virus moms talk about, which is the measles. How in the heck are measles getting stuck in the guts of autistic kids?

DR. JERRY: It gets very complicated.

JENNY: Try me; I'm all ears.

DR. JERRY: Let's take a look at how we are typically exposed to viruses. If somebody coughs or sneezes, the viral droplets will end up near our nose or our mouth or even in our eyes. From there they travel on into our body and eventually get presented to the lymph tissue. The lymph tissue is part of the immune system. Right there, the immune system starts working on first deciding that this is a pathogen (germ). This is an invader. This is worthy of destruction. How do we destroy it? It's a very complicated process that is still not fully understood. What we do know is that the immune system tags these little viruses as an entity to be destroyed. The germ starts setting up shop in our bodies. Before we even know we're sick, our immune system generally has a handle on it and is already taking care of it. It happens that vaccines that contain viruses are injected directly into the muscle tissue, bypassing the normal route of exposure. We put three or four live viruses directly into the bloodstream in the form of a shot.

JENNY: Called the MMR or MMR-V.

DR. JERRY: If the immune system isn't able to work well, such as demonstrated by a child who has recurrent ear infections, then it may have a real problem with this vaccine load of live viruses. So a common scenario may have a child on Augmentin, Zithromax, or some other antibiotic at one year of age when the child receives vaccines for mumps, measles, rubella, and varicella (chicken pox). The body—more specifically, the immune system—has already declared it is having trouble with bacterial infections. The hypothesis is that there is a mishandling of one or more of these viruses. They can trigger autoimmunity. They may, as in the case of the measles virus, set up a latent state with replication in the bowels. The measles virus has the capacity to spread into the spinal fluid and into the brain. The measles virus can spread into the gut. How do we know? There are published studies looking at the biopsy findings. They demonstrate that there is, indeed, measles virus in the bowels. Spinal taps have also demonstrated the measles virus in the spinal fluid of autistic individuals. The immune system is not able to mount an appropriate response, and so these viruses keep perpetuating themselves. In some children, then, you're going to have a problem with chronic inflammation in the bowels. The gastroenterologist will often note "ileo-lymphonodular hyperplasia" at these sites. What this means is that there are swollen lymph nodes at the end of the small intestines. This usually indicates an ongoing disease process and, in our children, most likely it's viral in origin.

JENNY: Which is all throughout the *Mother Warriors* book! So many moms I talked to had that problem with their child.

DR. JERRY: Where the GI doctors get into trouble with this is, they say, "But we see lymphoid-nodular hyperplasia in almost all of the kids we scope," and can falsely conclude that it is a normal variant. The problem here is that they are not scoping healthy children, so they are becoming complacent about this abnormal finding.

JENNY: I've had parents mail me photos of their child's scope showing their intestinal walls with measles all over them.

DR. JERRY: No, you don't see the measles! If you look at a zit, you don't see the bacteria that are causing it; you see the inflammation caused by the bacteria. When you see the "grape-like" clusters of the bowel, you are seeing the inflammation of the lymph nodes there. That inflammation will most probably turn out to be measles-virus-induced—when all the studies are done.

JENNY: So, major sores.

DR. JERRY: You are seeing some major owies in the gut. And they hurt. Just like those little canker sores that we get in our mouths. Look at the pioneering work of Dr. Arthur Krigsman with his pill camera. In his studies, a child swallows a pill that holds a camera. This camera, with built-in "auto flash," is able to take two to four pictures per second. These pictures are transmitted to a "buddy pack" that is clipped on to a belt and is worn around the child's waist. These photos have demonstrated that many children have ulcerative sores in the small intestines. No wonder that these children are crying all of the time, waking up in the middle of the night, or head banging.

JENNY: This isn't the case for all the kids, correct?

DR. JERRY: No, not in all children. Remember, autism is a collection of metabolic disturbances, and one child's issues are not necessarily the same as the next child's. This is why we have to be careful when we talk to the specialists. Those who are really involved with thimerosal believe that autism is primarily caused from mercury. But those people who are involved with viruses will say that some virus is the cause. Each doctor is going to develop a protocol that helps his patients, based on his clinical expertise and historical findings. Yes, I think viral exposure in vaccines contributed to the development of autism in a certain group of children. I think measles virus contributed to the current autism epidemic.

JENNY: So a simple explanation would be that the immune system is dysregulated and the vaccine comes in like the MMR and instead of doing what the vaccine hopes it does, the immune system says, "I can't deal with you right now." And the measles say, "Well, then, I'm going to go find a great environment called the gut and stay there."

Testing for Measles in the Gut

DR. JERRY: That's right, especially the terminal ileum, that is, the last part of the small bowels. There are places where the measles virus has a certain predisposition to hang out. At least that's what we know so far. There may be other areas. But that's an area that we can biopsy. It takes a tremendous amount of work to actually deduce that there is a measles virus in a biopsy specimen. Furthermore, more work has to be done in order to deduce whether that measles virus is vaccine strain or is a wild type. "Wild type" refers to the measles virus that is "caught" out in the community, not the vaccine strain. Keep in mind that although the vaccines mumps, measles, and rubella are live viruses; they have been attenuated, which means changed, so they don't cause the real disease. Our body makes antibodies to these viruses—little Patriot missiles that are specifically designed to blow them up should we come in contact with the real McCoy. Though measles gets a lot of press lately, we are also finding some immunological abnormalities with the immune response to rubella as well. So . . . there's more to follow on that story. One last point that often gets confused: The preservative thimerosal was never placed in any live viral preparation.

JENNY: Like the MMR.

DR. JERRY: That's correct.

JENNY: Any final words on virus?

DR. JERRY: Abnormal immune response to viral loads should be considered with every child with autism. This takes some blood work, and the actual laboratory work is "routine" with most labs (like LabCorp and Quest). We need to do a complete immune system evaluation as well as look for individual viral titers. Finally, a treatment plan must be put into place with frequent follow-ups to evaluate how the child is doing.

JENNY: Let's talk about bacteria. I had a doozy of a bacterial infection that I recall crying to you about on the phone, thinking I was going to die. The only nice thing about bacteria is that you can kill it with an antibiotic whereas with a virus, you have to wait it out, right?

DR. JERRY: We do have some wonderful antibiotics that kill bacteria relatively quickly! Usually, within twenty-four to forty-eight hours, the patient is much better after starting an antibiotic. On the other hand, it is true that most viral infections just have to be watched. Let the body's immune system remove them. Remember, you cannot treat a virus with an antibiotic!

JENNY: What type of bacterial infections do you most often see in our kids?

DR. JERRY: Believe it or not, by the time the children come and see me, I treat bacterial infections of the gut the MOST often. Sinus infections follow next, then the ears! The general pediatrician will see a slightly different picture. He will see these children and most commonly will treat ear infections, then sinus, and lastly lung infections (pneumonias, bronchitis, bronchiolitis).

JENNY: Are there bacterial infections that don't present themselves with fevers and lie dormant in the body?

DR. JERRY: It is true that bacterial infections do not seem to always cause fevers, but they never seem to lie "dormant" in the body. They are always mischievous, but we may not attribute behaviors or abnormal body functions to them. For example, obsessive-compulsive behaviors may be due to a streptococcus (type of bacteria) infection or the chronic diarrhea (often dismissed as "toddler's diarrhea") may be due to a bacterial overgrowth in the bowels.

JENNY: What are clues that our kids have a bacterial infection and not a virus?

DR. JERRY: Abnormal stools (that is, anything *not* normal) are always a huge tip-off that there is abnormal bacteria growing. Fevers that come and go is another clue that something is just not right. Persistent nasal congestion, persistent cough, and as mentioned earlier, behaviors that are not normal can all raise suspicion that a bacterial infection is present.

JENNY: Do you have a favorite antibiotic you use for bacterial infections in our kids? And what dosage?

DR. JERRY: First of all, I like to use what is known as a "compounded" prescription. This is where a special pharmacy, known as a "compounding pharmacy," will take the pure antibiotic powder and make a dye-free, gluten-free, dairy-free, sugar-free suspension (as some children can react poorly to those ingredients).

For upper airway infections (ears, sinuses): Azithromycin is my choice. There are dosing guidelines that doctors use when prescribing this, based on weight.

For gastrointestinal infections (bacterial overgrowth, chronic diarrhea): Metronidazole Benzoate, Clindamycin, and Gentamycin are all good choices as well. Again, there are well-established dosing guidelines to follow when prescribing these medications.

Reminder to use an antifungal with antibiotics.

ADVICE

Chronic viral and bacterial infections should be considered in every child with autism. The laboratory workup should include:

- CBC with differential
- Viral infections:

    —Viral IgG and IgM titers to: HHV-1, HHV-2, HHV-6, CMV (cytomegalovirus), and an Epstein-Barr viral panel. Consider Lyme disease panel.

- Bacterial infections
- Inflammatory markers: erythrocyte sedimentation rate, C-reactive protein, platelet count
- Streptococcus markers: ASO titers, Anti-DNase antibodies
- Stool cultures
- Urine cultures
- Urine organic acid testing

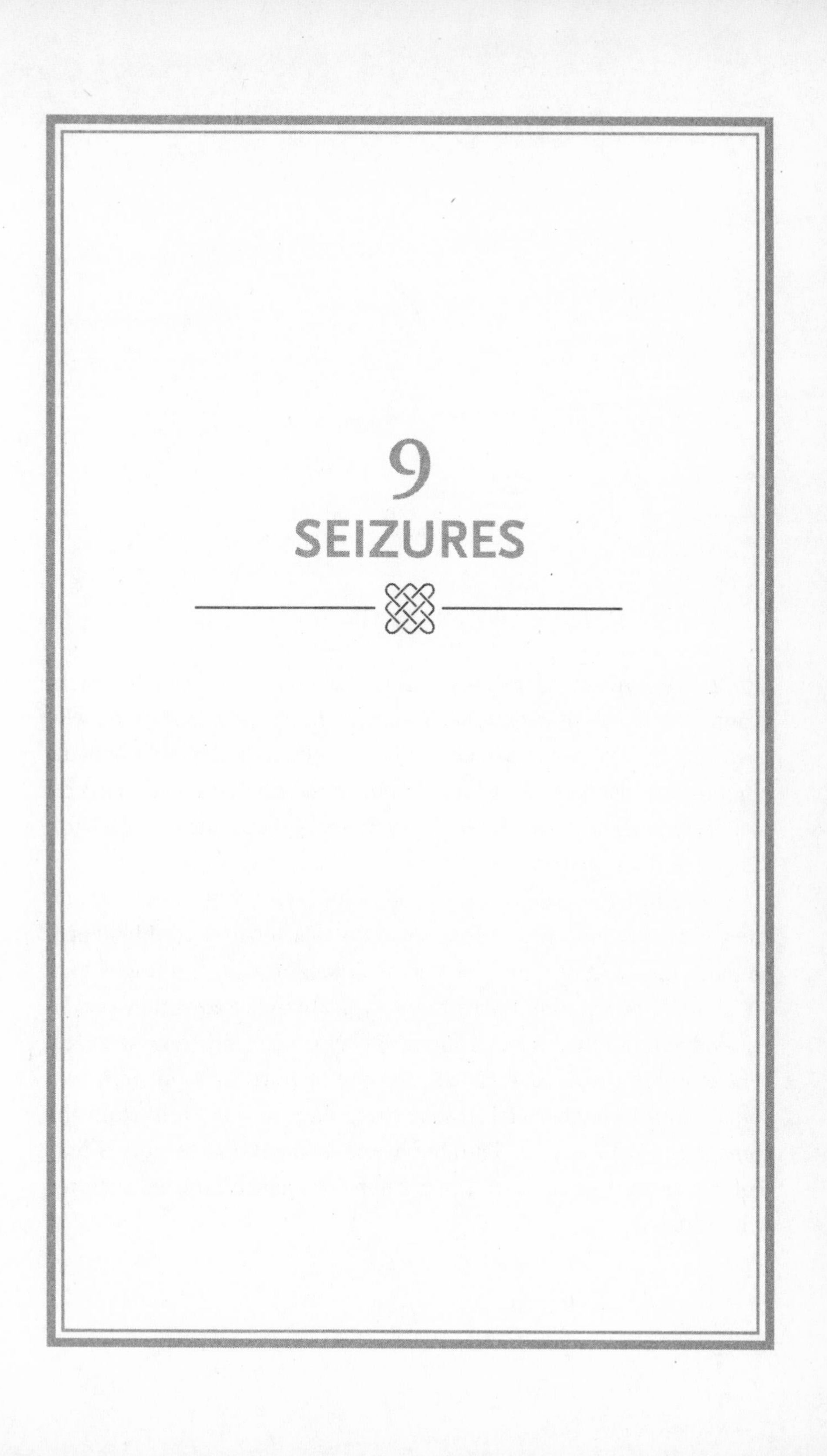

9
SEIZURES

DON'T PASS THIS CHAPTER UP even if your child is part of the lucky group who does not experience seizures. Thirty percent of kids who have autism experience seizures. I believe that percentage is actually higher—it's just that many times moms don't catch them. Staring off in a deep daydream sometimes is a seizure and our autism spectrum kids do that all the time.

I continue to have late-night cries about watching Evan's eyes dilate and seeing his body lifeless. I had no idea seizures could kill people, and the mortality rate for kids with seizures is climbing. There are some kids who don't react to the typical medications they give in the hospital, and we haven't found a way to shut off their seizures. When nothing worked for Evan, we had to purposely put him in a coma using Phenobarbital. It took three days to wake him from the coma, and to this day I'm haunted by the next possible seizure. I pray that the more I detox him, the greater the chance that his seizures will disappear.

WHAT IS A SEIZURE?

JENNY: I hate this topic.

DR. JERRY: I can understand why.

JENNY: Can you explain what happens in the brain that causes a seizure?

DR. JERRY: A seizure is a wildfire of electrical activity that starts in one area of the brain and either stays localized or can spread throughout the whole brain. People having seizures get that fish-out-of-water look: They are on the ground flexing and extending their arms, making grunting sounds. Very often they're drooling and their eyes are rolled up in their head to one side or the other. One minute can feel like two hours. This is what people usually think of when they hear the word "seizure." But seizures can be very subtle, such as staring off and not responding, or an eye tearing, or just a finger twitching. Most people can recognize what a major seizure looks like.

JENNY: I hate that I know exactly what that looks like. Can they swallow their tongue?

DR. JERRY: They cannot swallow their tongue. It is firmly "planted." The best thing to do with a child having a seizure is to lay her on her side, as this will offer more protection to the airway in the event of vomiting.

JENNY: Most parents get an autism diagnosis for their child between two and three. Do seizures have an age that is most common?

DR. JERRY: The first onset of the seizure can happen at any age. There seems to be a cluster around two to three years of age and again between eleven and thirteen years of age.

JENNY: It's so scary and seems so unfair that so many people have to deal with hardships of autism on top of seizures.

DR. JERRY: Seizures are very frightening. It's probably one of the hardest things that a parent can watch her child go through. It's an overwhelming fear of being totally out of control and not knowing what to do, mixed with the dread that this is a "picture" of their child dying (which, of course, it is not).

JENNY: Do seizures cause brain damage?

DR. JERRY: Generally, it is not a harmful event for the brain. They are not going to lose brain cells every time they seize. Most of the time, seizures resolve before the paramedics come. If this is the first seizure, it may be a good idea to go to the hospital to make sure that there is nothing more serious going on. The laboratory work is almost always normal and the child will be discharged from the emergency room with the recommendation to follow up with the family physician and to have a neurological consult. Rarely, as in Evan's case, the seizures remain severe and they have to admit the child and use medications to stop the seizure.

JENNY: Yes, and when they told me they were going to put him in a coma, I was actually grateful because then I couldn't watch him convulse past the seven-hour mark!

DR. JERRY: Placing a child into a coma protects the brain. Seizures that go over forty-five minutes, though very rare in general, can actually do damage to the brain cells if not treated. There is some evidence that recurring seizures may contribute to nerve cell damage. This is why prevention is so important.

JENNY: Prevention has really helped us. I've done my best to keep his autism and seizure triggers as far away as possible. Evan's seizures are triggered by getting a fever, having a stomach flu, staying up late, having too much yeast in his system, being dehydrated, and becoming overheated. Based on his triggers, I've decided to home-school Evan. Flu season in a regular school would drive me to the liquor cabinet. Forget it, it's too scary.

TESTING FOR SEIZURES: EEG

DR. JERRY: A lot of parents, after reading this, may wonder if their child does indeed have a seizure disorder. Many seizures may present with much milder symptoms, such as staring off in space for seconds to minutes. If this is the case, I would definitely recommend obtaining an EEG.

JENNY: Can you explain an EEG?

DR. JERRY: An EEG is a test to measure brain wave activity. It's done in the hospital with an EEG technician. We know what normal brain wave activity looks like and what seizure brain activity looks like. It is interesting to note that children with normal EEGs can still have seizures, and children with abnormal EEGs may not have seizures. The EEG may only be a twenty-minute recording and during the twenty minutes the brain will be functioning well. If the concern is great, there are twenty-four-hour (or longer) EEGs, and even EEGs with video monitoring. There are some more extensive ways of looking for seizure activity as well. Many children will not tolerate the EEG procedure very well because of all the wires and electrodes placed on the scalp.

JENNY: Now let me give you the Jenny version of an EEG.

DR. JERRY: Uh-oh.

JENNY: It sucks so bad. It's so difficult for parents because the doctors and nurses expect us to hold down our kids while they "superglue" like sixty electrodes to their head. Most of these kids don't let you brush their hair, let alone glue metal clips with wires hanging off of them. Some EEGs are an hour, and some are three days. I recently went in to do Evan's three-day EEG and it was like someone was cutting off his legs—the entire time. It was hell, BUT I knew it had to be done. I just want parents to be prepared that they need to bring rewards and DVDs to play during a test like this, especially if it's the three-day EEG. I should also tell parents that it doesn't hurt the child in any way. There is no pain. The only pain is in our hearts seeing our kid having wires glued to their head and watching them scream while trying to pull them off.

DR. JERRY: Well, I'm glad you're not endorsing an EEG machine, because they would fire you as a spokesperson.

JENNY: Should every child with autism get an EEG?

DR. JERRY: Any child who has the diagnosis of autism and could tolerate the test without too much wear and tear should have one done. Even if a child is not having seizures, it's good to get a baseline and to make sure that we're not dealing with something that we don't see. If we do see something, we can discuss the pros and cons of seizure medication.

JENNY: What about those seizures that you don't really see?

DR. JERRY: We call these subclinical seizures, that is, they are not obvious to the observer. Seizures come in all different flavors. Tearing seizures, vomiting seizures, rage seizures, staring spells, just to name a few. These are all signs of a possible seizure disorder.

Type of Seizure	**Duration**	**Behavior Displayed**	**Post-Seizure Symptoms**
Generalized: Absence (petit mal seizure)	2 to 15 seconds	Staring Eyes fluttering Automatisms (such as lip smacking, picking at clothes, fumbling) if prolonged	Amnesia for seizure events No confusion Promptly resumes activity
Generalized: Tonic-Clonic (grand mal seizure)	1 to 2 minutes	A cry Fall Tonicity (rigidity) Clonicity (jerking) May have cyanosis	Amnesia for seizure events Confusion Deep sleep
Generalized: Atonic		Head drops Loss of posture Sudden collapse Often occurs shortly after waking	
Generalized: Myoclonic		Rapid, brief contractions of body muscles Usually occur at the same time on both sides of the body	
Simple Partial	90 seconds	May remain alert and aware Sudden jerking Sensory phenomena (hear, smell, taste, see, or feel things that are not real)	Possible transient weakness or loss of sensation

Type of Seizure	Duration	Behavior Displayed	Post-Seizure Symptoms
Complex Partial	1 to 2 minutes	May have aura Automatisms (such as lip smacking, picking at clothes, fumbling) Unaware of environment May wander	Amnesia for seizure events Mild to moderate confusion Sleepiness
Subclinical		NOT obvious to the observer Shows no noticeable clinical signs or symptoms	
Status Epilepticus	Longer than 20 to 30 minutes	Prolonged in a series Patient is unconscious	Confusion Headache Exhaustion Sleepiness
Nonepileptic Seizures	Many minutes	Convulsive limbs Patient can be conscious or unconscious	

ANTISEIZURE MEDICATIONS

JENNY: As awful as the EEG was, I am grateful for the test because it showed me that Evan did need to start antiseizure meds.

DR. JERRY: Usually the neurologist will not start a child on antiseizure medications after the first seizure. Especially if it's a small seizure that lasted under three or four minutes. But if the seizure is over twenty minutes, or if there is something abnormal on the EEG, a seizure medication may be started.

JENNY: I want to get a little more into different antiseizure medications, but I can't name the ones I hate or love, for legal reasons—which sucks, because Evan went psychotic on one and then turned into a zombie on a different one. Finally, our third try was successful and Evan didn't experience any side effects. I'm so happy with it that I would endorse it if it weren't made by the same vaccine makers that screwed him up in the first place.

DR. JERRY: Any medication can have serious side effects. When a child is placed on a new medication, as happened with Evan, side effects have to be monitored and the medication stopped and switched immediately. Side effects such as hyperactivity, irritability, "spaced out" or "zombie-like" behaviors have to be addressed immediately, as these side effects do not seem to fade away. With seizure medications, there are follow-up labs that must be done to make sure the liver is "happy" with the new medications. Whenever we give kids drugs long-term we want to monitor how their body reacts to it, so we watch the liver panel. Parents should ask their doctor to keep checking the Comprehensive Metabolic Profile. It gives you salts, kidney function, and liver function. In addition we get a Complete Blood Count (CBC) to make sure the bone marrow is okay too. And we test for blood levels of the seizure medication itself if it's a med that's measurable.

In addition, one thing that many neurologists don't do is a follow-up EEG. I won't do another EEG if the child had a horrible experience with the first EEG, but if I can, I would like to know if the seizure activity has diminished.

JENNY: I agreed for Evan to have his second EEG just to make sure his new dosage was working.

DR. JERRY: A seizure is disorganized electrical activity of the brain that generates meaningless impulses. Areas of the brain involved with seizure activity can be very small and noticeable to very large and easily noted (for example, a child on the floor shaking violently). Seizures can be very short in duration, or quite long, and can occur many times a day, or they can be very rare events. Seizures are disruptive to the area of the brain being affected and prevent it from functioning as it should. Now, it's very interesting to note that many children start speaking after they begin taking antiseizure medication. That may be because the medication is suppressing seizure activity. If this abnormal brain wave functioning was indeed contributing to their inability to speak, then by removing this activity it may allow language to spring forth. So, in some cases, the seizure may not necessarily be all bad. Fixing them helps us. Suppressing seizure activity may improve language.

NATURAL TREATMENTS

JENNY: What can we do to help minimize seizures from a natural point of view?

DR. JERRY: I really like high doses of B_6 and B_{12}. I think that really helps to stabilize cells. I work under the premise that sick cells seize and healthy cells don't. If we can make these cells healthier, we may see some definite improvements. Many of the seizure medications deplete folic acid (a B vitamin), so we have to be on top of this.

JENNY: What do you mean by "high doses"? How much should we be giving them?

DR. JERRY: Depending on the weight of the child, they should be taking between 50 to 200 mg of B_6 per day, and between 1,250 mcg to 5,000 mcg of B_{12} per day. This will be more than is recommended in the supplements section, but this is the upper limit of the total amount recommended.

JENNY: When I toured around the country talking to moms, I was amazed at how many of them said that hyperbaric chambers lessen the severity and frequency of their child's seizures or even caused it to completely disappear.

DR. JERRY: I like using *mild* hyperbaric oxygen therapy (HBOT, in which oxygen is introduced in a pressurized chamber) on children with seizure disorders.

JENNY: I have a whole chapter dedicated to it (beginning on page 233), so we're not going to get into it now, but I encourage parents to be open to this amazing therapy for our kids, especially kids with seizures. Aren't you kind of baffled by these severe seizures that some of these kids endure?

DR. JERRY: Yes, this is the only group of children—that is, children with autism and a seizure disorder—that I've seen on two to three different types of seizure medicines at the same time. In fact, a lot of these children have been dismissed by the neurologist because there is nothing left to offer the child or the family to help control the seizures.

JENNY: What about the mortality rate of kids with seizures? Of course, witnessing it firsthand with Evan makes me think it happens all the time.

DR. JERRY: It is increasing. I've lost two children to seizures already in my practice. Pediatricians do not typically lose their children unless there is cancer involved.

SEIZURE PREVENTION

JENNY: What can a parent do to prevent seizures?

DR. JERRY: We know that there are certain conditions that can make it easier for the brain to have a seizure. This can be referred to as "lowering the seizure threshold." Some well-known conditions, such as a fever or dehydration, can make it easier for the brain to have a seizure. Each child will "teach" us about their particular triggers. Evan taught us that fevers and dehydration are definitely his triggers. Something as simple as giving him ibuprofen and fluids intravenously will keep him seizure-free. Another trigger I have found has been severe constipation. The children who have several seizures per day seem to have far fewer when completely cleaned out. This probably works with the whole notion of lowering the total body burden of toxins.

JENNY: The Web site for Lamictal (lamotrigine) is www.lamictal.com, which is Evan's seizure control medication, lists some common seizure triggers, although it does not list all and triggers will vary from person to person. Below is information on what to do to possibly prevent a seizure, depending on the common seizure trigger:

JENNY: Can I tell you one of the things I started doing that I also think helped Evan during fever time besides getting him an IV?

Common Seizure Triggers	How to Possibly Prevent Seizures
Inconsistency with medication: New seizures occur most often when one stops a medication completely	Stay on top of prescribed medications, always consult your doctor, and ask questions about what can and cannot be taken with the medication and what to do if you forget to give a dose
Being ill or sick (ie: viral infection or high temperatire)	Rotate between Motrin and Tylenol (dye-free) every 3 hours
Poor sleep	Create a regular sleeping schedule
Bright lights	Avoid to the best of your ability
Dehydration	Drink plenty of liquids
Any type of medication (i.e., over-the-counter, new and continuing prescriptions, vitamin supplements, or natural/herbal medication)	Read all labels and speak to your doctor about using medications while taking others
Stress on the body or emotional worry (these can be seen in the form of constipation or diarrhea)	Supplementation, use of laxatives and digestive enzymes, monitor food/diet
Bad diet	Eliminate certain foods

DR. JERRY: Well, I think you should, considering I'm his doctor and we are writing a book about it!

JENNY: I give him 5 mg of Ativan orally. Since this is what they give him if he seizes, I might as well give him one on his tongue during a fever.

DR. JERRY: That is a good point, Jenny. For our children, especially those who can have life-threatening seizures, this "preemptive strike" with a very mild antiseizure medication is a great move, and if nothing else, Evan's just going to have a very calm illness.

Also, let's not forget to mention alternating Tylenol (acetaminophen) with Motrin (ibuprofen). Most physicians who deal with autism cringe when they hear about the use of Tylenol because Tylenol does reduce levels of glutathione (your body's natural antioxidant). However, when you have a child who is prone to having high fevers, and Motrin may only last for three to four hours before the fever starts to rise, you can alternate Tylenol with Motrin, giving one, then the other every three hours. True, we may be losing glutathione with this regimen, but it just may keep the child out of the intensive care unit. On the other hand, we can always give the child more glutathione (for example, a transdermal cream) during an illness, as some studies suggest that there is a correlation between low glutathione in the brain and seizures.

JENNY: But most parents, who don't have seizure kids, don't have to fight a fever that hard, right?

DR. JERRY: No, they don't have to fight as hard. Fever is basically inhibiting the replication of the virus or the bacteria. These germs do not replicate at elevated body temperatures. Fever is protective. But to a child who seizes with fever, aggressive therapy may prevent another seizure.

SEIZURE AND DIET

JENNY: I've heard parents say, "I put my kid on the Specific Carbohydrate Diet and he stopped seizing and then when I took him off of the Specific Carbohydrate Diet, he started seizing again." Do you have any idea why that would happen?

DR. JERRY: Anytime you remove anything that the body views as toxic, like the grains you suggested in the Specific Carbohydrate Diet, then the result will be fewer seizures. Also the ketogenic diet works for children with severe seizures. That diet consists of low carbs and high fats. Epilepsyfoundation.org has more information on the ketogenic diet.

JENNY: If puberty can trigger seizures, what is this young generation of kids gonna look like when they hit puberty? Are they all going to be seizing?

DR. JERRY: Once again, we are looking at this dilemma real-time. As we advance the concept of biomedical interventions, we may have a very large impact on these children. So when they launch into puberty, they will not experience an increase in seizures.

JENNY: What do you mean?

DR. JERRY: If we start detoxifying a child from a young age, by cleaning up his diet and removing the chicken nuggets, sodas, and high-fructose drinks, and start the child on supplemental nutrients, like the ones we discussed earlier, consisting of vitamins, minerals, and omega-3 fatty acids, we may see many positive changes. For example, a child who has been working with a physician for many years with the incorporation of a nutritious diet, normalization of bowel movements, toxic materials, and metals removed, I think we will find a child free to enter puberty without the worry of having seizures.

JENNY: Should the more toxic kids be more worried?

DR. JERRY: I think those children are going to have a much lower seizure threshold. We are going have to look and see what happens to the two groups as they mature, and you will have to ask me that question in ten years.

JENNY: I'll be forty-six in ten years.

DR. JERRY: What does that have to do with it?

JENNY: Absolutely nothing. It just made me think of how old I was gonna be in ten years.

DR. JERRY: But you will be toxin-free and look as good as you do now!

JENNY: It won't help the boob sagging that's going on.

DR. JERRY: That's a different book and a different doctor.

BECOMING SEIZURE-FREE

JENNY: So, back to seizures. Will Evan ever be able to get off seizure meds? Is it possible with his type of seizures?

DR. JERRY: Eventually when Evan has been seizure-free for four or five years and has a normal EEG, you're going to say, "I think we need to start weaning his medication."

JENNY: That seems so scary to me.

DR. JERRY: In the meantime, if the EEG returns to normal, you will feel more reassured weaning the medication.

Another strategy is to let Evan outgrow his dose. In other words, Evan will stay on the same dose as he grows. As he gets bigger and bigger, the dose, relative to his body weight, becomes smaller and smaller.

JENNY: Have you seen kids become seizure-free?

DR. JERRY: Oh, yes. I have had children in my practice become seizure-free. I hope Evan will be one of those kids. Though this has not been proven yet, I believe vitamins B_6 and B_{12} are instrumental in raising the seizure threshold. Again, once our kids' EEGs return to normal, they may be telling us they are finally ready to come off the seizure medications.

ADVICE

- Get an EEG.
- If seizure activity starts, consider antiseizure medication. Common ones (not listed by favorite, but maybe they are, hee-hee):

  —Lamictal
  —Depakote
  —Neurontin

- During a fever:

  —Rotate Tylenol and Motrin (ONLY DYE-FREE) every THREE hours.
  —Continue to offer fluids to ensure adequate hydration.

- Keep up on vitamins B_6 and B_{12}.
- Hyperbaric oxygen chamber (go to www.oxyhealth.com for more information).

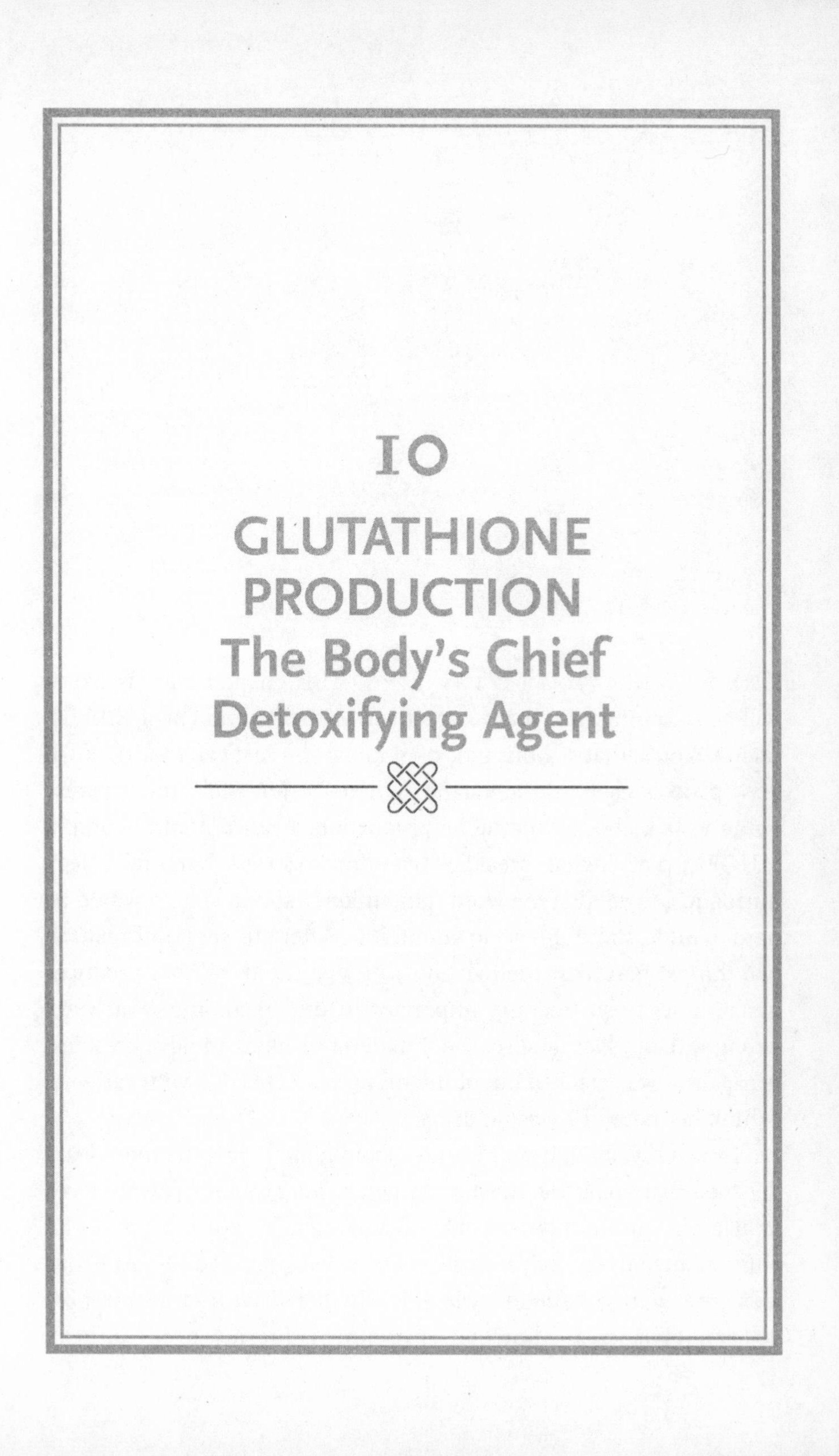

10

GLUTATHIONE PRODUCTION
The Body's Chief Detoxifying Agent

I KNOW WHAT YOU'RE THINKING. This chapter sounds like it will be so boring. Not that I expect you to rejoice and cheer with the poop chapter (that's coming next—I know you just can't wait), but at least poop is easy to understand. When Dr. Jerry told me we were going to talk about glutathione production, I ran out and bought a HUGE cup of English breakfast tea to make sure I didn't fall asleep during it. I think just the word "glutathione" sounds like it would be hard to understand. I have to admit, it is. After our session I realized two things: first, that methylation pathway, the thing that produces glutathione, is so freaking important in understanding what went wrong with our kids, and second, I'm never drinking English breakfast tea again. I was cracked out of my mind. It's LOADED with caffeine. I think he thought I was on drugs.

I must say, though, as I learned about glutathione, the more I understood that this is the most important substance our body produces to help our immune system fight off bad guys. It's our most powerful antioxidant and our body's most powerful detoxifier. Sadly, most of our kids are low in glutathione, which is why they have so much trouble detoxing vaccines, medications, environmental toxins, toxins in food, and why they have so much trouble fighting infections and diseases. The more you educate yourself about glutathione, the more you'll want to raise glutathione levels in your child so his or her immune system is capable of doing its main job, which is kicking the bad guys' asses!

METHYLATION PATHWAYS AND GLUTATHIONE PRODUCTION

DR. JERRY: You seem bright and cheery today!

JENNY: I'm ready to ROCK glutathione production and methylation pathways, baby!

DR. JERRY: Well, let's get right into it.

JENNY: Woo-hoo!

DR. JERRY: Glutathione is produced through methylation. Methylation is the movement of a carbon atom, which is called a methyl group (hence the name "methylation pathway") down a chain of chemical reactions until it ultimately produces glutathione. Each new compound made, by the addition of a methyl group, has its own specific characteristics and job descriptions.

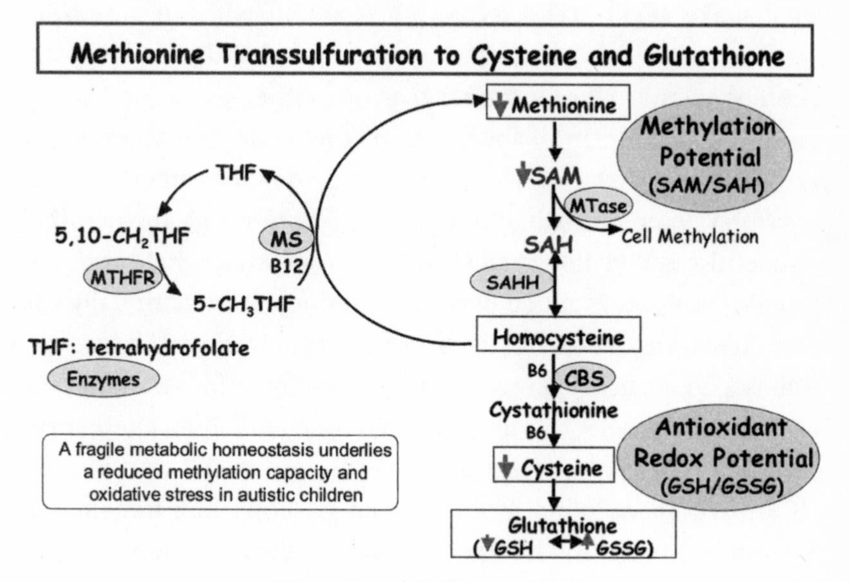

Chart courtesy of Jill James, Ph.D.

JENNY: This arrow graph you made me put in looks like hieroglyphics. And, when you say, "That's how we build things," what exactly are we building?

DR. JERRY: Limiting our discussion to the methylation pathway, we really, really want to produce glutathione, as this is our body's chief detoxifying agent. Let's start with methionine, which is an essential (meaning we have to take it in through our diet, we cannot make it ourselves) amino acid. It is found in meat, fish, dairy (which we often eliminate from autistic children's diets) and, to a lesser degree, in fruits and vegetables. You can see in the diagram that methionine is eventually converted to homocysteine by the process of methylation. Homocysteine now has a decision to make: Either continue down the road and form the glutathione, or join with a very special form of folic acid (denoted by CH_3THF) and regenerate methionine to restart the cycle. So in this case, Jenny, we are trying to build glutathione.

JENNY: Okay, I'm gonna hang in there with ya, but I gotta tell ya, it's already a little hard.

DR. JERRY: It's going to get a little more confusing, and then I think it will make sense. Let's recap. You start off with an amino acid called methionine and then it becomes SAH and then it becomes homocysteine. Homocysteine that can either go around joining with a special form of folic acid to regenerate L-methionine, the amino acid we started with, or it can go down another branch to make cysteine and glutathione. Now, before we go further, that's what this methylation is all about. These are cycles that continually spin in our bodies much like transmission gears continually spin. And like transmission gears, they don't spin by themselves—we're talking about this pathway being like one gear in a transmission, but you know one gear abuts another one and abuts another one, so they spin together. So if any one of the gears isn't working, well, it impacts many other processes that go along in a transmission and in our body. You'll hear "folic acid pathway," "biopterin pathway," and now you are familiar with the *methylation* pathway.

These pathways tend to be, as we have it figured out in biochemistry, interrelated cycles—each gear, if you will, turning another.

The overall function of this methylation pathway is under genetic control and this is how entire families can be impacted. You can have a family of "poor methylators." In other words, genetically you didn't get all of the methylation pathways working at full capacity. Another point to make here is that these pathways are excruciatingly sensitive to environmental toxins, such as mercury. Now you can see the disadvantage a person may have who is already undermethylating and exposed to a toxin, say, mercury. This system will really slow down under those circumstances. Remember, this whole pathway was designed, among other things, to make the super-strong detoxifying agent, glutathione. Then, as you can see, we get into a vicious cycle where the body cannot detoxify agents coming into it and they keep poisoning the pathways.

SIGNS OF IMPROPER GLUTATHIONE PRODUCTION

JENNY: Are there signs that show who is undermethylating?

DR. JERRY: Well, that's where I'm going. If you come from a family that has poor methylation, what you'll see in that family history is depression, bipolar disease, schizophrenia, suicide, constipation, attention deficit disorder, alcoholism and, of course, autism. So when I have a set of parents sitting in my office and a mom looks at me and says, "My gosh, you just described both our families," then I know that this child comes from a poor methylating family—it's in the genes! This is the genetic component. Now, this history can be very important in the medical management of our children as well as in understanding, perhaps, how these medical problems came to be.

The purpose of the methylation pathway is for detoxification from toxic exposures. We talk a lot about mercury exposures because we understand this problem, but keep in mind there are many toxins that enter the body. Recent umbilical cord blood analysis of infants revealed more than two hundred chemicals known to cause cancer, neurological problems, and endocrine dysfunction. Our methylation pathways better be up and running when we are pregnant, because once our children are born, they are exposed to many potential toxins just from breathing, eating, and receiving vaccines. It is all cumulative, and there seems to be a definite tipping point in many of our children.

JENNY: Wow, I think I get that. I mean it's still hard, because methylation is so intertwined, but at least I can see now what happens to people who don't methylate well.

DR. JERRY: We can inexpensively test for products of this methylation. We can ask the lab to assay the amount of cysteine and glutathione in the blood. A more expensive way to look is directly at the genetics of some of the controlling enzymes of the pathway.

Bottom line, when the methylation pathway is spinning, it is making glutathione, it is making cysteine. Cysteine can be converted to metalthioneins, which bind to metals such as mercury, thus protecting the tissues and enzyme systems that would otherwise be poisoned by mercury. Cysteine can be converted to glutathione in the liver. Glutathione can also be generated in the brain by specialized cells utilizing cysteine. (Interesting note: Glutathione made in the body cannot cross the blood-brain barrier and go into the brain and thus glutathione in the brain is made by brain cells.) You can think of glutathione as a garbage truck that goes around and detoxifies debris. So it's very important to have normal levels of glutathione and cysteine. We have standards and we know what's normal and abnormal.

JENNY: Where else do you see glutathione being low and causing disease?

DR. JERRY: In the most recent literature, they're looking at schizophrenia as being a low-glutathione disease. You can also find references of a low-glutathione state and depression, bipolar disease, dementias, and alcoholism, among other diseases.

BOOSTING GLUTATHIONE LEVELS

JENNY: Let's talk about raising these glutathione levels so that our kids can detox properly.

DR. JERRY: We know from the literature that we can positively impact glutathione levels. Jill James's research clearly demonstrated that by adding methyl B_{12}, TMG, or DMG, and folic acid, one could increase the total glutathione measured. That is just what we do, and many children clearly benefit. We sometimes add the essential amino acid methionine because that is part of the pathway and is not in sufficient levels (as by direct blood measurement or by taking a dietary history). We also add folic acid, another cog in this pathway that seems to be deficient.

See the supplements chapter on page 53 for methyl B_{12}, TMG, or DMG dosage information and protocol.

JENNY: If this works for kids with messed-up methylation pathways, won't it work for the parents who might be suffering from depression or alcoholism?

DR. JERRY: While treating the child, I often recommend that the rest of the family treat themselves in much the same manner. We can give the family members many of the same things we're giving the child. Mom will often report back later, saying, "You know, I feel like I'm eighteen years old again," and Dad says, "I've got my game back, I'm a lot more consistent." And Mom's nodding her head, saying, "He is so much better when he gets his glutathione and his B_{12}."

This is how the methylation pathway affects people. We're doing it to help the body rid itself of toxins. We're doing it to get the glutathione levels up. Glutathione or cysteine can be given orally, but may promote yeast growth. We can give glutathione transdermally, in a cream that is absorbed through the skin, and this works well. In addition, we can give glutathione with a nebulizer, which is a way to turn it into a mist that the child breathes in; and we can give glutathione intravenously. This can be done by doctors who treat kids biomedically, or who are well-acquainted with glutathione protocols.

JENNY: I had a glutathione IV from your office last week.

DR. JERRY: How did it make you feel?

JENNY: Overall, it made me feel great! How often do you give glutathione to a patient?

DR. JERRY: I do what the child and the parent tell me works best for them. So if Mom says, "I am giving glutathione once a month but I only have two great weeks," this would be an indication that the child would benefit from twice-monthly infusions. Another scenario could be a child who does great for about eight hours following an infusion, but then regresses back to baseline. This would be an indication to consider twice-daily dosing of glutathione with a nebulizer. A nebulizer allows us to place glutathione in a specialized cup and generate a mist that the child breathes in. Sometimes, a transdermal (a cream that takes the medication in through the skin) glutathione is all you need. In addition to this, we can give B_{12} injections that include both folic acid and cysteine. All this can be done with your doctor. Some children do better with more, some children do better with less.

JENNY: Can kids be born with low glutathione?

DR. JERRY: We are all born with different capacities to detoxify substances that we are exposed to. One of the body's best detoxifying agents is the glutathione, as we have just discussed, and its availability is genetically influenced. We won't know if it is low unless we start doing screening on babies before they are exposed to numerous toxins. Basically, the genetic predisposition here is that these children were not good methylators to start with. They were a setup and the cumulative exposures to toxins overwhelmed their metabolic capacity to neutralize them. Disease then follows, and in the case of children, we call their collective symptoms autism.

JENNY: So, in my cartoon drawing, the metabolic pathway can look like gears and if one's not working, it's not going to make the other ones turn?

DR. JERRY: That's right. When we try to teach this, we speak of each concept as if it stands by itself, like little individual squares in a waffle. Actually, though, all these squares are so interrelated, it looks more like a plate of spaghetti. When you tug on a noodle over here, you don't know how it's going to affect the meatball at the other end of the plate. So when we start the B_{12}, B_6, DMG, glutathione, folic acid, and N-acetyl-cysteine, we can sit back and watch what happens to a child when toxins are neutralized and removed by the body. We often see a child start blooming and doing great in ways that Mom didn't expect but hoped for.

JENNY: You mentioned DMG a little bit earlier but didn't say what it was. What is it and what does it do?

DR. JERRY: DMG is the abbreviation of dimethylglycine and is a supplement, but it is also found in grains and meats. We supplement it to our kids because it enhances mood and energy levels along with chemical metabolism and enzyme production.

JENNY: How can parents go to their pediatrician and ask for the test to see if their child has low glutathione?

DR. JERRY: If we want to look at what is happening genetically, LabCorp has a test called Methylenetrahydrofolate Reductase (MTHFR) Thermolabile Variant, DNA Analysis (test number 511238). I recommend this test, as most insurance companies will cover the cost. There are more commercially available testing that is more extensive, but insurance will usually not cover them. Glutathione and cysteine can also be directly measured at LabCorp as well. These tests are blood tests and will need a doctor's prescription. Other labs that assay glutathione and cysteine would include Genova Diagnostics and Vitamin Diagnostics.

Genova Diagnostics
800-522-4762
www.genovadiagnostics.com

Vitamin Diagnostics/European Laboratory of Nutrients
732-583-7773
www.europeanlaboratory.com

JENNY: Do you typically see good results from raising glutathione levels?

DR. JERRY: Raising glutathione levels clearly benefits two-thirds of our children. Keep in mind, this therapeutic intervention, like any other, does not work on every child. Methylation may not be a problem in some. In others, I have seen language develop over the next twenty-four hours following an IV infusion of glutathione. It is just one more tool in our tool chest we use to work on these children with broken and poorly functioning metabolic pathways.

JENNY: Anything else about methylation pathways before we move on?

DR. JERRY: There is so much more. What we know can get very complicated, and there are some really great books available that deal just with methylation as we know and understand it today. We have to keep in mind that science is a daily event, making history at every turn. What we know now will be a drop in the bucket in just a few years.

JENNY: So this is for sure a "to be continued."

DR. JERRY: Absolutely. Bottom line: We have to help the body maximize glutathione production.

ADVICE

- Support for the methylation pathway is support for the production of glutathione, one of our body's most important antioxidants.
- Methyl B_{12} injections
- Raise glutathione: intravenous, transdermal, nebulized
- Folic acid (see page 53 in the supplements chapter for dosage)
- TMG or DMG
- N-acetyl-cysteine

II

POOP
The Whole Story on Constipation, Diarrhea, and Your Kid's Behavior

You still don't think we should test this, huh, Doc?

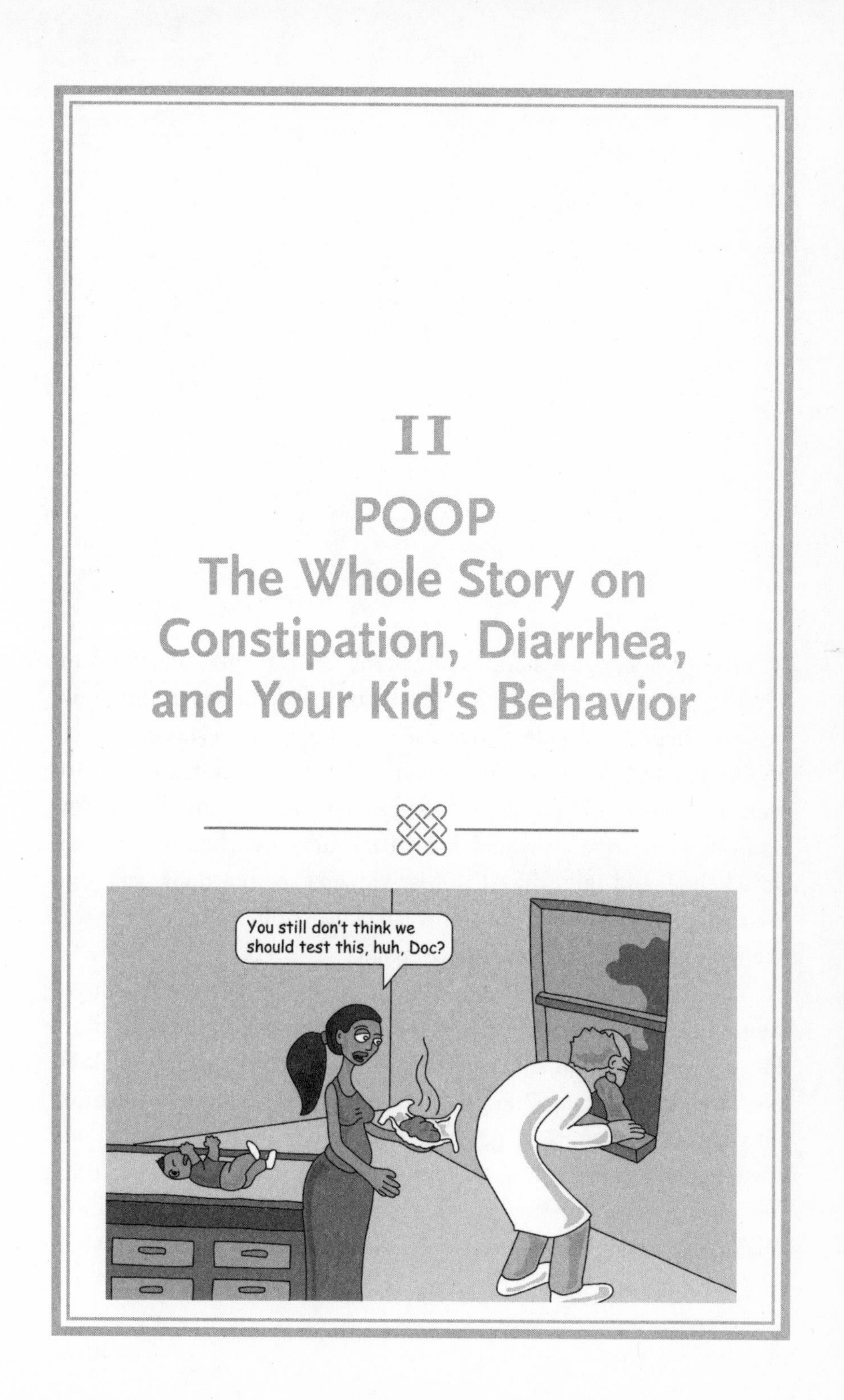

WITHOUT A DOUBT, poop is one of my favorite topics to talk about because I'm so fascinated by it. Once you have autism in the home and you begin biomedical treatment, poop samples become your hobby. Besides the insane foul smell, our autism spectrum kids also seem to have whole pieces of food in their poop. I couldn't understand how the noodle would form back into a curlicue after Evan would chew and then digest it. I would also see hot dogs back into their original shape because he wasn't digesting it properly. It was like magic, but not a good kind of magic.

The actual poop is only part of the story. Getting it to come out of them is the other part, because sometimes it's stuck in there for more than a week. Then we all have to deal with the constipation, the laxatives, and the diarrhea. One thing I have learned is that our kids must have consistent poop to get better. Anytime there are nutritious wastes entering the colon, there will be an increase in yeast/fungi and anaerobic bacteria that break down this waste. By now you know what the behavior consequences can be for this. So, no matter what, get your kids to poop!

CONSTIPATION

JENNY: Let's start with constipation. I was constipated my whole life and thought it was normal to go poop only once every fourteen days. It wasn't till I moved out to L.A. and met with a nutritionist, Dr. Bo Wagner, that I realized how bad that was. I thought Evan inherited it from me, but there was another culprit I called the "vaccine-induced gut damage" that was blocking him up.

DR. JERRY: Constipation in our children can be simply defined as not completely emptying the bowels daily. Obviously, having a bowel movement every other day or once a week is indeed constipation. One can also be constipated even with a bowel movement every day. If the body makes, for example, eight inches of poop a day, and six inches per day is removed with each bowel movement, then two inches of stool per day will keep accumulating. Parents will say, "There's no way he can be constipated. He's pooping once or twice a day." But my question is, "Is he eliminating all of the waste material when he has a bowel movement?"

JENNY: Kids with autism have the same type of poop, don't they?

DR. JERRY: Constipated stools vary in their "presentation" from child to child. Some can look like little rabbit pellets or can be huge, grapefruit-sized poop that will not flush down the toilet. All the while one wonders how a four-year-old was able get that huge mass of stool out of his little body.

JENNY: Evan would push a grapefruit-sized poop out so many times that his butt would bleed afterward. He would scream so badly that sometimes I had to dig it out of him. It was hell.

DR. JERRY: Sadly, that story is very common with kids who have autism.

JENNY: Now anyone can say poop in general smells bad, but I would like you to confirm that our kids' poop smells unbelievably horrific!

DR. JERRY: The stools these children eliminate can be incredibly foul-smelling. In addition, they can be just about any color: white, gray, and all shades of green, yellow, and orange.

JENNY: I've seen orange.

DR. JERRY: These are clues that digestion and bowel motility (movement of the stool through the colon) are not working properly. Another problem here is that the stool material is decomposing organic material that is kept warm, moist, and dark. It quickly becomes fertile growth material for bacteria and yeast. Our children are not digesting foods well, so even more proteins, fats, and sugars become available to be used as "fertilizer" in the stool. The breakdown of proteins by bacterial organisms is called putrefication. This is the etymology of the word "putrid" and why we associate it with an *intense* foul smell. If the bowels are moved regularly and completely, then the overgrowth of putrefying bacteria will be kept at a minimum. If not, many untypical bacteria and yeast will proliferate, creating a situation commonly referred to as dysbiosis. Many parents will confess that they just want to take off all the clothes and the diapers and take them right out of the house and into the trash can. They do not even want to wash the clothes. It smells like an animal crawled up there and died. That is putrefaction. Now, there are other types of bad-smelling stools. Some stools can smell like a bakery, stale old beer, or even have what has been described as a chemical smell.

JENNY: I've learned why poop is so important, but I need YOU to give your doctor's input on the stinky matter.

DR. JERRY: It used to be, back in the old days, pediatricians were always pictured wearing a bowtie. They could not wear a long tie, as part of an examination of a sick child would include examining the stool and no one wanted the lower third of their tie in the diarrhea! The analogy of this is simple. If you get behind a car and it's choking out blackish-blue, foul-smelling smoke, you don't have to be a mechanic to figure out that there's something wrong with that internal combustion engine. It's not doing its job properly. The stool is what comes out of the child's "exhaust pipe" and can be very revealing before we even send it to the lab. For example, everyone is aware that stool does not have a pleasant aroma, but parents have described many different smells: like a dead animal, like a bakery, like "chemicals," or even acrid-smelling. The colors of stool: white, tan, yellow, green, orange, all shades of brown, and even black. It can float, sink, or flake when it hits the water. It can be huge in size, both in diameter or length, or small and squiggly like worms. It can be oily or dry, be easy to wipe off the bottom, require a tremendous amount of wipes to remove the goo from the bottom. It can be watery, and then just about every other consistency has been described to me (soft-serve ice cream, peanut butter, and even "frothy"). So, by examining the stool, one can get a good idea of what the problem is before the stool is even sent to the laboratory.

Constipation and Behavior

JENNY: I've noticed that poop always had an effect on Evan's behavior. To this day if Evan is constipated, he won't talk most of the day, and as soon as he poops, it's like, BAM! He doesn't shut up.

DR. JERRY: That is a good point. I have parents who say their child is at his absolute worst prior to a massive bowel movement. Then, this child becomes a really cool kid for the next four to six hours or longer, until the backup of stool recurs and starts the cycle of behaviors over again.

JENNY: I've heard doctors say that this poop problem is just part of being autistic, that autistic kids are willfully holding their poop. How do you respond?

DR. JERRY: What animal on God's green planet willfully holds his poop? They are not willfully holding on to their poop to teach us a lesson, to demonstrate to us that this is the only thing "they" have control over, or some other such psychobabble rap. They may not want to have a bowel movement because it hurts too much. They may not have a bowel movement because they don't have the control to move it. They may not have a bowel movement because of dysmotility, in other words, the bowels just don't move. There IS a very good reason they are not able to move their bowels, and I assure you, it is anything but "voluntary."

JENNY: How come the bowels don't move?

DR. JERRY: Stool moves much in the same way you move soap up one hand into another. Remember when you were a kid and you would take a bar of soap in the shower and squish it up in one hand and into the next? That's how the bowels are moved. We call that peristalsis. The colon squishes and squeezes the poop until it comes out. There can be many reasons the natural forward progression of stool is greatly hampered or even arrested. Some reasons may include neurologic disconnect, uncoordinated movement, poor muscle tone, pain, and partial obstruction caused by the fecal material itself.

Enemas

JENNY: I know it's hard to potty train our kids. Do you have a more medical reason besides them not understanding what we're asking them to do? Like, do they not know they have to go?

DR. JERRY: I'm glad you brought that up. Yes, it's called mismanagement of incoming stimuli. Whether it be Mom saying, "I love you," or Dad saying, "Go get your shoes," or the bladder saying, "I'm full," our kids can't process the message. There are stretch receptors, and as the colon is stretched, it's supposed to send a signal to the brain to go have a bowel movement. When you have a bowel movement, we don't talk about this as adults, but it sure does feel good. We get a "cookie" from our nervous system saying "job well done." We haven't a clue what autistic kids feel and that's why potty training is so difficult with them. So the first step is, we have to clean them out. And if you have a kid who's young enough, I recommend child-sized Fleet enemas that you can buy at the drugstore. Do one a day for five days.

JENNY: Why so many days?

DR. JERRY: Because you want to try to remove the cork, which can be quite long, and each enema will only remove a portion of it.

JENNY: Any tips on the enema technique?

DR. JERRY: Place the child on the toilet (if he will sit on the toilet, that is), and have him bend over and touch his toes, and then you go down the back side, find the anus, insert the enema, and gently infuse it in there. Then try to have the child stand up (so the enema does not come right back out) and congratulate him. It would be best to try to keep the enema fluids in for three to five minutes before sitting down again. If they're still in diapers, this can be done on a changing table or bathroom floor. It can get messy! Sometimes it takes two to hold or distract the child.

Now, of course we may not be able to do this with older children. They can be as strong as the Hulk and will absolutely, with all their strength, refuse this "intervention"! It is best not to force the issue in this case.

JENNY: I always did the surprise attack with Evan, like I was changing his diaper because he would lie on his back in the perfect position with his feet up in the air and I would put it in and out before he could do anything about it. Then I would put a diaper on him and let him push it out. Because he was so constipated, I knew it wasn't going to be loose, so I wasn't worried about a mess. I also always started with the baby-sized enema to see if that one would work and, to my surprise many times, that's all he needed. It also made it easier to insert. I know some kids might need otherwise, but I thought it was at least good information. What else can we do to clean them out?

Laxatives

DR. JERRY: For our children who do not move their bowels daily, we need to give them a push. We need to give them a laxative. There are all kinds of laxatives on the market. All claim great results. All claim the others are "toxic." In my ten years of managing severely constipated children, I have found the first line of attack is MiraLAX and its generic version, GlycoLax (both are corn-derived, and should not be used with children with corn sensitivities). It's available over-the-counter and available at most pharmacies. Once we establish daily bowel movements, we can always try other more "natural" alternatives. But, initially, I will bring out "the big guns." If the child is allergic to corn, Oxy-Powder is a great alternative.

JENNY: MiraLAX has done a great job with Evan.

DR. JERRY: There are a lot of preparations available that can be used to move the bowels. But this is always an urgent matter. If we have a child who's up to his eyeballs in poop, let's push it out with some GlycoLax, from "above," while from "below," we are relieving the stoppage with enemas. Parents are always amazed at how much stool can be expressed. I have had children who have severe abdominal pain and go to the emergency room for evaluation of appendicitis! An X-ray of their tummy reveals a huge amount of "fecal material." They end up getting a $200 enema (the usual copay for an ER visit) and the child greatly improves.

X-rays

DR. JERRY: Very often, I will get an X-ray of the tummy, called a KUB (Old World term for kidneys-ureter-bladder) just to see how backed up the child is. I have had parents tell me that the child had a massive BM in the toilet the day of the X-ray . . . but go and get the X-ray, anyway. The radiology report invariably comes back reporting that the entire colon has a moderate amount of stool, even though the child had a large BM before the X-ray.

Another indication for an X-ray of the tummy is to follow up the clean-out. Very often, the parent will tell me that the child is completely cleaned out yet still has lot of behaviors consistent with constipation. I will get a follow-up X-ray to prove to me that the bowels are cleaned out.

JENNY: Evan still poops enormous poops. We clog every time, not because he is constipated but because there is so much poop!

DR. JERRY: That means we still have a lot of work to do.

JENNY: Really?

DR. JERRY: Large amounts of stools *daily* indicate one of two things. Either the child is consuming too much food daily or the child is not able to digest and absorb the food that is consumed. Very often, these children are not growing well and not gaining weight. The proteins, fats, and carbohydrates are not being broken down and absorbed and end up in the colon feeding the bacteria and yeast and waiting for elimination.

We keep talking about proper digestion. Many children with autism do not produce adequate amounts of digestive enzymes for the digestive process. This has been published and here is just one article to illustrate malabsorption contributing to behavioral problems (note the reflux, too). Note this was published in 1999!

GASTROINTESTINAL ABNORMALITIES IN CHILDREN WITH AUTISTIC DISORDER

Horvath K, Papadimitriou JC, Rabsztyn A, Drachenberg C, Tildon JT. J Pediatr 1999 Nov;135(5):559-63. Department of Pediatrics, University of Maryland School of Medicine, Baltimore, USA. PMID: 10547242 [PubMed—indexed for MEDLINE]

OBJECTIVES: Our aim was to evaluate the structure and function of the upper gastrointestinal tract in a group of patients with autism who had gastrointestinal symptoms. STUDY DESIGN: Thirty-six children (age: 5.7 +/- 2 years, mean +/- SD) with autistic disorder underwent upper gastrointestinal endoscopy with biopsies, intestinal and pancreatic enzyme analyses, and bacterial and fungal cultures. The most frequent gastrointestinal complaints were chronic diarrhea, gaseousness, and abdominal discomfort and distension. RESULTS:

> Histologic examination in these 36 children revealed grade I or II reflux esophagitis in 25 (69.4%), chronic gastritis in 15, and chronic duodenitis in 24. The number of Paneth's cells in the duodenal crypts was significantly elevated in autistic children compared with non-autistic control subjects. Low intestinal carbohydrate digestive enzyme activity was reported in 21 children (58.3%), although there was no abnormality found in pancreatic function. Seventy-five percent of the autistic children (27/36) had an increased pancreatico-biliary fluid output after intravenous secretin administration. Nineteen of the 21 patients with diarrhea had significantly higher fluid output than those without diarrhea. CONCLUSIONS: Unrecognized gastrointestinal disorders, especially reflux esophagitis and disaccharide malabsorption, may contribute to the behavioral problems of the non-verbal autistic patients. The observed increase in pancreatico-biliary secretion after secretin infusion suggests an upregulation of secretin receptors in the pancreas and liver. Further studies are required to determine the possible association between the brain and gastrointestinal dysfunctions in children with autistic disorder.

Digestive Enzymes and Other Supplements

JENNY: Okay, proper digestion will help them to poop more regularly?

DR. JERRY: Yes, and just as we mentioned in the Digestive Enzymes and Protein section on page 63, digestive enzymes are one more tool we can use to help the digestive and elimination process.

JENNY: Okay, let's name a few more things that clear up the bowels while we are still on the topic.

DR. JERRY: I also use Oxy-Powder, which works very well. This is another nonaddictive supplement to help the bowels move. A product I use in conjunction with a laxative is George's Aloe. Depending on the weight of the child, I typically use anywhere from two to six ounces per day. Fiber is also very important for normalizing bowel function, and the product I like to use is called Fibersure. I recommend one to two teaspoons per day. This formulation goes into any drink and is colorless, odorless, and tasteless.

JENNY: Will removing certain foods from their diet stop constipation in these kids?

DR. JERRY: Some foods in individual children can be constipating. I have found that rice can be constipating in some children. Other foods include dairy, gluten, potato chips, meat, and sugar.

JENNY: Wait a minute. Meat too? Can these kids eat ANYTHING?

DR. JERRY: Parents shouldn't try to take their kids off meat, but they should be aware that all meat—red meat, chicken, fish—is constipating. It just means you have to add fiber, especially insoluble fiber: Fibersure is great. You'll want to include a high dose of vitamin C, 2,000 to 6,000 mg of buffered vitamin C per day depending on weight and age. Add magnesium as well—between 400 to 800 mg per day depending on age and weight. Follow magnesium blood levels as well.

UNDIGESTED FOODS AND WHAT THEY MEAN

JENNY: What about seeing whole pieces of the food they ate in their poop? It's very bizarre. I mean, I know corn comes out the same way that it goes in, but a freaking hot dog?

DR. JERRY: That's another sign that the bowels aren't quite working and you need digestive enzymes. I've had parents tell me that they can see the bite marks in the French fries. Keep in mind, though, some foods are not digested well even under the best of cases, such as corn.

JENNY: You could probably use nuts and corn as a good way of telling how long it takes to come out of your kid? It would take Evan seven days before I would see the watermelon seeds I gave him a week prior. And if it's taking more than a day, you know your kid isn't digesting properly.

DR. JERRY: Nuts, corn, seeds, raisins are all good markers. In other words, if you give your child corn tonight and you don't see that in the stool for five or six nights, then you know there is a definite delay in motility. Depending on age, the time from swallowing to the time of elimination is eight to twenty-four hours.

DIARRHEA

JENNY: What about diarrhea in some kids? Many parents will say that their child will have ten loose stools a day and the doctor says nothing is wrong with that.

DR. JERRY: If you have a doctor that's a little slow to help you, the best thing to do is bring in a loaded diaper full of the nastiest-looking poop and just open it up while you're waiting. The visual of the diarrhea plus the impact of the smell can be very convincing to a pediatrician to help. Merely describing the situation at home will often result in the pediatrician announcing this is merely a case of toddler's diarrhea and being reassured he will outgrow it. Trust me, with the visual and the smell, they won't try to convince the parent of the normalcy of what will take the rest of the day to clear the smell out of their office.

JENNY: That's a great idea for moms to do. I love that! What about the doctors who still insist toddler diarrhea is normal?

DR. JERRY: Let's look at all of God's creatures. What other animal walks around with diarrhea cascading down the "derriere"? For any other animal, it means they are sick, and if NOT treated, they will die. In fact, if a newborn calf gets diarrhea, it'll be dead in three days. That's why cow's milk is so full of colostrum for newborn calves; if they do get sick, they will die. Diarrhea is never normal. Constipation is never normal.

COMMON POOP TESTS

JENNY: What are common tests that you do with poop? What exactly are you looking for when you make moms dig through their kid's poop and ship it to labs?

DR. JERRY: Here is the list:

1. Stool for blood
2. Stool for white blood cells (WBCs)
3. Stool for culture and sensitivity (looks for bacterial organisms)
4. Stool for fungal elements (looks for yeast)
5. Stool for C. diff toxin (a toxin from a bacteria named clostridium difficile)
6. Stool for ova and parasites (looking for parasites and eggs)
7. Stool for reducing substances (sugars in stool)
8. Stool for quantitative fecal fat (how much fat is in stool)

JENNY: I could talk about poop forever.

DR. JERRY: (Laughs) I'm sure you can.

JENNY: It's so fascinating. Thanks, Doc.

ADVICE

- Constipation: Bowel movements must be daily and complete. Many children need daily help (not just "once in a while"). Consistency is the name of the game if you're looking for improvements in language, behavior and ability to connect socially.
- Dietary considerations: Removal of gluten and casein.

—For more information, go back to the diet chapter (page 29).

1. Clean out: Daily laxatives may be needed to enhance motility

   —GlycoLax/MiraLAX available at a pharmacy
   —Sold over-the-counter at most major and small pharmacies, drugstores, and health food stores

2. Oxy-Powder to help the bowels move

   —www.oxypowder.com

3. Fleet enemas (one daily for about five days)

   —Sold over-the-counter at most major and small pharmacies, drugstores, and health food stores

4. May need an X-ray to determine the extent of the problem

   —Ask your doctor for one.

5. May need a "blast" from magnesium citrate, also a laxative (given over two days)

   —Informational site: www.drugs.com/ppa/magnesium-citrate.html
   —Purchasing site: www.organicpharmacy.org

6. May try a short course of MOM (milk of magnesia)

   —Sold over-the-counter at most major and small pharmacies, drugstores, and health food stores
   —Purchasing site: www.magnesiumdirect.com

7. Expect to be vigilant for six months to a year

- Fiber

  —Fibersure (1–2 teaspoons daily) http://us.fibersure.com/index_flash.shtml
  —You can also place your order at www.drugstore.com

- Nutritional healing

  —Zinc
  - 20–40 mg daily
  - Zinc supplements are available for purchase without a prescription, at almost all major and small drugstores, pharmacies, health food stores
  - Fact Sheet—http://ods.od.nih.gov/FactSheets/Zinc.asp
  - Dosing information: www.lenntech.com/recommended-daily-intake.htm
  - General information: www.mayoclinic.com/health/drug-information/DR602313

  —George's Aloe
  - 2–6 ounces per day
  - Warren Laboratories
    www.warrenlabsaloe.com
    Office: 254-580-9990
    Fax: 254-580-9944
    Online purchasing also available at Natural Nirvana
    http://store.naturalnirvana.com

- Probiotics

  —Kartner Health (Dr. Jerry's supplements)
  www.kartnerhealth.com or call 866-960-9251

—Kirkman Labs
www.kirkmanlabs.com or call 800-245-8282
—Klaire Labs
www.klaire.com or call 888-488-2488

- Diarrhea

    —Remove offending foods.
    - Most common are juices/fruits/dairy products.

    —Treat bacterial infections.
    - Antibiotics depend on bacteria. Have to get stool studies as outlined.

    —Treat parasitic infections.
    - Antiparasitic agents such as Alinia or metronidazole are excellent choices. Since parasites may be hard to discern on stool cultures, may have to treat empirically (as a "trial").

    —Treat nutritionally—much the same way as constipation.
    - Zinc
    - Fiber
    - George's Aloe
    - Probiotics
    - Digestive enzymes

- Have to treat infections! Have to remove offending foods!

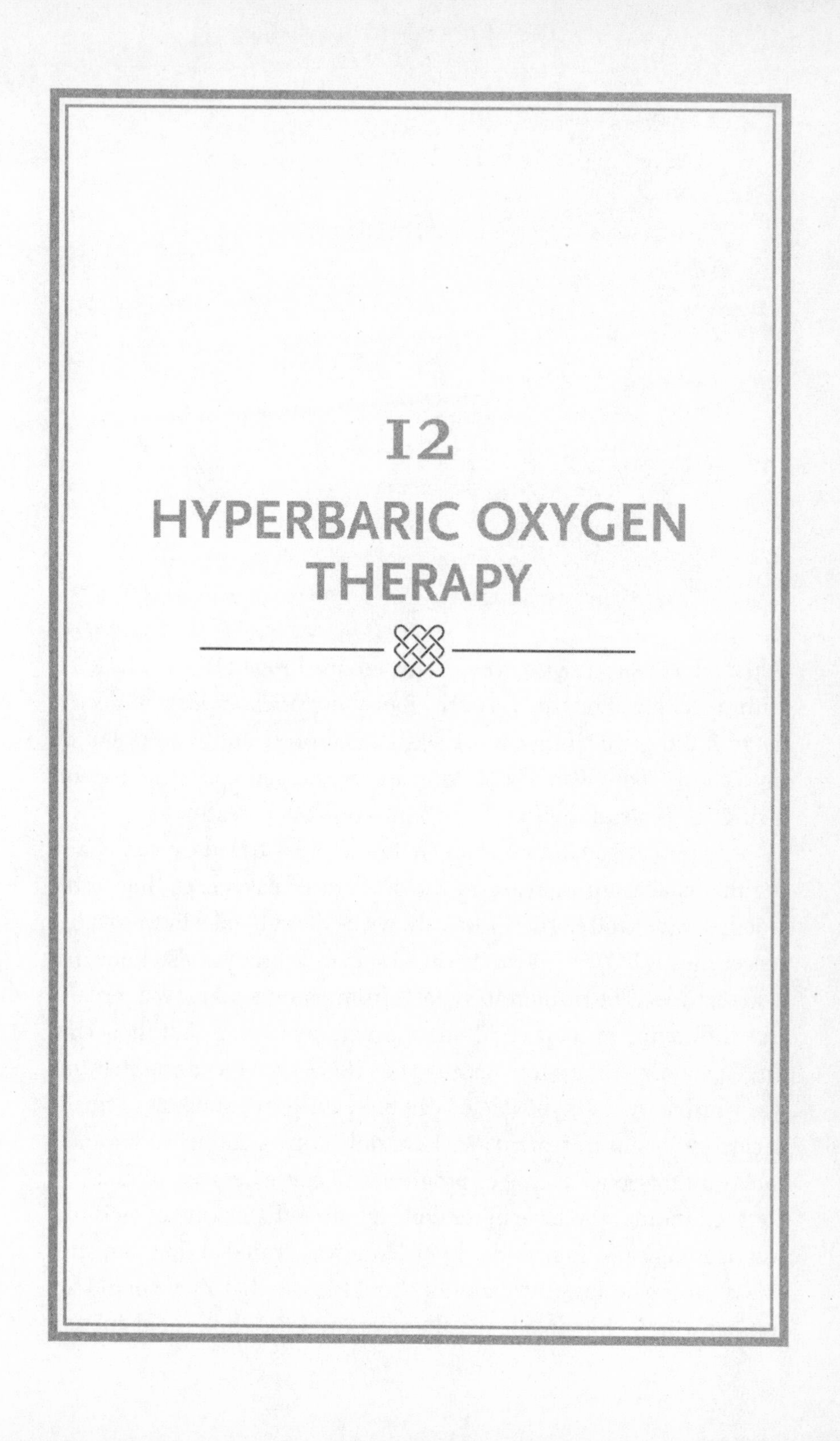

12

HYPERBARIC OXYGEN THERAPY

When I first heard about hyperbaric oxygen therapy (HBOT) I immediately thought, *Isn't that something Michael Jackson does?* I heard it did great things, but I wasn't sold on it until I went out on my *Louder Than Words* book tour and witnessed countless parents giving accounts of their children's progress after treatment.

A hyperbaric chamber is an enclosed, pressurized oxygen chamber that causes an increase in the amount of oxygen getting to the blood, organs, and tissues. I was always hesitant to take Evan because sometimes HBOT is known to cause seizures, but it is also known to heal seizures. The numerous reports from parents that saw a remarkable difference in their children, and parents stating that their children are now seizure-free because of HBOT convinced me that this was worth a try. So that Evan too can be seizure-free someday, I finally decided to begin treatment. We have only done a couple so far and I can't wait to see what type of progress will come because of it.

I tell moms who have never done it before that it kind of feels like you're going camping inside a tent. Evan was scared at first, but after two minutes he loved it. Parents should know that they should accompany their child inside the chamber until the child is old enough or comfortable enough to go in alone. For now, just enjoy the cuddle time with your child and know that oxygen is an amazing healing agent, especially for kids with autism.

JENNY: So many mothers have approached me with numerous success stories because of hyperbaric chamber therapy. Can you explain what a hyperbaric chamber is?

DR. JERRY: A hyperbaric chamber is a closed container, in which the child (and usually a parent) sits or lies down, which is gently pressurized. The child will breathe in additional oxygen during the pressurized session.

JENNY: Why do kids with autism need this therapy?

Jerry: Special CT scans of the brain, called Single Positron Emission computed tomography, or more commonly referred to as SPECT scans, often reveal decreased blood flow in the brains of both children and adults with autism. This decreased blood flow is called hypoprofusion and is most commonly noted on both sides of the brain, bitemporally. So, if we know that we have decreased blood flow to the brain, wouldn't it be wise of us to add oxygen so those areas can have a normal flow of oxygen in those tissues? HBOT can increase the flow of oxygen to the brain, so I believe it is wise to use it as a treatment.

HYPERBARIC CHAMBER AND OVERALL IMPROVEMENTS

JENNY: It has also been known to help the immune system. How does it do this?

DR. JERRY: The immune system works with oxygen. Cells kill pathogens (germs) with an oxygen burst. If you increase the oxygen supply to the small and large intestines, those bacteria are not going to do very well in an environment that's richer in oxygen than they're used to. Inflammation appears to decrease. There are numerous studies of HBOT and inflammation and the positive effects HBOT has on inflammation, which is a big issue for kids on the autism spectrum. Many of them have chronic, low-grade infections from viruses and bacteria. When that's going on, the body protects the brain by reducing nourishment so that the virus or bacteria doesn't get into the brain and make it swell. HBOT can reduce this effect.

JENNY: What are some of the great results you see in these kids?

DR. JERRY: One of the first improvements we see is change in the child's sleep patterns. After treatment, children have a much easier time getting to sleep and many start to sleep through the night. The second improvement is that a child overall becomes calmer. The therapists will tell us that acquisition of skills is faster. Wherever they were at, they start improving those skills. So we see a nice jump.

HOW MANY TREATMENTS DOES IT TAKE?

JENNY: Many parents have said that after forty dives (treatments), they noticed an increase in the children's language. Why do they say to do forty dives and not, say, fifty? Where did that number come from?

DR. JERRY: Forty dives is the number of treatments that demonstrated new blood vessel growth following a stroke. There's nothing special that connects the forty dives to the poor blood flow seen in our children. Some children start improving after the first dive. I've had some children who didn't make any improvement until after their 82nd or their 103rd dive. So it takes a while. There are some children who actually regress a little bit. We usually see this type of regression in our clinic between dives seven and fourteen. The children are actually getting a little bit more edgy, hyper, and a little bit more irritable.

JENNY: And then do you stop?

DR. JERRY: No, we keep going.

JENNY: You push through?

DR. JERRY: Absolutely. We cannot say what is actually happening here, but within a week, any symptoms of regression improve. This, in itself, is no reason to stop.

SEIZURES

JENNY: I've heard that hyperbaric chambers can trigger seizures even though it can also heal them. In Evan's case, because his seizures have been so severe, it scares the crap out of me.

DR. JERRY: When we initiate hyperbaric oxygen to a child who has a history of seizures, we do it very, very carefully. We certainly do not want to have any seizures triggered by the addition of oxygen. The addition of oxygen should never trigger seizures at low pressure. Hyperbaric means increased pressure, that is, an increase in pressure that one would normally experience at the ocean (sea level). Terminology would call this pressure at beachside a "1," or 1 atmosphere of pressure. When a child with a known history of seizures comes in for HBOT therapy, we slowly increase the pressure from 1 to 1.1 atmospheres, and then slowly work up to 1.3 atmospheres of pressure. This is equivalent to the pressure one would feel at the bottom of the deep end of an eleven-foot-deep pool. The seizures that have been published in conjunction with hyperbaric therapy are due to oxygen toxicity. This oxygen toxicity can occur when pressures are at 2 atmospheres of pressure for too long a time period. That is why we purposely place our children at 1.3 atmospheres (much less than 2!).

Our protocol for a child with seizures is first to introduce the oxygen for a few days. If I have a child who's willing, I put him in a face mask and let 10 liters per minute run for half an hour first day, an hour for the next day and get him used to breathing pure oxygen to make sure it isn't going to trigger seizure. Then I'll place him in the chamber with just a little "nubbin" of pressure and, in the course of the week, bring him up to 1.3 atmospheres of pressure. This is not at all a painful experience. In fact, most kids love it and sometimes even fall asleep in there.

JENNY: Have you ever had any kids increase the amount of seizures they had because of hyperbaric chamber treatments?

DR. JERRY: I can tell you that my partner, Dr. Buckley, and I have never had a child increase their seizures. Sometimes, the therapy doesn't change a patient's condition, but usually we do see the seizure episodes decrease with hyperbarics. So it's very exciting.

TREATMENT COST

JENNY: Why isn't everyone in a hyperbaric chamber? Since it helps with delivering oxygen, which in turn helps the immune system, why don't hospitals stick sick people in them all the time?

DR. JERRY: Because it's very expensive. Nobody is looking for ways to increase the cost of health care. If you think about it, if you have a stroke or if you have a heart attack, by definition that's an impaired flow of oxygen to that tissue. The first thing I tell my wife is, if I have a stroke, make sure my treatment plan includes HBOT ASAP! It is imperative to restore oxygen to tissues. Insurance is starting to pay, in some instances, for HBOT. As more and more studies come out, this should one day be part of mainstream interventions. Remember, any tissue, in order to heal, requires oxygen.

TREATMENT PROTOCOL

JENNY: Do parents need to prepare their child in any way before they commit to hyperbarics?

DR. JERRY: Well, as with everything else, you have to have a good foundation before you are going to be able to assess whether a child will respond. There will be no obvious response if the child is eating cupcakes, French fries, pizza, juice, and milk. Hyperbaric oxygen therapy is not a silver bullet. It is just one more tool to help with increasing oxygen delivery to the brain. You will have to clean up your child's diet first and begin the detox and supplement protocol. All of theses treatments work together. For the most part, none of them work magic by themselves. Sometimes one can work magic and you'll hit the healing jackpot, but most of the time it's a combination of things.

BEFORE HYPERBARIC TREATMENT

Begin the diet and supplement protocol, and help your child detox first. Be aware of all the risks (you can check out www.genoxinc.com, www.hyperbaricsupport.com, www.oxyhealth.com, or www.performance-hyperbarics.com for some good information).

Here are the supplements to focus on:

Antioxidants
Vitamin C (1,000 mg per day)
Vitamin A (5,000 IU per day) minimum

JENNY: What kind of minerals and vitamins should people be consciously aware of, to be up on, before they even consider hyperbaric?

DR. JERRY: I'd recommend that they all be on some antioxidants, because we're putting them in an oxygen-rich environment. Vitamin C (1,000 mg per day), vitamin A (5,000 IU per day) would be the very minimum. There are a lot of protocols that other physicians would say are a "must." Since HBOT is physician-directed, they will have the protocol that should be just right for the child. Ask your biomedical doctor.

JENNY: Is there any danger in doing hyperbaric chamber?

DR. JERRY: It's a medical intervention, and just like anything medical, there's always risk. The most common complaint is ear pain and occasionally some sinus pain. We call it sinus squeeze. Often, we work through this by teaching the children how to equalize the pressure in their ears. They learn very quickly it's like going in an airplane. In San Antonio, Texas, where I did my training in HBOT, they had put horses (expensive racehorses) into HBOT to accelerate healing. It was amazing to see how they could equalize the pressure in their ears.

JENNY: How many days a week?

DR. JERRY: Five days a week, one-hour sessions. If the child is willing or can be conditioned, we like to use a face mask to deliver the oxygen. Otherwise, the oxygen tubing can be "near" his face.

JENNY: The estimated cost for an hour, one session, runs between $50 an hour to $100, and to buy a chamber is $12,000 to $20,000—correct?

DR. JERRY: Depending on the manufacturer or clinic, that is a pretty good estimate.

JENNY: A tanning spa session nowadays runs $35 for seven minutes, so it's really not that far off.

DR. JERRY: You're kidding.

JENNY: It's expensive to be a woman, Doc. We pay a lot to try and look good sometimes.

DR. JERRY: Well, moms should know that when they get in the chamber with their child, not only are they healing their child but they're healing themselves, too. It can help Mom's PMS and is also good for antiaging.

JENNY: Has this been one of the most exciting treatments for autism that you've seen in the last few years?

DR. JERRY: I wouldn't say it's one of the most exciting. I look at each treatment that helps our kids as being thrilling. Anything that recovers a child to me is exciting. I mean, who would call a gluten-free, dairy-free diet exciting? But as far as what it can do for some of the kids, it's terribly exciting. From my point of view, it's one more tool, and let's see what happens. When other doctors and parents are telling me a treatment is fabulous, I'm excited, whatever that tool is.

ADVICE

Insurance coverage depends on your plan, but please look into it, because it has been covered for some people. You can get more information at International Hyperbarics Association, Inc., www.ihausa.org.

Where You Can Buy or Rent a Hyperbaric Oxygen Chamber

OXYHEALTH
877-789-0123
www.oxyhealth.com
3224 Hoover Avenue
National City, CA 91950

Prices to Rent ($ per month):

(Small $1,500)
(Medium $2,000)
(Large $3,000)

Prices to Buy:

(Small $10,500)
(Medium $16,900)
(Large $20,900)

HYPERBARIC SUPPORT
866-937-9755
www.hyperbaricsupport.com
6015 University
Cedar Falls, OH 50613

PRICES TO RENT ($ PER MONTH):

(Small $1,895)
(Medium $2,395)

PRICES TO LEASE:

(Small $200 per session)
(Medium $400 per session)

PRICES TO BUY:

(Small $7,998)
(Medium $13,995)

GENOX INC
678-957-0156
www.genoxinc.com

PRICES TO RENT ($ PER MONTH)

(Large $2,500)

PRICES TO BUY:

(Small $9,450)
(Medium $15,210)
(Large: $18,810)

PERFORMANCE HYPERBARICS
888-456-4268
www.performance-hyperbarics.com
372 Hopalua Drive
Pukalani, HI 96768

PRICES TO RENT ($ PER MONTH):

(Small $2,000)
(Large $2,650)

PRICES TO BUY:

(Small $12,900)
(Large $16,900)

WHERE YOU CAN GO FOR HYPERBARIC OXYGEN CHAMBER SESSIONS

To find out where you can go for hyperbaric oxygen treatment, there is a great list, arranged alphabetically by state, for centers in the United States at www.geocities.com/aneecp/hbocent.htm.

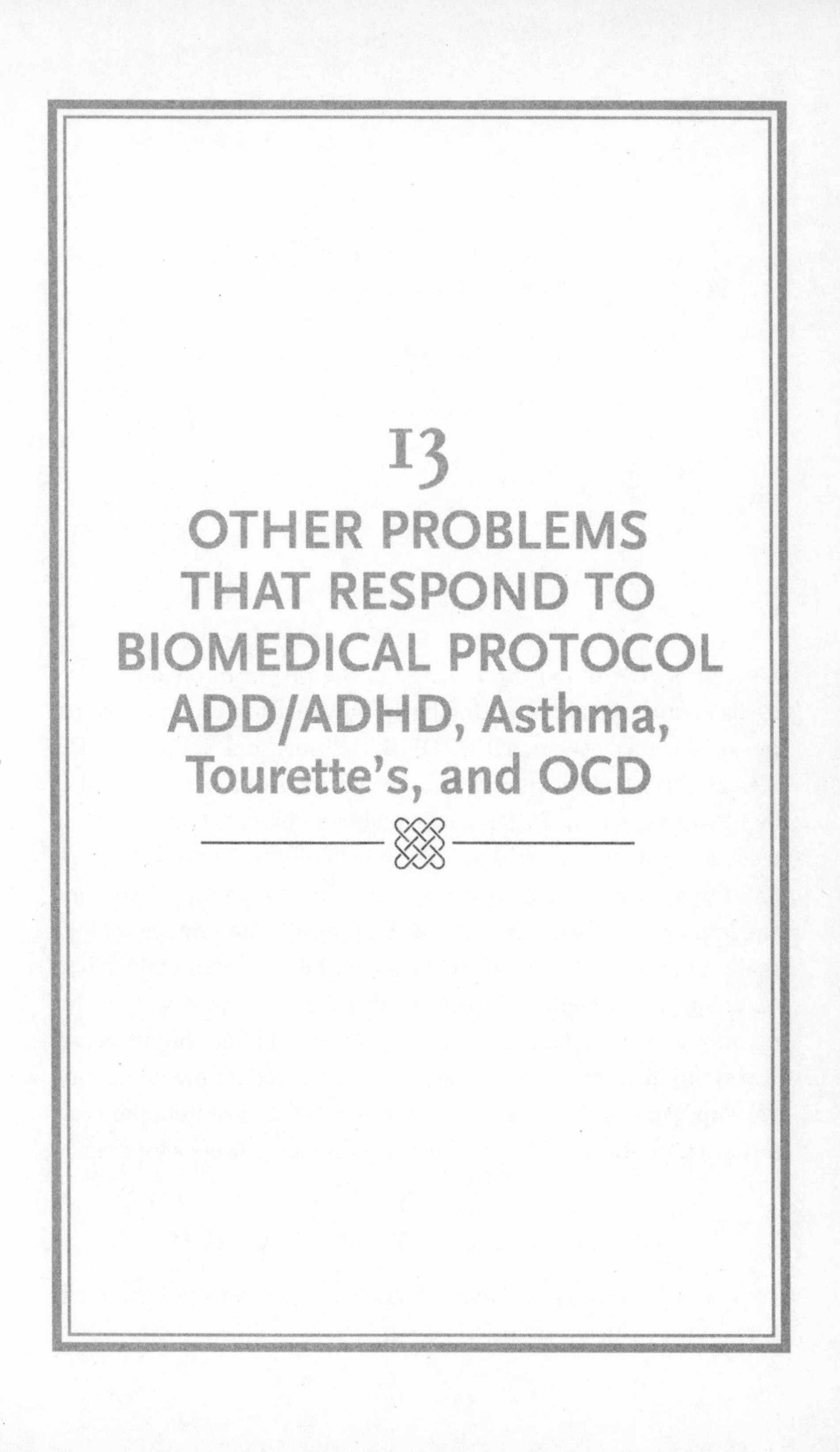

13
OTHER PROBLEMS THAT RESPOND TO BIOMEDICAL PROTOCOL
ADD/ADHD, Asthma, Tourette's, and OCD

We all know that autism is on the rise from the amount of media attention that it's getting lately, but we also need to pay attention to the increase in ADD/ADHD, asthma, and Tourette's. The sales of Ritalin or Ritalin-like substances are given to 20 percent of the nation's children. Doctors are convincing parents that their child needs a stimulant to get through the school day. I strongly believe that if these kids were treated biomedically through diet, detox, and supplements, like we treat autism, they would not only get off the Ritalin but many of them would lose their label. If your child is having attention problems and you're allowing one sip of soda in his mouth, you are adding fuel to the fire. If your child has high-fructose corn syrup in anything he or she eats, you are adding fuel to the fire. Wake up, Mom and Dad, and realize you play the most important role in your child's healing. You're the one doing the grocery shopping.

ADD AND THE AUTISM SPECTRUM

Jenny: Would you consider attention deficit disorder with hyperactivity on the same spectrum as autism?

DR. JERRY: In one corner you have your child with autism. He is rocking, biting his wrist, and he doesn't know Mom or Dad, he doesn't even know when he's hungry or not. In other words, all information coming into this child's brain is nonsensical. Thus, he is not able to participate in our world. Now, at the other end of this spectrum we have the child with attention deficit disorder. He has great use of language, a sense of humor, makes friends, and is proficient on the soccer field. The problem is that when he is in his third-grade classroom and his teacher explains that George Washington was the first president of the United States, fought in the Revolutionary War, and married a wonderful lady named Martha, he seems to miss "it." When he is tested on this material the following week, he does not have a clue what was taught. In other words, yes, he makes sense of most stimuli coming in, but when it came from the teacher, he wasn't able to assimilate it and be able to recall it. These children tend to have problems with focus, concentration, and recall, which, like autism, is another type of inappropriate management of everyday stimuli. So this child and the child with autism in this example do indeed have something in common: the mismanagement of incoming stimuli. For the child struggling in the classroom, it is the "teaching" stimuli. For the other child, it seems all stimuli are grossly mismanaged.

JENNY: It drives me NUTS when people say that the only reason there is an increase in all of these childhood diseases is because we know how to diagnose it better, that the increase is actually an illusion.

DR. JERRY: Not only have we seen a huge increase in autism, but also allergies, asthma, and attention deficit disorder, what Dr. Kenneth Boch refers to as "the Four A's of Childhood." Now, you have to keep in mind, we are not any better diagnosing ADD in 2008 than we were in 1970. The inattentiveness, the inability to recall information, the inability to follow through with tasks have always been easy to recognize. The difference now, of course, is the increased numbers of children who are being diagnosed with ADD.

ALLERGIES ON THE ADD SPECTRUM

JENNY: We know that our kids with autism have a tremendous amount of allergies. But what about kids with ADD, ADHD, and asthma? Do they also have more allergies?

DR. JERRY: Absolutely! The increase in allergies and mortality from asthma attacks has been dramatic over the past twenty years. Children are being diagnosed with allergies and asthma at a far greater rate than only twenty years ago. What's more, these diseases are far more complicated than they were twenty years ago. One can go to the mall and easily see children with dark circles under their eyes, or big red cheeks or red ears, which is a huge sign that they are suffering from allergies and/or sensitivities.

OTHER ALLERGIES TO LOOK FOR

Besides hay fever, also consider perfumes, hair sprays, dryer antistatic treatments, and animals. Watch for red ears, red cheeks, dark circles around the eyes—sure signs of allergies.

DIET CHANGES THAT HELP KIDS ON THE SPECTRUM

JENNY: Why do you think so many parents opt for mood-stabilizing drugs like Ritalin and Prozac over changing a child's eating habits? Is everyone that brainwashed into thinking those are magic pills?

DR. JERRY: The Surgeon General actually acknowledged that one in six children have a diagnosable mental disease, which includes, of course, attention deficit disorder. Parents are very busy with their work and home schedules. When they hear from school that their child is not doing well, they will next go see the very busy doctor. Both the parent and the doctor have a common goal: Fix the problem as quickly and easily as possible so both can go on with their hectic schedules. The pill is the quickest and easiest way to get the child back on track, so they say. Ritalin or another, similar drug, is prescribed, and out they all go. There is no discussion of diets, past history of antibiotics, allergic symptoms, home and school environments, etc.

JENNY: Why don't doctors take the time to give alternative treatments?

DR. JERRY: I really believe it has a lot to do with time constraints and productivity, for both the parent and the physician. This would require a minimum of an hour of the doctor's time to obtain a thorough history and physical exam. There is some blood and stool work to do. Some preliminary dietary considerations will need to be made. A follow-up in one week will need to be scheduled in order to review the lab studies. Then, a discussion of the alternative treatments will need to take place. This is another hour-long appointment. A pediatrician could have seen five to eight patients in that hour. What he could have brought into the clinic, financially, is far greater than what he could charge the insurance company for the one "ADD" visit. From the parent's perspective, "wasting" two hours with a pediatrician versus picking up some Ritalin is a no-brainer. They want the quick fix. The only winner here is the manufacturer of the Ritalin. This is why, in mainstream medicine, alternative treatments are rarely discussed. Obviously, not all practices operate this way, as not all parents are concerned with cutting down time spent in a doctor's office. The important question, often missed, is: WHY do they need a "Ritalin-like" medication to make it through the day? Could food, artificial flavorings, or sugar be causing behaviors? Could environmental toxins and medications be putting our kids at risk? These are the questions that need to be examined. I think that ADD, ADHD, OCD, Tourette's, and asthma have causes that are similar to what's behind the autism epidemic. And I've seen evidence that the biomedical approach helps these conditions as well.

It comes down to priorities. If the parent is determined to solve a problem without medications, or at least the smallest amount of medications, it is going to take work and sacrifice. Some sacrifices may just be too difficult for some parents to make, such as giving up sodas and fast foods. The work may include having to hand-prepare meals that do not originate in a box, using fresh ingredients. The child may have to sacrifice video games and television. I am not saying this "tongue in cheek." I am serious. This is very hard to accomplish in today's society. For families that find this unacceptable, we have stimulant medications such as Ritalin to help control behaviors. I remember when I first started to practice medicine with "alternatives" I was excited to share my discoveries with a fourteen-year-old youth with attention deficit disorder and sugar addictions. He was so addicted that he ate a can of cherry pie filling every night before bed. I told him about dietary changes and limiting video play. He was rather unimpressed and left the office with his prescription.

JENNY: Can you please talk about the role of food in behavior?

DR. JERRY: When the majority of a child's calories are derived from sugary foods you are going to have a child with behavior problems. Keep in mind that foods that are not usually considered sugary can be! Such as French fries and breads. They are quickly broken down to sugar. With the amount of sodas, juices, and unhealthy foods our children are consuming, there is little wonder why they don't do well in school.

JENNY: Amen! But I do believe that foods didn't or don't necessarily cause ADD or ADHD. I believe that foods aggravate the disorder more. I believe that vaccines played a role in these conditions also. They just got lucky and didn't get autism. I call it "getting brushed by the bullet" and not a direct hit. Would you agree?

DR. JERRY: Yes, Jenny, it is my personal opinion that the environmental exposures, including vaccines, have the capacity to alter metabolic pathways and immune system response. The degree and severity of these alterations, combined with the individual's genetics, will produce the clinical manifestations that we may call autism, attention deficit disorder, asthma, allergies, autoimmunity, seizure disorders, and the list goes on and on! We have had children who are two and three years old coming to our clinic who have been placed on Ritalin for their attention deficit disorder. I ask, how do you diagnose attention deficit disorder in a two- or three-year-old? This is why autism is being called a spectrum disorder. There is a wide array of presentations. Thank God these children did not develop autism, but they did develop the attention deficit disorder just like many of our children with autism have. I would be one to say that's a very good theory and that it still has a long way to go to be validated.

PEDIATRIC AUTOIMMUNE NEUROPSYCHIATRIC DISORDERS ASSOCIATED WITH STREPTOCOCCUS (PANDAS)

JENNY: I want to talk a little bit about obsessive-compulsive disorders and Tourette's. Many times our doctors have found that autistic kids or kids with Tourette's actually have a bacterial streptococcus infection that we call PANDAS. Once you treat the strep, sometimes the Tourette's and the OCD behavior go away. Can you first talk about what PANDAS is?

DR. JERRY: PANDAS stands for pediatric autoimmune neuropsychiatric disorder associated with streptococcus. Dr. Susan Swedo did some pioneering work on this while at the National Institutes of Health (NIH). She found that OCD behaviors may follow a streptococcus infection. She also found that some of the children's OCD behaviors tremendously improved with plasmaphoresis, a procedure where plasma (the clear fluid part of blood) is taken slowly out of the body and replaced with new plasma and returned back into the body, and IVIG (which we have already discussed; see page 89). From this information, it appears even oral antibiotics such as azithromycin (Zithromax) can have a profound impact on OCD behaviors by its ability to kill streptococcus bacteria.

JENNY: I can't tell you how many parents have told me how their child's OCD behaviors went away from treating strep/PANDAS.

Also, some kids who were diagnosed with Tourette's lost their diagnosis. I almost think every child should be tested for it who has bad OCD or tics because it could be treated. What do these kids look like when they come in your clinic?

DR. JERRY: These children tend to have had numerous infections during the first two to three years of their lives. A very common cause of infections of the ears and sinuses is the streptococcus organism. Currently, the diagnosis of PANDAS is based on clinical findings and NOT laboratory findings. Thus, if a child has OCD behaviors or behaviors consistent with Tourette's syndrome, consideration of using an antibiotic may be warranted.

JENNY: And parents who are probably going to read this are going, "Well, how come my pediatrician doesn't know this—that he's got PANDAS?"

Dr. Jerry: Many doctors are now aware of PANDAS. They just may not know exactly what to do. As we have said, what they are taught in their training may be ten-year-old information!

- A parent can Google "PANDAS autism" and print some articles for the doctor to consider.
- We like to use a thirty-day course of Zithromax along with an antifungal.
- Keep a very good diary of how behaviors change.

ADVICE

Dietary changes

- Markedly reduce sugars, juices, carbohydrates (pastries, French fries, sweetened cereals, "healthy waters" that have flavorings/sugar, pancakes, waffles). Each meal and snack should consist of a protein, carbohydrate, and a fat. Meat is a nice combination of protein and fat.
- Follow a gluten-free and dairy-free diet.
- Completely remove food colors and dyes from all food, supplements, and medication sources.

—To find out about food dyes, go to:

- www.cfsan.fda.gov/~dms/col-toc.html
- www.thealmightyguru.com/pointless/fooddye.html

- Organic diet
- Antifungal therapy (see "The Best Antifungals and Course" on page 160 in the yeast chapter)

Supplements

(Please note that this is a separate set of recommendations for the conditions discussed in this chapter. The supplement recommendations on page 67 also work. This is in addition.)

- Vitamins: www.kartnerhealth.com or call 866-960-9251

—www.kirkmanlabs.com or call 800-245-8282
—www.klaire.com or call 888-488-2488
—High-quality multivitamin, vitamin D_3 (see page 70)
—Vitamin B_{12} in methyl form (injected subcutaneously every other night)

- Minerals: (Kartner Health, Kirkman Labs, Klaire)

  —Calcium (see page 67)
  —Magnesium (see page 67)
  —Zinc (see page 67)

- Oils: (Kartner Health, Kirkman Labs, Klaire)

  —Omega-3 fatty acids (see pages 68 and 71)

- Short-term medications, such as Ritalin, are a great Band-Aid until the cause of the inability to focus/concentrate is discovered.

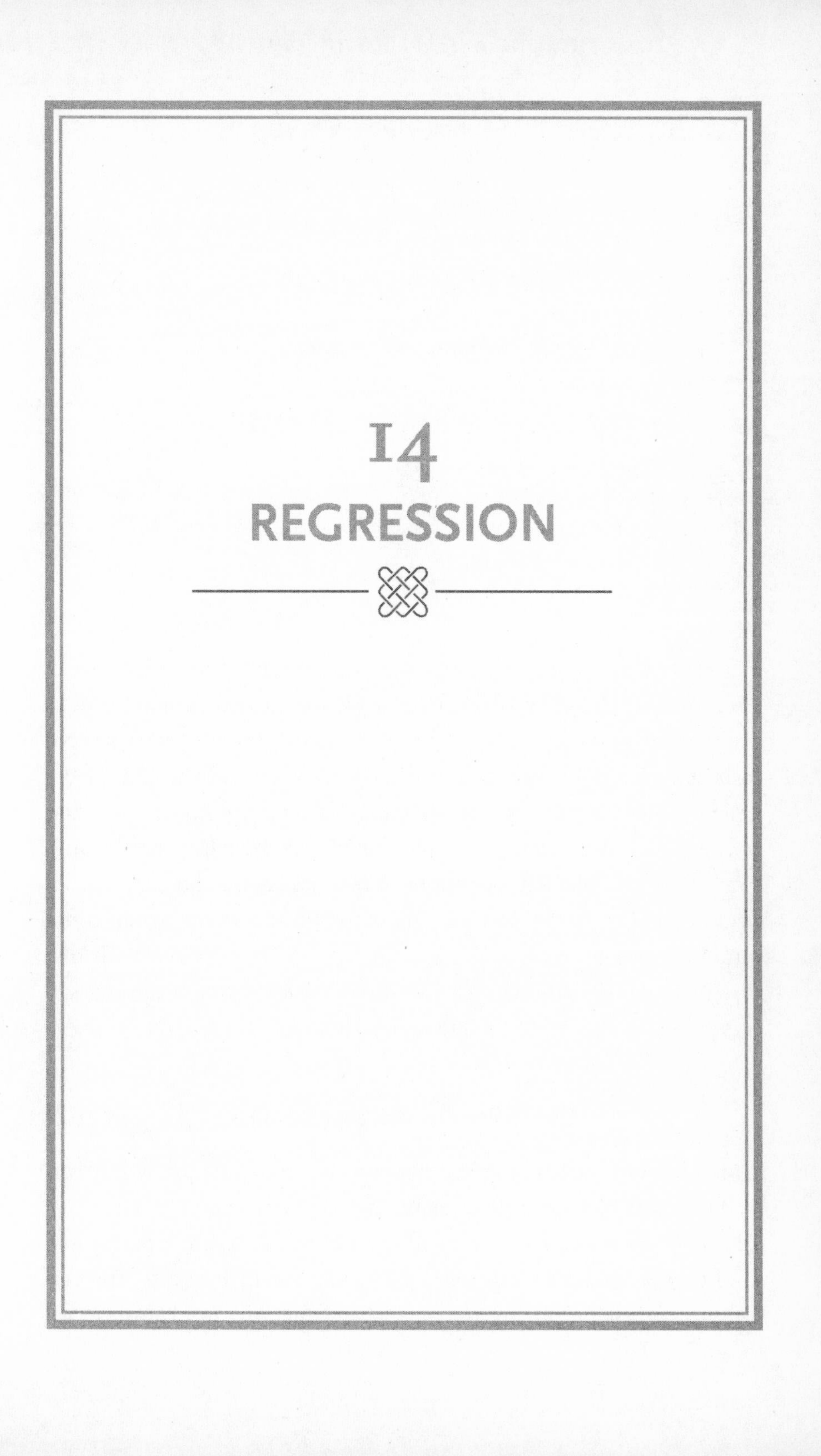

14
REGRESSION

I STILL GET A CHILL up my spine when I hear that word. "Regression!" It's inevitable that our kids do regress at one time or another because of getting sick or other factors, but they always seem to bounce back. I would get so frustrated when Evan would have a head cold and regress back to flapping his arms ten hours a day and not responding or talking. I would feel like all my hard work healing Evan had disappeared overnight. Then, once the boogers disappeared, the flapping of arms would dissipate and words would come out of his sweet mouth again. I wanted to ask Dr. Jerry about his history of watching kids regress and bounce back through the years. I was happy to hear what he had to say about it.

CAUSES OF REGRESSION

JENNY: Besides life-threatening seizures, regression is pretty high on the list of "Mom's greatest fears." Why do our kids regress?

DR. JERRY: First of all, on the road to recovery, there are lots and lots of bumps, and there are some pretty harrowing drop-offs. You can have regression during the spring and the fall. You can have regression when the swimming season opens up and the kid starts swimming in the pools and drinking the chlorinated water. You can have kids regress when they get a strep throat and are put on Amoxicillin. Regressions seem to be a part of the management of autism.

JENNY: Can you describe some things that happen during regression?

DR. JERRY: Whatever they have gained they can lose some part of, or even all. These losses include language, eye contact, understanding, and calmness. They may start jumping and clapping. I've had children who haven't spun and lined things up for three years and now they're doing just that. This is just horrifying for the parents to witness. But the good thing is, there's been a change. They don't "just" regress. The brain doesn't just melt away. Something changed, and if something changed, we can pinpoint what that change is and proceed to unchange it. For example, a parent might say to me, "Well, you know, we haven't been really monitoring his potty habits and he probably hasn't had a bowel movement in two weeks. Now he's flapping, jumping, spinning, he's aggressive, and he's clawing everybody." Although this is regression, we can figure out what might have caused it. A very common regression is when a child is placed on an antibiotic without an antifungal. My favorite is this one: "Well, he was doing so well and then we started letting him cheat on his diet when he goes to his sister's soccer practice, because there are always brownies or whatever and we didn't think a couple could hurt him." These are easy to fix. Harder ones to figure out may happen at school. They may start using different cleaning agents, pesticides may have just been applied, or even an aide with a delightful "bouquet" of perfume may be setting off our children. In the spring they will also start up the air conditioners when they haven't been running for six months and they have all that dust and mold that's accumulated blowing through the vents. These kids are chemically sensitive. These kids are allergic. These kids are still sensitive in their tummies to different foods. We can usually pinpoint why they've regressed when we take a good history. Therefore, it is very important for the parents to take good notes about behavior changes.

JENNY: Can you know ahead of time that a child is going to regress with a certain type of treatment you might start?

DR. JERRY: Yes. Let's say I have a child I suspect is yeasty and I put him on an antifungal. There is a good chance that while we kill the yeast, the child may develop flu-like symptoms, and may be crabby and irritable. This regression has a very interesting name, called a Herxheimer reaction. These children actually suffer for a few days as toxins are released in their body as the yeast dies off. This will appear to be a regression as the child becomes more irritable, cranky, and possibly lethargic. It'll be very disquieting for the parents. Some of the things that have to be considered are: Is the behavior change due to a die-off reaction or is the child actually having a bad reaction to the medication? For example, one of the medications we use to kill gram-negative bacteria is metronidazole. The metronidazole, in a few children, can cause some really significant stomach cramps. We need to consider if the child is howling, irritable, and up all night because of a die-off reaction or because the medicine is irritating the tummy.

REGRESSION DURING YEAST DIE-OFF

- Consider stopping the medication.
- Give a smaller dose of the medication.
- Add ibuprofen, charcoal.
- Give Epsom salt baths to help with the detoxification.

JENNY: I think many parents will agree with me that they're so scared that regression will happen and they'll never get their kid back to wherever he was. How often do you see that?

DR. JERRY: Almost never. Never say "never" in medicine. But we can usually figure it out in most cases.

JENNY: Great! Never! How comforting.

DR. JERRY: I do take care of some children who come from other practices, who may have been a little too aggressively managed and have regressed some. It may take six months to a year to reverse the regression. We have to keep in mind that these children have some of the most fragile metabolic systems. Small things can tip them into a regressive state. I have had children regress on cod liver oil, selenium, probiotics, and just about anything else we try. One child can absolutely thrive on one thing, and it can be a disaster for the next child.

PREVENTING AND DEALING WITH REGRESSION

1. Start one new supplement at a time, giving 3–4 days before adding another supplement/intervention.
2. Start with 1/2 the target dose for 1–2 days to see how it is tolerated.
3. Keep a diary.
4. Look for patterns of behavior changes:

    - Before or after bowel movements
    - Before or after eating
    - After a supplement starts
    - When starting or stopping a medication
    - With changes in school performance
    - When there is increase or decrease in tantrums
    - If you see an improvement in sleep, or changes in sleep
    - When using more or less language
    - If your child has more or less flexibility/OCD/perseverations/anxiety

15
PREVENTION OF HARM (Ensuring Your Baby Is the Healthiest Possible at Birth)

Congratulations! You're pregnant! Make sure you don't eat too much tuna. That mercury in fish is not good for the baby. Now give me your arm. It's time for your flu shot.

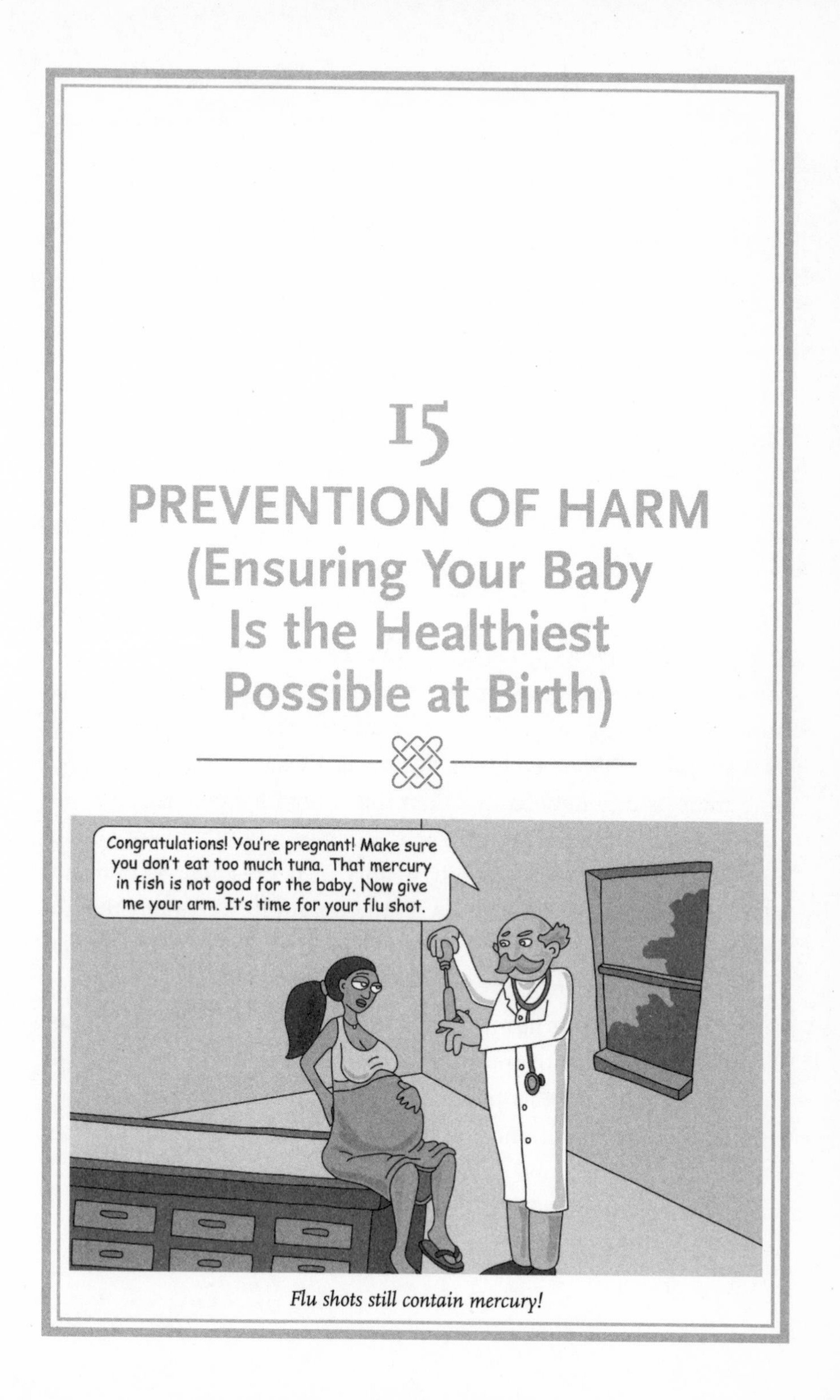

Flu shots still contain mercury!

I'M SURE MANY PEOPLE WILL SAY TO US, "Who do you think you are, saying you could prevent autism?" I have no doubt in my mind that the majority of cases of autism can be prevented. I've learned that for many children, autism is a toxic overload. Yes, I believe there is a genetic component, but only in the sense that you have a genetic vulnerability to toxins, such as a family history of autoimmune disorders or a family history of depression, alcoholism, ADD, schizophrenia (look at the family tree in this chapter) that indicates methylation pathway issues, and a glutathione deficiency. This would prevent the body from being a totally awesome detox machine. So look at your family history for depression, diabetes, lupus, rheumatoid arthritis, or many other diseases for warnings that your child could be vulnerable to autism. Thousands of parents, like me, have learned so much and the only reason we won't shut up is to teach YOU, so you don't have to walk in our shoes. Dr. Jerry and I want to arm parents with all the tools and information necessary to have the healthiest baby you can. The next generation of kids is counting on it!

ADVICE BEFORE PREGNANCY: METALS IN PREGNANT WOMEN

JENNY: Let's say a woman asks you, "Hey, I want to get pregnant and I want to know what some of the precautionary things are that I can do to help ensure my baby's well-being." Actually, that was the nice way of saying it; if it were me, I would be saying, "Dude, I don't want an autistic baby, help, what do I do?"

DR. JERRY: This will actually help with all issues, not just autism. It will help moms with chronic fatigue or any other ailments that are occurring in her because we will be detoxing her and filling her body with nutrients. But the first thing we can do for our moms-to-be who are considering pregnancy and want to give the baby the best start with the lowest amount of toxins in his system would be . . .

JENNY: Have your silver fillings removed from your mouth!

DR. JERRY: (Laughs) Yes, that is what I would start with. We call those amalgams. And this needs to be done by a dentist who is really well versed in mercury-free dentistry. In other words, he or she really understands the process of how to remove amalgams safely without making the person he's removing them from even more toxic through the drilling and the dropping of little pieces that can be inadvertently swallowed or inhalation of the vapors of the metals created while drilling.

JENNY: How far in advance should this be done before you get preggers?

DR. JERRY: At least a year. I would also recommend chelation (detoxification of metals from the body) during the procedure and for a while afterward. This has to be monitored by a physician. Do NOT do this if you are already pregnant. Again, I recommend doing this a year before conception.

JENNY: Aren't the fumes from removing the fillings the cause of the metal poisoning in the body?

DR. JERRY: That's right. During the drilling of the amalgams, the dentist will use special precautions to make sure to generate the fewest fumes during the removal, along with efficient vacuum devices that suck the fumes out of the oral cavity.

JENNY: If a woman were to chelate after removing amalgams, do they chelate the same way we chelate our kids?

DR. JERRY: Mercury-free dentists have different protocols for chelation. Some of them use oral chelators, in a pill form, such as DMSA. Some of them offer IV chelation. Some of them use a combination of oral and IV chelation along with multiple protective supplements.

JENNY: How long do you suggest someone stay on that?

DR. JERRY: I'd have them stay on it for at least two weeks after the removal. During this time, I recommend having the urine checked for toxic metals, as there may be a lot of metals being dumped in the urine; the patient may want to stay on a chelation protocol for several months in this case.

Fish

JENNY: What about the moms who have porcelain fillings, which are safer? Should they still be worried about metals in their body from, let's say, overconsumption of fish and the mercury it contains?

DR. JERRY: Well, once again it depends on how soon she wants to conceive. If she's just reading this and they're trying anytime, then it's best to leave it alone. Do not chelate and stir up the heavy metals. Wherever they're parked, leave them be. But you certainly don't want to add to them. And because you brought up fish, that's certainly the next thing that we'd want to talk about, making sure that we stop eating fish and shellfish. If we really want to splurge, there are a few companies that fish up near the Arctic Circle, and these fish have the least amount of toxins in them. You could consider them to be "mercury lite"! And you can purchase them through different companies over the Internet. Try Safe Harbor: www.safeharborfoods.com/stores.

JENNY: When I was pregnant, back in the day, no one informed me about mercury in fish, so I ate tuna salad and sushi constantly, which I'm sure didn't help things. So you would suggest now, in this age of autism, to just not eat fish during pregnancy?

DR. JERRY: Do not eat fish during pregnancy. There is a great Web site that looks at the content of mercury in fish: www.cfsan.fda.gov/~frf/sea-mehg.html.

JENNY: Do shellfish carry mercury?

DR. JERRY: They can. Crustaceans (like lobster and crab) are scavengers and eat dead and decaying material. Shellfish mercury content does tend to be lower than that in other fish. It is best to look up the fish or shellfish that you want to eat and look at the numbers. To be safe, it is best to avoid the majority of fish. Keep in mind that although fish can have very high levels of mercury, they do not seem to be affected adversely. The theory here is that they have a very good defensive system that protects them from the effects of the mercury. This defense mechanism includes selenium. Selenium prevents mercury from being toxic, but it isn't a cure-all.

Organic Food

JENNY: Since we are on the topic of food, what other things should a woman eat or not eat to ensure the well-being of her baby?

DR. JERRY: I feel strongly that we should eat food as whole and as organic as possible. Limit prepackaged items, frozen items, and boxed foods that have preservatives and artificial sweeteners. Sodas that contain aspartame are a really big NO! In fact, we really recommend decreasing all sugar sources (they can mess with blood sugars while pregnant, which could potentially cause gestational diabetes). If there is no history of dairy intolerance, allergies, eczema, asthma, and constipation, then organic dairy products can be recommended. Grains should be whole. While some physicians recommend starting out the pregnancy gluten-free, there is little evidence that this elimination would be beneficial during pregnancy, unless there is intolerance in the mother-to-be. Finally, significantly limit caffeine-containing beverages and eliminate all alcoholic beverages. Talk about a sign of the times, I don't know if I even have to put it in here, but seriously consider stopping all cigarette smoking during the pregnancy and, for that matter, the rest of your life!

JENNY: No fast food.

DR. JERRY: Fast foods are not nutritious. So, no fast foods! Start learning how to cook from scratch. As I speak with many young moms around the country, I hear all the time that they are "baking impaired" or "cooking disabled." Go organic with fresh colorful fruits and vegetables, nuts, seeds, and meats. Buy the best you can afford. This will reduce your exposure to pesticides, hormones, and other toxins.

Makeup and Perfume During Pregnancy

JENNY: I don't want to get too crazy and name every toxic thing a mom shouldn't have, but if we are talking about having the healthiest baby you can have, I think it's okay to ask about makeup and fragrances.

DR. JERRY: There are reports about lead in lipsticks and facial makeups. These lead-containing products slip in under the radar and we absorb the lead in them through our skin and into our cells. Moms just have to be aware that lead is a toxic material. These cosmetics are in an oil base and, when applied to the skin, can be readily absorbed. So we certainly want to make sure that our makeup is lead-free. The fragrances can be a real problem, too. By their very nature, they are in a gaseous form (so we can smell them) and can easily be inhaled into the lungs and trigger inflammation in the respiratory tree. Of course, a gas in the lungs can then easily be transported by the bloodstream. This has to be strongly considered when working around strong-smelling products such as nail treatments, hairsprays, and perfumes. There are airborne toxins in perfumes, dryer sheets, scented candles, air fresheners, cleaning products, fabric softeners, and laundry detergents. Another area I have to bring up is the chemicals and colorings we put on the scalp. The scalp easily absorbs many chemicals directly into the bloodstream.

JENNY: Wow, women are going to have to look like cavemen to ensure good health.

DR. JERRY: No, not like cavemen, just the smart women they are!

JENNY: To this day I go to the nail salon with a surgical mask on, and I couldn't care less what people think because the fumes are so bad.

DR. JERRY: Well, I'm not going to say go with the mask. I'm not going to go that far, because that's probably something that our moms aren't going to do. But we certainly don't have to walk into a place where you're knocked flat from the smell. That can't be good for the baby. Remember, everything that is getting into your body either through the lungs or through the digestive tract is going to be preferentially concentrated at the placenta. Remember that the placenta is the rich blood supply that nourishes the developing baby.

SUPPLEMENTS FOR PREVENTION OF AUTISM: PROBIOTICS

JENNY: Let's talk about taking probiotics, which by taking them you are basically putting good bacteria into your body. Is it an important next step for prevention and ensuring baby's well-being?

DR. JERRY: Again, taking probiotics is very, very important for all of us, but especially as we're getting pregnant. We're trying to build up our own host immune defenses so we don't have to go on antibiotics or antifungals while we're pregnant. So taking probiotics will be very helpful. Take vitamins—and there are some new ones that are now organic, which are very healthy and wholesome. Please refer to the supplement chapter for a list of probiotics and where you can get them.

Vitamins, Oils, and Other Healthy Nutrients

JENNY: What about taking vitamins and oils?

DR. JERRY: They make vitamins that are organic or derived from organic sources. Stick with a brand of vitamins that caters to the organic/vegan crowd. They tend to be high quality. But vitamin choice is rather a personal thing. Many vitamins can cause nausea or be constipating, despite what they promise on the label. It is good to acclimate your body to a vitamin before you become pregnant. If you are used to your vitamin regimen and then you start to experience nausea, you will know it's probably morning sickness and not the "new" vitamins you just started.

I recommend fish oils for all women who plan to get pregnant. You might say, "Hey, you just said don't eat fish." But now we're talking about the fish *oil,* which is very clean and has been obtained and processed in a way that is not going to have measurable concentrations of mercury or other toxic compounds. But we can't use just any old fish oil. Some preferred providers, like Nordic Naturals and Carlson, are great sources for fish oil. For flaxseed oil, I like Barlean's Flax Oil. Talk to your OB-GYN about these supplements. The omega-3s found in these oils are crucial during pregnancy.

PREFERRED OIL SOURCES:

- Nordic Naturals
- Carlson
- Barlean's Flax Oil

PREGNANCY AND YEAST

JENNY: What about killing yeast? I really believe that yeast in women is an epidemic right now. I'm not talking about just yeast in the vagina; I'm talking about candida in the gut!

DR. JERRY: Many OBs are now doing prepregnancy screening: lead, mercury, yeast, viral infections, etc. This is really a great idea because when pregnant, the immune system actually DOWN-regulates. That is, becomes less vigilant. This is life-saving for the developing baby, as there cannot be an immune attack on it. After all, it is a foreign body! Though great for the baby, for the mother it may mean three-month-long colds, viral flare-ups, and of course, yeast infections. Well, one can imagine what happens if yeast starts to bloom while the immune system is throttled back. The gas, bloating, and digestive trouble is a nightmare. Bottom line here is to get the yeast diagnosed and treated. In addition, as mentioned, stay on a low-sugar diet!

JENNY: Wouldn't you suggest every woman who wants to get pregnant should get tested, no matter what, for yeast?

DR. JERRY: The OB is mostly concerned with a vaginal yeast infection. Women can be more prone to these if they have been on the birth control pill, taken antibiotics, and if they are diabetic. The yeast can also be located in the gastrointestinal tract. Both sources should be tested. Diflucan, the main prescription that treats yeast, should **NOT** be used during pregnancy. So it is best to get this settled prior to conception. Again, I stress a low-sugar diet to prevent the recurrence of yeast. There are many healthy women who don't have yeast overgrowth, so these screening tests will be negative.

JENNY: There are healthy people out there? I don't believe it. I think they THINK they are healthy but if you turned them all inside out, they would have Starbucks running through their veins, not blood.

DR. JERRY: All I'm advocating is that we can easily reduce the colonies by lowering the sugar in our diet. In essence, we are making it harder for yeast to grow.

HOUSEHOLD TOXINS

JENNY: Let's get into more preparation for baby into a nontoxic environment. Let's talk about household toxins.

DR. JERRY: This is a great topic: the home environment. We are now going to consider changing many things around the house that we have grown up with. We will need to consider nontoxic alternatives for cleaning agents and nontoxic alternatives for indoor pest control. I really understand the need for insect-free homes. I live in Florida! We had one child (in our practice) who was exposed to massive amounts of pesticides. When the company came in to spray for termites, they used long wands that are stuck into the dirt and infuse pesticide. In this child's case, they inadvertently penetrated the big silver ventilation tubes and sent termite spray into his room. He then developed brain cancer but survived brain cancer and the surgeries. Then they gave him all of his vaccines because he was behind, and he developed autism.

JENNY: What about paints? Every about-to-be mom wants the nursery painted.

DR. JERRY: Nesting, as my wife calls it, is a fun time! No-guilt painting can be done with what is called nonvolatile organic compound paints. Though a little more money per gallon, these paints will not be off-gassing toxins. Many paint stores offer low-VOC paints, but look for NO VOC paints. Home Depot has a great line of NO VOC paints and NO VOC dyes (coloring agents).

JENNY: What about carpeting?

DR. JERRY: Our children with autism generally do not do well with carpets. The carpets, along with their foam padding, off-gas volatile organic compounds. They can also be a source for house dust mites. Children may also be sensitive to the synthetics as well. If there must be carpeting, a real budget buster is 100 percent worsted wool (no glue on the back of this type of carpet) with a "green" pad or jute. Make sure the dyes used are low or no VOC.

JENNY: Why are these things important for all "about to be" families?

DR. JERRY: Well, if we're going to be nesting, and we're going to be redoing our home, it is best to do this once, rather than step by step, as I did things. My son's room was full of pressboard furniture, which he is sensitive to since it contains formaldehyde. I had the pleasure of selling it on Craigslist for pennies on the dollar (Goodwill for some). One must strongly consider thoughtful planning about purchasing nontoxic products. Seems like a novel idea these days. Even hardwood has stains and varnishes. They, too, will off-gas.

JENNY: Yikes! What if the furniture is old?

DR. JERRY: If it's old, it has off-gassed already. But you definitely don't want to use pressboard. And thank God we have oak. Oak is cheap. And oak doesn't off-gas. Remember, if you use pressboard, there's formaldehyde in there. New homes are notorious for off-gassing, and I have taken care of many children who were fine and then things started falling apart medically shortly after moving into the new home.

VACCINES AND RHOGAM

JENNY: Continuing with pregnancy, I would say not to vaccinate while pregnant—would you nod your head to that?

DR. JERRY: To ensure the least amount of toxic exposures to the baby during pregnancy, I would not have my daughter-in-law get vaccinated during her pregnancy. It's a key point. I also would not recommend that moms get an MMR vaccine (measles, mumps, and rubella) after delivery for any reason. If the baby is going to breastfeed, I would not want any of the live virus vaccines passed to her child in her breast milk.

JENNY: The Rhogam shot?

DR. JERRY: Rhogam is important in that it does protect you from what they call Rh incompatibility. This occurs when the mother has a negative blood type, like O-negative or A-negative, and the developing baby has a positive blood type, like O-positive or A-positive.

The positive contribution here would be from the father, but he too must have a "positive" blood type. If the father has a negative blood type, such as O-negative, there is no chance for the baby to have a positive type unless there was laboratory error in testing the dad, or the man who thinks he is "dad" is not! The OB or midwife will usually insist on giving the Rhogam injection because she can't really be certain who the dad is. But if you're certain who the dad is, then you don't need a Rhogam shot if your husband is Rh negative. Otherwise, it is very important to receive this particular shot, and the good news is that the formula no longer contains mercury.

JENNY: How does the Rhogam shot work?

DR. JERRY: Rhogam is a shot that interferes with the production of antibodies to the Rh-positive blood the baby might have. If the mother is, for example, O-negative, she will make antibodies to O-positive blood (if sensitized, which is a complicated topic). If the dad has a positive blood type, the baby has a chance for a positive blood type too. Rhogam blocks the formation of antibodies the mother would normally make against O-positive blood. If this was not blocked, these antibodies would pass right through the placenta and blow up all the baby's blood cells, which can be fatal. Now, I am O-positive and my wife is O-negative, so she did have to have the Rhogam shots, because she would have made antibodies against the baby's blood. Unfortunately, this was twenty-two years ago and the average shot had 25 mcg of mercury per injection, given at a time when there is crucial nervous system formation.

JENNY: There are so many moms who have had Rhogam shots and have kids with autism. Do you think there's a correlation?

DR. JERRY: Definitely. They all have had 25 mcg or more of mercury per shot, and they get it at six weeks and at delivery. So by the third or fourth baby, the mother has had quite an exposure to mercury from the Rhogam she received.

JENNY: Is this still a problem today?

DR. JERRY: Now they've taken out the thimerosal from Rhogam, so it's a safe thing to do in this country, but I don't know about Rhogam in other countries, if it's still preserved with thimerosal or not.

JENNY: So the Rhogam shot is a yes if you need it?

DR. JERRY: You do need that one if you have a different Rh type, more specifically, if the mother is Rh-negative and the father is Rh-positive.

JENNY: Should pregnant women get flu shots?

DR. JERRY: Absolutely not.

CLEAN LIVING

JENNY: Moms need to eliminate all their exposure to alcohol, drugs, and smoking. This includes secondhand smoke.

DR. JERRY: Yes, yes, yes.

JENNY: God, I just feel like I want everyone to be so sure their body is the best it can be before they get pregnant and test for everything.

DR. JERRY: Well, testing gets expensive.

JENNY: So the best advice is to clean out the toxic barrel as best as you can?

DR. JERRY: I think that is the best advice. Clean out the toxic barrel. Do the best you can with your home. Think about your internal environment and the foods you put into your mouth. Avoid plastics and if you are going to microwave, use glass. Avoid cooking in Teflon. Think about your external environment, where you sleep (toxic materials in bedding and the off-gassing from the "memory foams") and where you live. Don't forget about your clothes. Avoid dry cleaning. If you need to, then unwrap them from the plastic they come in and let them air out for a day. And if you're otherwise healthy, I think it would just get very frustrating trying to get a doctor to do a yeast test and put you on an antifungal when you have no symptoms. Now, if you have rashes, if you have eczema, if you have some funky breath odors or body odors, then yes. Absolutely clean out your toxic barrel!

FOOD SENSITIVITY

JENNY: Do you think a mom should get tested for food sensitivity?

DR. JERRY: By detecting what foods she is sensitive to, it makes removal of certain foods and rotation of others a whole lot easier. If there are a lot of symptoms that go along with her diet, such as constipation, bloating, excessive gas production, cramps, dull feelings, and fatigue, for example, a food sensitivity profile could be quite revealing. But even without testing, in this particular case, I would definitely recommend removing all dairy and all gluten-containing grains. If you remove dairy, make sure you're taking calcium, magnesium, and vitamin D supplements.

JENNY: If a mother is super cautious like me, can she send her breast milk in to get it tested for things like metals or other garbage?

DR. JERRY: The milk is going to reflect what you're eating as well as what is going on inside your body. If a mother has elevated mercury in her body, it will be positively assayed in her breast milk.

JENNY: So if we live in a highly polluted place where autism is off the charts, like Jersey or California, as a mom, I go, "Gee, this air sucks. I should test my breast milk because I'm breathing in crap." That would still be a good thing to do?

TESTING BREAST MILK FOR TOXINS

DR. JERRY: Testing breast milk for toxins is a whole new field with tremendous ramifications. The CDC clearly states that it has not established normal and abnormal levels to aid in clinical determinations. First of all, one has to determine what is "normal." The next step is to determine what toxin levels are "acceptable." Where does one collect that type of data? How is a parent going to determine whether the potential toxin risks outweigh the benefits of breast-feeding and breast milk? This whole chapter has been dedicated to cleaning up the internal environment as well as the external environment. Doing so will decrease the toxins in the new mother's body and thus will translate to the lowest amount of toxins in her breast milk.

Keep in mind, formula milks have toxins in them, too! Cows are prone to many pollutants and this will be expressed into the milk as well.

One last point here is to maximize the ability for the body to remove toxins:

- Drink lots of water.
- Assure daily regularity.
- Exercise regularly and sweat those toxins out of your skin!

JENNY: All right. Let's talk about what to do after a baby has been born!

DR. JERRY: Well, that will bring us right into vaccines!

JENNY: I renamed them, ya know.

DR. JERRY: To what?

JENNY: You won't let me swear in this book, so I can't say.

DR. JERRY: All right then, I'll move on. I think it is very important for parents to understand a major medical intervention called vaccination. Each parent should understand the vaccines offered and decide for their child if it is appropriate for them or not. There are two excellent books on this subject: *What Your Doctor May NOT Tell You About Children's Vaccinations,* by Dr. Stephanie Cave, and *The Vaccine Book: Making the Right Decision for Your Child,* by Dr. Robert Sears.

JENNY: If you don't mind, Doc, I would like to end with a note directly to the parents reading this.

DR. JERRY: Please do.

JENNY: I hope all parents out there come to realize that YOU are in control of YOU and of your child's health. YOUR voice is the one your child is counting on. Please educate yourself fully and make the best decision for YOU. The life you are bringing into this world is counting on it.

DR. JERRY: Well said!

16
VACCINES

Why do those indigenous people keep running away from us? We are here to help them.
They said these shots were making their kids retarded.
expired vaccines

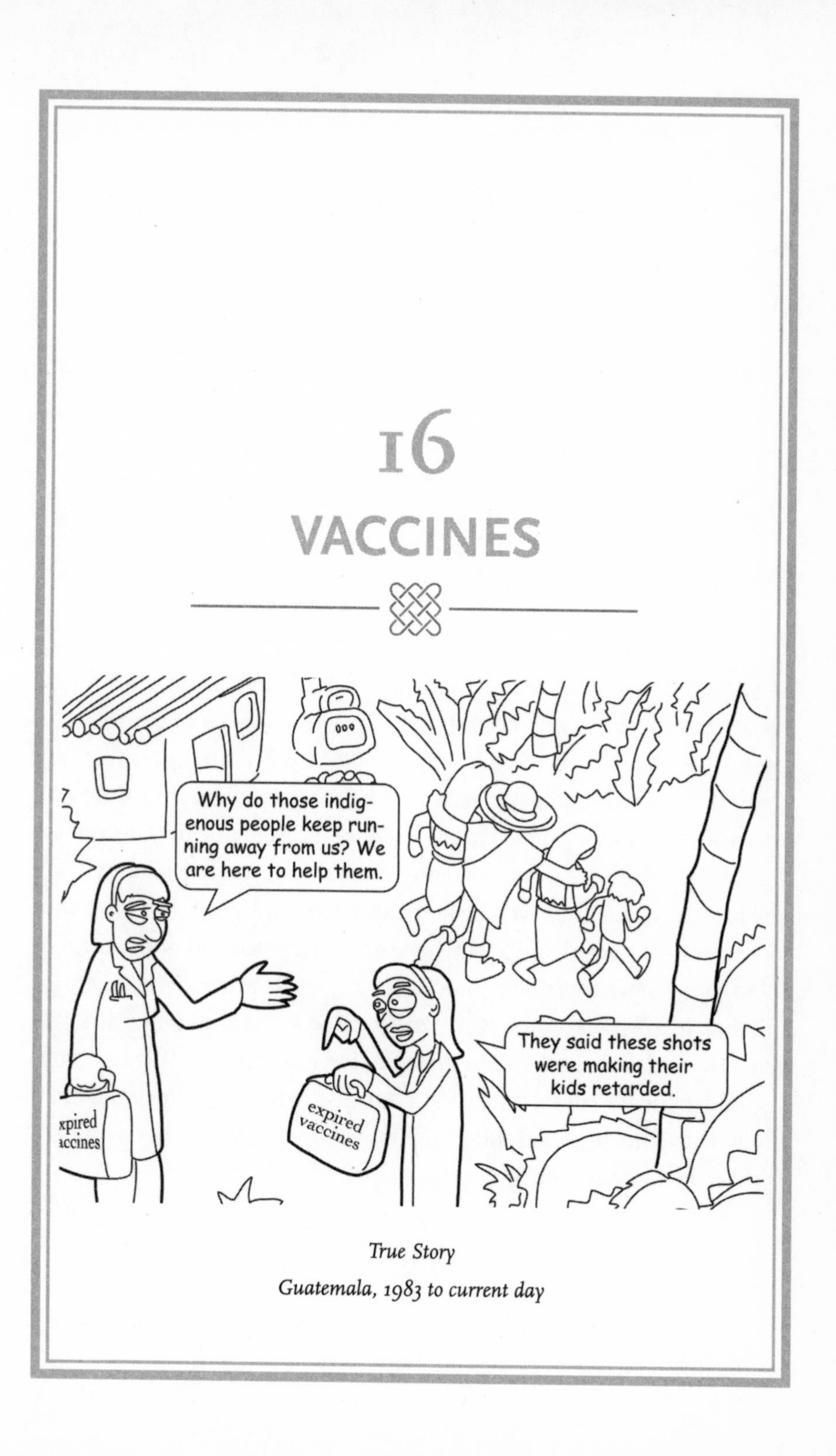

True Story

Guatemala, 1983 to current day

MANY PEOPLE ASK ME if I had to do it all over again with a new baby, would I vaccinate? The answer is no. Hell no. Most parents who know they have a vaccine-injured child usually are that adamant about it. There are many parents who haven't walked in our shoes yet and are still scared to vaccinate but also scared not to vaccinate. I don't blame them. It's so confusing to hear your pediatrician tell you not to worry and then you watch the news and read articles about moms who are screaming they have a vaccine-induced autistic child. So what's a new mom left to do? Despite what anybody thinks, I'm still not against vaccines. I'm really pissed off about the amount given these days and the crap that's inside of them. So, if I were you, I would educate myself on each shot and what it protects against, along with the possible side effects. I hope this chapter with Dr. Kartzinel helps you make the right choices.

VACCINES GIVEN AT BIRTH

JENNY: So you push your baby out and he comes into this new world and immediately gets injected with what?

DR. JERRY: There are three medical interventions the newborn will be subjected to. The vitamin K is the first injection to greet the newborn.

JENNY: Yeah, what is the vitamin K shot supposed to do?

DR. JERRY: The vitamin K shot is given to prevent the hemorrhagic disease of the newborn. About 1 child out of 100,000 will be born with insufficient levels of vitamin K that can contribute to the possible outcome of uncontrolled bleeding. Depending on the baby's weight, either 0.5 mg or 1.0 mg of vitamin K is injected into the thigh of the newborn. There is some concern about the association of vitamin K injections and birth and the development of childhood leukemia. An alternative to a very large dose given at birth may be giving one-fifth of the vitamin K intended for injection, orally! This way, the newborn is not flooded with a huge amount of vitamin K, but rather gets one-fifth of 1 mg given orally once weekly for five weeks . . . so the total dose is the same, just given over five weeks. Another consideration is to ensure that the mother consumes vitamin K–rich foods (Brussels sprouts, broccoli, cauliflower) during her pregnancy. The parents should research these different ways of giving vitamin K and put them into the birthing plan.

The second intervention the newborn will be greeted with is antibiotic ointment for the eyes. Erythromycin ointment is administered to prevent potential eye disease caused by three bacteria: gonorrhea, syphilis, and chlamydia. Some states have laws about this mandatory administration, but this can be waived by the parents. Side effects are very rare, the most common being chemical irritation.

JENNY: Yes, and the third?

DR. JERRY: I knew you were going to ask! It is the hepatitis B vaccine.

JENNY: They never even asked me if I wanted Evan to have it. They just gave it to him without me knowing. That happens to most people.

DR. JERRY: Hep B is given anywhere from within the first hour of life to just prior to discharge from the hospital. Unless the mother is a hepatitis B carrier, there is no other reason to vaccinate with hepatitis B. Hepatitis B is a viral infection that can be transmitted by contact with infectious blood, body fluids such as semen, having sex with an infected individual, sharing contaminated needles to inject drugs, or from an infected mother to her newborn. Thus hepatitis B mainly occurs in sexually active heterosexual adults with more than one sex partner in the prior six months or a history of sexually transmitted disease; homosexual and bisexual men; illicit injection-drug users; persons at occupational risk of infection, such as surgeons; hemodialysis patients; and household and sexual contacts of persons with chronic hepatitis B infection.

Obviously, this just does not seem to be a concern for most of our newborns. Let us be very clear here. Hepatitis B is a very serious disease that can cause liver damage and liver cancer. Since we cannot tell which newborn is going to make poor lifestyle choices, the American Academy of Pediatrics mandates that we must vaccinate every child (much to the glee of the pharmaceutical industry, no doubt).

The risk to people receiving the vaccine can be very great. In fact, the French stopped mandating its use in school-aged children in 1998.

This study looks at the Hepatitis B Vaccine in adults:

CHRONIC ADVERSE REACTIONS ASSOCIATED WITH HEPATITIS B VACCINATION

David A Geier, Mark R Geier, M.D. Ph.D. *The Annals of Pharmacotherapy*, 2002: Vol. 36, No. 12, pp. 1970–1971. PMID: 12452762 [PubMed—indexed for MEDLINE]

In conclusion, our study demonstrates that adult HBV is statistically associated not only with acute neuropathy, neuritis, myelitis, vasculitis, thrombocytopenia, gastrointestinal disease, multiple sclerosis, and arthritis, but some of these patients go on to develop chronic adverse reactions that persist for at least 1 year following HBV. These types of chronic adverse reactions following adult HBV should be discussed with patients contemplating being immunized with HBV and should be included in the differential diagnosis of those who develop them following adult HBV.

After the approval and licensure of the vaccine, additional conditions developed that are now included in the manufacturer's hepatitis B post-marketing report (http://us.gsk.com/products/assets/us_engerixb.pdf):

Hypersensitivity: Anaphylaxis; erythema multiforme, including Stevens-Johnson syndrome; angioedema; arthritis. An apparent hypersensitivity syndrome (serum sickness–like) of delayed onset has been reported days to weeks after vaccination, including: arthralgia/arthritis (usually transient), fever, and dermatologic reactions such as urticaria, erythema multiforme, ecchymoses, and erythema nodosum (see CONTRAINDICATIONS)

Cardiovascular System: Tachycardia/palpitations

Respiratory System: Bronchospasm, including asthma-like symptoms

Gastrointenstinal System: Abnormal liver function tests; dyspepsia

Nervous System: Migraine; syncope; paresis; neuropathy, including hypoesthesia, paresthesia, Guillain-Barré syndrome and Bell's palsy, transverse myelitis; optic neuritis; multiple sclerosis; seizures

Hematologic: Thrombocytopenia

Skin and Appendages: Eczema; purpura; herpes zoster; erythema nodosum; alopecia

Special Senses: Conjunctivitis; keratitis; visual disturbances; vertigo; tinnitus; earache

So, we are asking newborns to take all the risks for a hepatitis B vaccine, without realizing any true benefit.

JENNY: So, would you suggest waiting until maybe the child is twelve years old to give hep B?

DR. JERRY: Yes, I would put it down for consideration at a later age. There are risks for anyone, at any age, to get this vaccine. Let's be truthful here. This is a vaccine that protects the recipient from contracting hepatitis B from lifestyle choices. Let's also talk rationale here. This vaccine was designed to block the contraction of hepatitis B from sexual activity and IV drug use, as well as to protect those who care for individuals with hepatitis B. The bottom line: Many individuals are going to have some serious medical consequences to being vaccinated against hepatitis B. Again, though, it is a totally unnecessary consideration for newborns except for those born to mothers infected with hepatitis B.

VACCINES GIVEN TO INFANTS

JENNY: Then, the next shot they'll give is a few weeks later.

DR. JERRY: The next shots are at the two-month, four-month, and six-month visits. Here is a list of vaccines they receive at each visit:

The Center for Disease Control's Recommended Immunization Schedule for Persons Aged 0–6 Years—United States 2008

Vaccine ▼ Age ▶	Birth	1 Month	2 Months	4 Months	6 Months	12 Months	15 Months	18 Months	19-23 Months	2-3 Years	4-6 Years
Hepatitis B1	HepB	HepB				HepB					
Rotavirus2			Rota	Rota	Rota						
Diphtheria, Tetanus, Pertussis3			DTaP	DTaP	›		DTaP				DTaP
Haemophilus influenza type b4			Hib	Hib	Hib	Hib					
Pneumococcal5			PCV	PCV	PCV	P				PPV	
Inactivated Poliovirus			IPV	IPV		IPV					IPV
Influenza6							Influenza (Yearly)				
Measles, Mumps, Rubella7						MMR					MMR
Varicella8						Varicella					Varicella
Hepatitis A9							HepA (2 doses)			HepA Series	
Meningococcal10										MCV4	

Range of recommended ages

Certain high-risk groups

Source: www.cdc.gov/vaccines/recs/schedules/downloads/child/2008/08_0-6yrs_schedule.pdf

JENNY: What is the DPT?

DR. JERRY: Those are three different vaccines in one shot, and that's why they call it DPT, or DTaP. The D stands for diphtheria, the T stands for tetanus, and the P stands for acellular pertussis.

Diphtheria is a bacterial infection that has been very rare since World War II and the introduction of the diphtheria vaccine. I have seen one case during my training years.

Pertussis is also known as whooping cough. The whole cell pertussis vaccine was very "reactogenic." This means it caused some unfortunate immune system responses. It subsequently was pulled off the market in favor of the new and improved version called acellular pertussis. The only cases of whooping cough I have managed were among previously fully immunized children! For more information on pertussis specifically, I recommend the book by Harris Coulter and Barbara Loe Fisher, *A Shot in the Dark*.

Tetanus is a disease cause by *Clostridium tetani*. These bacteria liberate toxins that lead to muscle paralysis. This is a very rare disease and, according to the CDC, there are about forty-three cases per year.

Now here is the dilemma. If vaccines were without risk, it would be a no-brainer to receive these vaccinations. Unfortunately, this is not the case. With one in six school-aged children having a diagnosable "mental illness," and one in eighty males currently being diagnosed with autism, we have to consider the very real possibility that vaccines have had a role in this. In 1983 we had ten shots on the vaccine schedule. Autism was one in 10,000. Today there are thirty-six vaccines given and autism is nearing one in 100. With that said, we try to balance the risk of the vaccine on one side with the disease we are trying to protect the child from. Consider, for example, the chance of contracting tetanus. Directly quoted from the CDC with regard to tetanus: "the average annual incidence was 0.16 cases/million population." In other words, if there is a reasonable concern that the current vaccine schedule is contributing to the burgeoning numbers of ill children, parents may choose to consider alternatives to the current vaccine schedule. That is, some may choose to delay the vaccines, pick and choose which ones they want (i.e., zero concern for hep B vaccine and great concern for tetanus), and, of course, they may choose no vaccines.

JENNY: What's haemophilus influenzae type B?

DR. JERRY: Haemophilus influenzae type B (HIB) is a potentially fatal disease in children, especially if they are less than one year old. In my first two years of training, I took care of several children with this potentially life-threatening disease. Since the introduction of the HIB vaccine in 1987 (the improved form that can be given to two-month-olds), I have rarely seen a case of HIB disease. The reported number of cases of HIB disease went from 40–100 cases per 100,000 children to 1.3 cases per 100,000 children. This sounds great initially. It is interesting to note that since the routine use of this vaccine, childhood diabetes type 1 has increased dramatically. Here is just one article I have excerpted to demonstrate this concern:

CLUSTERING OF CASES OF INSULIN DEPENDENT DIABETES (IDDM) OCCURRING THREE YEARS AFTER HEMOPHILUS INFLUENZA B (HIB) IMMUNIZATION SUPPORT CAUSAL RELATIONSHIP BETWEEN IMMUNIZATION AND IDDM.

Classen JB, Classen DC. Autoimmunity. 2003 May; 36(3):123. PMID: 12482192 [PubMed—indexed for MEDLINE] Classen Immunotherapies Inc., 6517 Montrose Avenue, Baltimore, MD 21212, USA. classen@vaccines.net

OBJECTIVE: The hemophilus vaccine has been linked to the development of autoimmune type 1 diabetes, insulin dependent diabetes (IDDM) in ecological studies. METHODS: We attempted to determine if the Hemophilus influenza B (HiB) vaccine was associated with an increased risk of IDDM by looking for clusters of cases of IDDM using data from a large clinical trial. All children born in Finland between October 1st, 1985, and August 31st, 1987, approximately 116,000 were randomized to receive 4 doses of the HiB vaccine (PPR-D, Connaught) starting at 3 months of life or one dose starting after 24 months of life. A control-cohort included all 128,500 children born in Finland in the 24 months prior to the HiB vaccine study. Non-obese diabetic prone (NOD) mice were immunized with a hemophilus vaccine to determine if immunization increased the risk of IDDM. RESULTS: The difference in cumulative incidence between those receiving 4 doses and those receiving 0 doses is 54 cases of IDDM/100,000 (P = 0.026) at 7 years (relative risk = 1.26). Most of the extra cases of IDDM appeared in statistically significant clusters that occurred in periods starting approximately 38 months after immunization and lasting approximately 6–8 months. Immunization with pediatric vaccines increased the risk of insulin diabetes in NOD mice.

CONCLUSION: Exposure to HiB immunization is associated with an increased risk of IDDM. NOD mice can be used as an animal model of vaccine induced diabetes.

THE SHOT SCHEDULE

JENNY: Let's talk more about the shot schedule.

DR. JERRY: Okay. The shot schedule printed above is said to be "mandatory" but it is not really! It is almost ALWAYS up to the parents to decide which if any vaccines they would like to have administered and when they want them given. Only two states do NOT allow the parent any say-so in the matter: Mississippi and West Virginia. They have very strict medical guidelines and only a physician may sign the waiver.

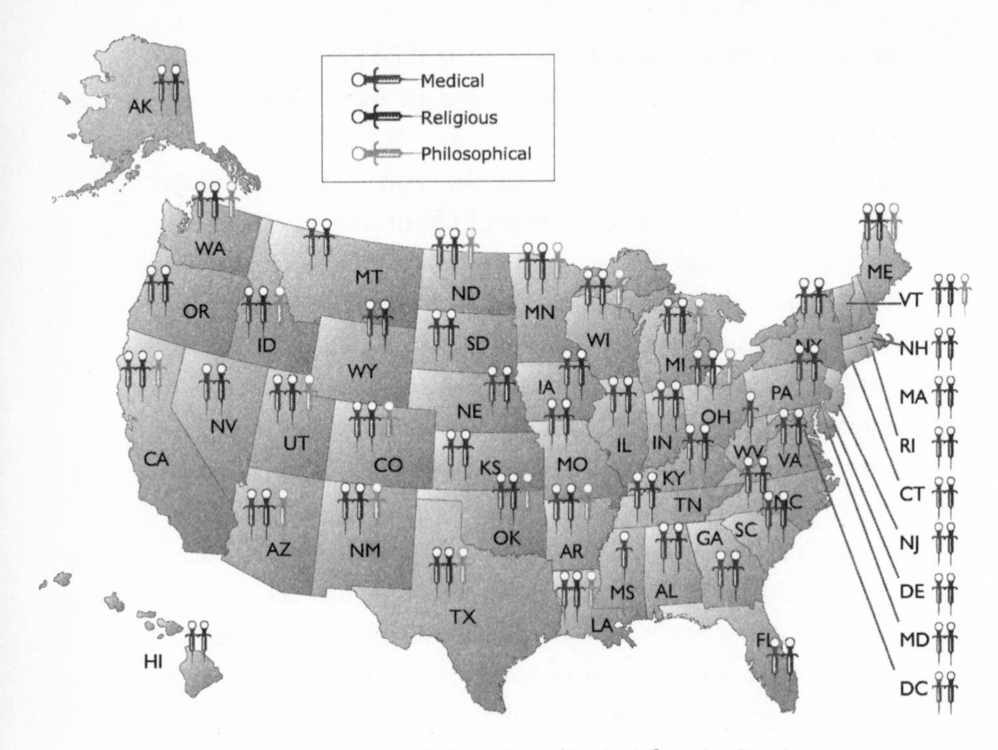

Courtesy of www.NVIC.org (National Vaccine Information Center)

WHEN TO VACCINATE

DR. JERRY: We never want to vaccinate when the baby is sick or is currently on antibiotics. Recurrent infections such as ear or sinus infections, eczema, or allergies may be a big red flag when it comes to vaccinations.

We should establish a period of normalcy of growth and development, as there is no rush to get the shots. (Normalcy being hitting milestones and a child having a healthy immune system—that would mean no chronic infections from birth to three years old.) There's no rush unless you're in an environment in which your child is exposed to disease from, say, kids in daycare, or you're living in a third-world country. Then you have to think carefully. But another thought here: Why do we need to give so many shots over and over? Many children may not need the kindergarten shots. They may still have full protection from their last set of immunizations. One can easily check this by doing a titer test.

JENNY: Explain titers again in case anyone is, like, "What?"

DR. JERRY: Titers are a blood test to see if antibodies are being made toward a specific agent, such as a particular food, or a disease like chicken pox. If you were to measure my titers to chicken pox that I had over forty years ago, the results would come back as "elevated," meaning I am still protected from chicken pox. These titers can check to see if an individual is still protected from tetanus, mumps, measles, rubella, diphtheria, pertussis, polio, hepatitis B, and whatever else!

JENNY: So everyone should just test titers instead of vaccinating for the same disease again and again.

DR. JERRY: Titers do make a lot of sense. If the child is protected from a particular disease, what is the point in giving a booster?

JENNY: Sadly, titer tests can sometimes be so expensive. I still think it's worth it in the long run, but they sure don't make it easy on parents. Now let's talk about shots between six months and a year.

DR. JERRY: As one can see on the schedule, the vaccines are more of the same! Let's recap, looking at the recommended vaccine chart for 2008; up to now, our child has had the DTaP, IPV (polio), hep B, pneumococcal, HIB, and rotavirus vaccines. The rotavirus is a very common viral cause of diarrhea that is just a mild disease. It is less of a concern to breast-fed babies who stay at home and more of a concern to bottle-fed babies who attend daycare. Where the problem lies, as with any disease process, there will be a few devastating cases of rotavirus that can land the child in the hospital for dehydration and IV fluids. But any disease can do this! Let's take strep throat, for example. I had a patient who went camping with her girlfriend and parents. Both girls were nine years old and healthy. They pitched the tents on Wednesday; on Thursday, the girlfriend had a bit of a sore throat and just wanted to hang in the tent for the day. On Friday, she had passed away during the night. Cause of death: streptococcus. My illustration here is that there will always be a few devastating cases that will be "reported" to justify the need of this vaccine or that. Don't get me wrong here, every life is precious, and if there were really few if any risks to vaccines, I would be 100 percent supportive of vaccines without any alterations to the schedule. What I am concerned about is the trading of an incredibly rare outcome (such as a child contracting hepatitis B, for example, and passing away from liver failure) for a very real concern over causing complete dysregulation of the immune system for our sensitive kids.

For example, polio is definitely not a disease to be trifled with. The only polio in the U.S. for nearly thirty years has been caused by the ORAL polio vaccine, that's why it was switched to a safer form to give children the inactivated polio virus (IPV). There is no debate as to whether this vaccine has been effective. But let's look what is in a typical IPV injection:

Manufacturer	**Aventis Pasteur**
Microorganism	Polio-virus types 1, 2, and 3
Licensed	12/21/1990
Recommendations	5 injections at 2, 4, 6 months, and boosters at 18 months and at 4–6 years of age. Booster dose prior to international travel.
Ingredients	Formaldehyde, neomycin, 2-phenoxyethanol, polymyxin B, streptomycin, stopper vial may contain dry latex rubber, bovine (cow) serum, virus: polio.

The problem is, again, more environmental toxins being pushed into our children's bodies.

JENNY: I'm gonna give a whole list of ingredients and side effects at the end of this chapter. Has there ever been a study done of vaccinated versus unvaccinated children and their history of ear infections?

DR. JERRY: No, but that would be a great study. A study like that would cost $250,000 to $500,000. What pharmaceutical company would invest money into a study that would most likely demonstrate that there are far fewer ear infections, or other diseases, for that matter, in children who do not receive vaccines? In fact, what if they also found that the unvaccinated group has very few cases of attention deficit disorder, allergies, and asthma? Now, follow this thread. Fewer vaccines might imply less illness, and thus a marked decrease in the need for medications (and, of course, a much lower need for vaccines). This would also equate to fewer trips to the pediatrician. Let's face it, if not for the "vaccine schedule," how many of us would be stepping into the pediatric office five times in the first year of life with our new baby?

JENNY: Generation Rescue, the nonprofit autism organization that I work with, funded a study simply asking if there were more cases of autism, ADHD, and neurological disorders in the vaccinated group of children compared to unvaccinated children. Let's look at the results:

ALL VACCINATED BOYS, COMPARED TO UNVACCINATED BOYS:

- Vaccinated boys were 155 percent more likely to have a neurological disorder (RR 2.55).
- Vaccinated boys were 224 percent more likely to have ADHD (RR 3.24).
- Vaccinated boys were 61 percent more likely to have autism (RR 1.61).

Older vaccinated boys, ages 11–17 (about half the boys surveyed), compared to older unvaccinated boys:

- Vaccinated boys were 158 percent more likely to have a neurological disorder (RR 2.58).
- Vaccinated boys were 317 percent more likely to have ADHD (RR 4.17).
- Vaccinated boys were 112 percent more likely to have autism (RR 2.12).

Granted, in this study, only autism, ADHD, and neurological disorders were queried. I think the next study, asking about infectious disease (ear infections, allergies, asthma, etc.), would be most telling.

For more information on the Generation Rescue study, go to: www.generationrescue.org.

MMR

JENNY: So now we are at a year in the shot schedule; what's going on there?

DR. JERRY: At a year, they get their mumps, measles, rubella, written as "MMR," and chicken pox (varicella) vaccine. That's four live viruses in one shot (ProQuad) or in two injections, the MMR being one, and the varicella being the second. Consider this: We are purposely injecting four live replicating viruses at one time directly into muscle tissue. The human body is usually exposed to viruses through the respiratory tree, specifically the nose or the mouth. There is a very complicated series of events that then involve antibodies IgG and IgA as other mechanisms that are designed to tag the offending agent for destruction. With injections, we actually inject the viruses right into their bloodstream via muscle tissue, thus completely circumventing the respiratory immune defenses. Now, if the immune system is compromised in any way, such as having real difficulties with recurrent infections, it may not be able to handle that set of four viruses that have been introduced in an artificial manner. These viruses will then be transported by lymph fluids and blood to their target tissue, where they will establish their infection.

It is interesting to note a study published by Dr. Andrew Wakefield in the *Lancet*, concerning a series of children who developed behavior symptoms (per the parents' report) following the mumps, measles, and rubella vaccine. All twelve children, who underwent endoscopy, were found to have intestinal abnormalities ranging from swollen lymph tissue (lymphoid-nodular hyperplasia), inflammation of the colon, and small sores (called aphthoid ulcerations). Dr. Wakefield suggested that there was an association of gastrointenstinal disease and developmental regression in previously normal children with a possible environmental trigger. Note, he did NOT suggest (at this time) that it was the MMR vaccine. It was the parents who associated that relationship.

Measles virus also appears to have a predilection to spinal fluid. Working with my previous partner, Dr. Bradstreet, we did a series of spinal taps in children with distinct regression following the MMR. We published these findings in the *Journal of American Physicians and Surgeons*, volume 9, number 2, Summer 2004: "Detection of Measles Virus Genomic RNA in Cerebral Spinal Fluid in Children with Regressive Autism: A Report of Three Cases."

We found that there was evidence of measles virus RNA in spinal fluid in the three cases and that there was a possibility of damage to the immune system (we called it immunopathology).

JENNY: I'd like you to reiterate that it's not just the MMR. A lot of people think, like I did when I told the doctor that I didn't want Evan to have the MMR because that's the autism shot, that it's not necessarily the case. It could be any shot that pushes your child over the toxic threshold.

DR. JERRY: I have plenty of children who seemed to have hit that "tipping point" at four months. They were doing great until their four- or six-month vaccines. Another scenario is that the child was doing great at six months, but somewhere between six months and nine months, the child stops developing normally and starts ever so slowly beginning to lose eye contact and withdraw. Parents notice subtle changes of not playing patty cake, not pointing, not having words, loss of eye contact, and changing patterns in sleep behavior. When brought to the attention of the pediatrician at the one-year well-baby exam (maybe not so well), these concerns are just "blown off." The MMR just seals the deal and all of a sudden, the child's issues become very obvious.

JENNY: And that's when the immune system begins to break down and can't rid itself of, let's say, the measles that were inside the MMR shot. It'll just kind of find itself a great host, called the gut.

DR. JERRY: The gut is a great host. And, we suspect now, the spinal fluid and the brain are also the hosts for some children, causing neurological problems.

JENNY: Okay, if a mom is going, "Well, I still want to get it," would you say wait at least until after two for that MMR? If you were to do it again?

DR. JERRY: We just don't know, Jenny. It may not be just a matter of timing. It may be the wrong intervention for the wrong child. Look, it does not matter when you give my wife a shot of penicillin, or if you "half" it. Her immune system is set up in a way that she will have such a severe reaction to it that she will die within five minutes of receiving it. The wrong medical intervention for a child can have a disastrous outcome.

JENNY: What if they separated the MMR shot? What if we get each component, the mumps by itself, the measles by itself, and the rubella by itself?

DR. JERRY: It sounds good, but I don't have any data to tell you that is any safer to do. We've had parents in our clinic who have split them up, and they ended up with an autistic kid. If you have the genetic predisposition, that's fine. But if you're exposed to the trigger, and it is pulled, you are going to get whatever comes out of the "genetic barrel." The more environmental triggers, the more disease we are going to see. The particular disease will be determined, of course, by your genetics. Some will do fine with the vaccines. Some will not. The question is: How do we identify the children who will not have a good outcome before the vaccines are given? I can tell you that may not be such a difficult screen. But, this screening device will not come into practice UNTIL the medical community realizes that vaccines can do real damage to some children.

PARENTS, DOCTORS, AND VACCINES

JENNY: I'm trying to arm parents with at least a couple of things, especially when they say, "My doctor won't budge." Can I tell them to at least demand spacing them out or not giving eight shots in one visit? I know you said there are no studies to prove that even doing that will prevent problems, but isn't it better than doing nothing?

DR. JERRY: Jenny, we just don't know. I don't want to give a parent a false sense of safety here. Even if you have one shot, there may be four vaccines in the "jab" along with a whole host of additives.

Why didn't you say in the first place? We could have used this new all-in-one vaccination rather than the traditional multiple injections. Oh well! We'll do it this way next year . . .
How about that!
Emma Hollister 2005

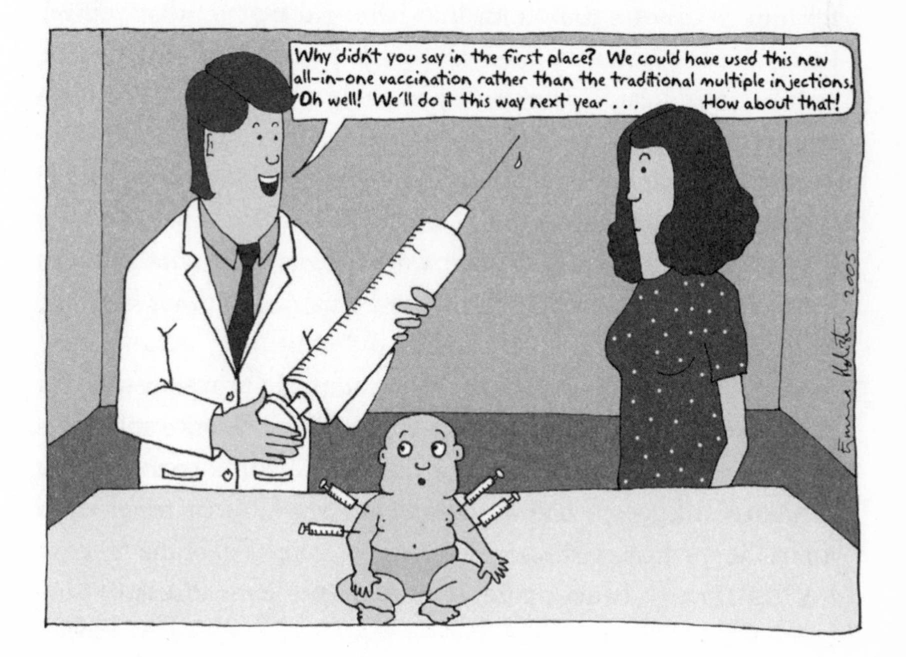

So we have parents, like you, who have been shouting, "There are too many shots." So the other side says, "Let's put more things in the shot, but we can tell the parents it's only one shot. It has twenty-five different things in it, but at least it's only one poke!"

JENNY: Why don't doctors report on reactions from vaccines?

DR. JERRY: Let's talk about a few things that are going on. First the DTP, the diphtheria, pertussis, and tetanus, that's three things, then polio's number four; and the hepatitis B is number five; and the haemophilus influenzae type B is number six. Pneumococcus and rotavirus make eight different "diseases." Then you have all the preservatives, adjuvants, and stabilizers. They are going to feel ill. They will have a fever. The shot sites will be hot, red, and painful. There will be crying, diarrhea, increased or decreased sleep, and possibly a rash. So when you call the pediatrician's office, all they can say is, "That is normal." A four-month-old girl in our city this year received her four-month shots at ten a.m., cried all day, was given Tylenol throughout the day per the physician, and by ten p.m., she died. All the pediatric office heard was "crying, fussy" and felt this was normal. Bottom line here: No matter what you tell them, the response would be, "That's to be expected." Another response I have heard: "They were just going to come down with that, anyway. They just happened to get vaccines that day."

JENNY: Or they're ignoring it. They know, and they just don't report it.

DR. JERRY: And the reason the pediatrician doesn't is because he's afraid if he admits fault, in other words, he gave the shot and now the kid's not doing well, then he can be named in the lawsuit. So instead, he insists, "I didn't see it, it didn't happen, I didn't document it, and so you can't hold me accountable or responsible for it." I have seen the medical records from other doctors' offices that do not record the mother's concerns in the medical record. As far as the record goes, whatever complaints were voiced never show up in the medical record.

JENNY: Let's pretend I'm a paranoid mom and feel like I have to at least get a couple of shots, just a couple. Which are the essential shots you would recommend to her?

DR. JERRY: For the really concerned mom who desires to vaccinate, but just with the most medically essential, I would first recommend the HIB shot to protect against the haemophilus influenzae bacterial infections—but only in the first year of life. Children are very susceptible to this disease the first year of life. So, if someone who is reading this has a two-year-old, this would not be as necessary. The second vaccine would be the tetanus shot, but there is little reason to administer it prior to two years of age.

JENNY: Hasn't the pertussis vaccine been linked to asthma and the HIB been linked to juvenile diabetes?

DR. JERRY: There are studies that suggest haemophilus influenzae type B to juvenile onset diabetes, and the pertussis vaccine with asthma.

JENNY: So the HIB and tetanus would be the only two you would recommend for moms still wanting to vaccinate. The other ones, you would say no.

DR. JERRY: That's correct.

JENNY: And if they want to give those, should they wait a little longer to give them?

DR. JERRY: The HIB vaccine can start at four months. Breast-feeding, if only for four to six weeks, can really help the child to remain disease-free. Breast-feeding longer just provides more protection. In the breast milk are antibodies that fight infection. You might think of this as a "temporary vaccine"! Now I know I made a lot of docs and researchers cringe when I said that . . . but lighten up, you know what I mean.

PREGNANCY WARNING SIGNS

JENNY: Are there any warning signs during pregnancy that would indicate a mom would have an autistic child?

DR. JERRY: Nothing I have seen yet. This supports the notion that these children were born normal, and were later damaged. There are many concerns shared by mothers. I have heard moms share concerns about premature delivery of infants: "We had premature babies and they have autism." Well, it wasn't the prematurity. I think it was getting vaccines at even a younger age, at a younger and a lighter birth weight (less "body" to distribute the vaccine load to). So I don't think it was the prematurity. I don't think it was the Pitocin, the epidural, the C-section, or the in-vitro fertilization. I really believe it is the sum total of all exposures working with their genetics to clear the toxins. If the toxins build up past a certain point, there will be repercussions.

JENNY: I've heard pediatricians say it's even more important to vaccinate if you have a preemie because they have a greater chance of developing these diseases.

DR: JERRY: And they are right, at least partially. I seriously doubt there is going to be a problem with polio or diphtheria. HIB? Yes. RSV? Yes. The only disease a preemie is going to be more susceptible to, in this country, would be the respiratory syncytial virus (RSV). Almost all children have had this disease by age two. It can be life-threatening in children with lung disease, and many preemies have chronic lung disease (from the breathing machine required to keep them alive). There is not a vaccine for RSV yet, but there is an antibody preparation that can be injected monthly (per physician recommendation) that will kill the virus should it enter the body.

FLU SHOTS

JENNY: Let's talk about the flu shots, which still contain mercury in a major way!

DR: JERRY: Let's talk about the flu shot. Every year the anticipated flu "epidemic" is the deadliest one ever and we will need to be hyper-vigilant and see that everyone gets his or her flu shot. Our elderly and children are going to die. Then, every year, for some reason, they publicize that there is a shortage of the flu vaccines.

JENNY: Always.

DR. JERRY: So what do Americans do whenever they hear there is a shortage?

JENNY: They line up around the block to make sure they get "theirs" before it all runs out.

DR. JERRY: And then every year, after the flu comes in, they'll say, "Well, you know, it's not quite the flu virus we anticipated!" They are then quick to add that the flu shots they sold everyone will have some effectiveness. You see, they're working right now on next year's flu, but they really don't know what strain it's going to be, so they're hoping there's going to be some cross-reactivity.

JENNY: The flu season starts in November or something like that, right?

DR. JERRY: It does tend to start in November and wrap up in March. Flu vaccines go on sale in September in order to get the antibody production well under way before the season actually hits.

JENNY: But in February I always hear the biggest advertisement to go get your flu shot. It's like they're trying to pawn off their supply. Don't they know by February that they got the wrong strain?

DR. JERRY: Absolutely. But they're already committed and they need to sell their flu shots so they can make their profits and fund next year's flu adventure.

Three-quarters of the flu shots available still have mercury in the form of thimerosal as a preservative.

JENNY: How do you not lose your mind? Because I'm losing mine. I mean, that's why I'm doing this. That's why I'm sitting here. It just makes me crazy why people don't get it. And I see those old people lining up around the block, and I'm thinking, "If Alzheimer's is associated with aluminum, what in the hell do you think that flu shot containing mercury is doing to Grandma?"

DR. JERRY: That's right. We just have to say no to flu shots as they are currently being made and marketed.

TITERS AND REVACCINATING

JENNY: I know we briefly touched on titers earlier, but I want you to explain to parents how it can be a good idea to test for titers instead of revaccinating.

DR. JERRY: Parents have said, "Look, he's going off to camp, we need to make sure his tetanus is good." Instead of just giving a tetanus shot again, we can draw some blood and see if there are still tetanus-fighting proteins called tetanus antibodies. The lab report is easy to read (the doctor will use the word "interpret") and either there are enough antibodies to protect a person, or there are not. A tetanus-"only" booster can be very hard to come by. It has sporadically been available, but it usually comes with the diphtheria, called a DT (diphtheria-tetanus) booster. Even if the diphtheria is not wanted, or even needed, you get it with your tetanus shot.

ALLERGIES AND VACCINES

JENNY: Do you think it's smart once the baby's born to immediately check for allergies of any sort?

DR. JERRY: Allergies are reactions of antibodies that the child creates to something outside the body. At birth, all the antibodies circulating in the child's body are derived from the mother. So allergy testing shortly after birth is not helpful. We can look at some of the genetics along with the family history and get some insight there. Allergy testing is all immune-based, and the newborn really is just a reflection of what was going on in the mother's immune system.

JENNY: Oh, so you won't see a true allergy test until when?

DR. JERRY: It depends on exposures. The earliest allergy that an infant can possess would be a cow's milk or even human milk allergy. So, shortly after birth, the infant is capable of making an immune response, and allergies may show up with different symptoms.

JENNY: Like what?

DR. JERRY: Some signs are really obvious. Red rings around the eyes, dark circles around the eyes, red ears, red cheeks, scaly rash or eczema, scales on the scalp, reflux, and vomiting.

JENNY: You just described Evan at two months old. I wish I could have read this book back then. I had no idea it was a warning. My pediatrician told me eczema was normal and to go buy some lotion. What an idiot. Please continue with other things a baby might show us that are warnings.

DR. JERRY: They can be colicky, irritable, poor sleepers, and quite often they're spitting up a lot! They may require constant motion to keep them happy (battery-powered swings, for example). Pediatricians might just say they are teething or it's normal to be colicky. How can you have twenty-four-hour-a-day colic? You can't. There's no such thing as twenty-four-hour-a-day colic, so it must be something different.

JENNY: I want to talk about the methylation tree and the autoimmune tree for a moment. These are amazing tools for parents to look at so they can if they have a family history of something from either tree.

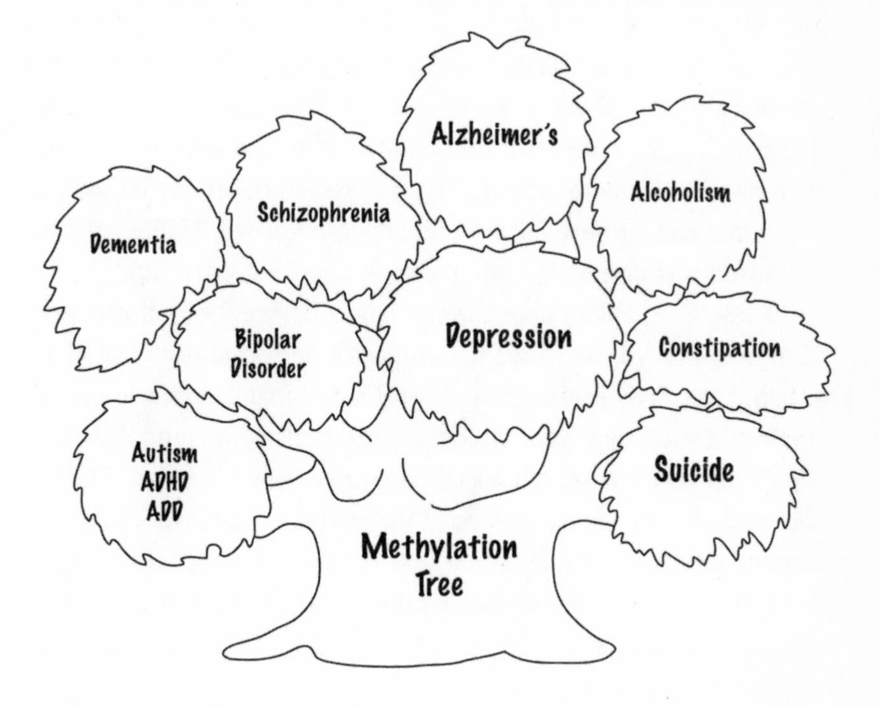

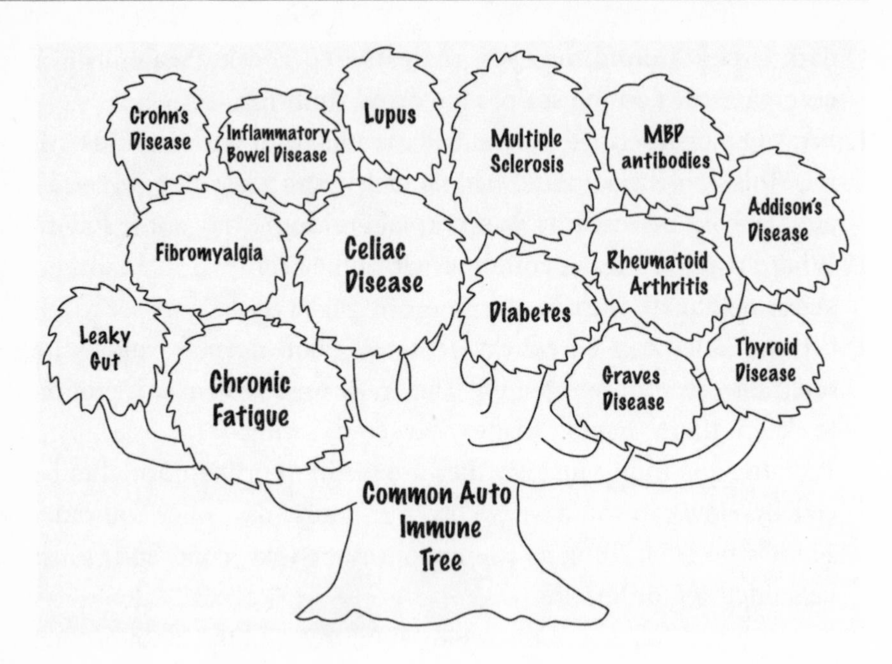

When I look at these two trees side by side I can clearly see where my family history of illness comes from. My dad has arthritis, my grandparents had diabetes. I came from the autoimmune tree. Looking back I wish I would have had this tree to look at as my warning that Evan might have a problem with detoxing and his immune system. When I showed this tree to my girlfriend, who also has a child with autism, she pointed to the methylation tree. Her dad had suffered from depression his whole life and her grandma was bipolar. These trees are your first warnings.

I know we talked about methylation before, but tell me again if there are any tests to see if a child is a poor methylator at birth?

DR. JERRY: Yes, we can do a genetic evaluation that can clearly demonstrate if a child may have difficulty with methylation, and thus trouble detoxifying the body. It doesn't require very much blood. This test will actually look and see which of the enzymes that drive the methylation pathway may be lacking. It has not been done yet to newborns. Everyone can be poisoned; just some are easier to poison than others.

JENNY: Well, you're damn right. If I heard that, I'd be out testing for it.

DR. JERRY: But I think we can get a lot of red flags from the family history, which is why those trees are so good for people to look at.

JENNY: So have you seen this family tree history thing come to life? I'm a firm believer after witnessing it with Evan and talking to other parents with kids with autism. They all belong to at least one tree.

DR. JERRY: There are distinct patterns that we can be alerted to in the family history. During my initial work-up of a child, I try to figure out which tree the autism came from (in some cases, both trees are heavily involved). In doing so, this will help me decide my treatment approach.

WARNING SIGNS TO STOP VACCINATING

JENNY: I know it might seem like I'm repeating myself a bit, but I just want this information to sink into everybody's head. Will you repeat some of the physical warning signs babies might exhibit that should make parents stop vaccinating?

DR. JERRY: These are some of the warning signs to stop vaccinating:

- Chronic ear infections
- Eczema
- Cradle cap
- Recurrent fevers
- Seizures
- Constipation
- Diarrhea
- Sleep issues
- Tantrums
- Lining up things
- Reclusiveness
- Transition issues
- Red ears
- Red cheeks
- Puffy eyes
- Poor growth

JENNY: Mercury poisoning is very similar to autism. Take a look at the side-by-side symptoms for mercury poisoning and autism. This came from www.generationrescue.org.

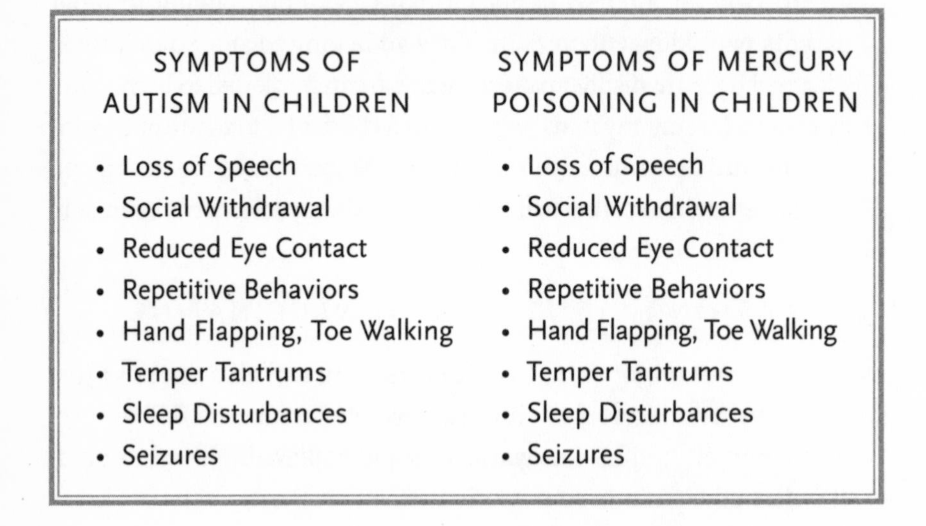

SYMPTOMS OF AUTISM IN CHILDREN	SYMPTOMS OF MERCURY POISONING IN CHILDREN
• Loss of Speech	• Loss of Speech
• Social Withdrawal	• Social Withdrawal
• Reduced Eye Contact	• Reduced Eye Contact
• Repetitive Behaviors	• Repetitive Behaviors
• Hand Flapping, Toe Walking	• Hand Flapping, Toe Walking
• Temper Tantrums	• Temper Tantrums
• Sleep Disturbances	• Sleep Disturbances
• Seizures	• Seizures

THE PREVENTION WINDOW

JENNY: What is the oldest normally developing child you have seen autistic behaviors come up?

DR. JERRY: I had a twelve-year-old girl who was developing normally after having a mild regression with the kindergarten shots. This mother knew that vaccines damaged her daughter at five years of age, albeit minimally. At the twelve-year-old checkup, it was time for her DTaP and flu shot. The next day, this twelve-year-old girl was rocking, had minimal language, and just reentered the nightmare of autism. Mom was crying, "I knew better. I shouldn't have done this."

JENNY: What do you do with a child who gets a wound, goes to the emergency room, and they want to give him a tetanus shot?

DR. JERRY: The child should have antibodies in the bloodstream to fight a potential tetanus infection. When you get a vaccine, any vaccine, it may take several weeks to induce antibody formation. It doesn't happen overnight. In other words, if you take somebody who's never had a tetanus shot before and he's twelve and you give him a tetanus shot today, you can't expect if you were to draw his blood the next day to see protective tetanus antibody titers. Now if we think that a child has a nasty wound that's tetanus-prone, he will probably need what's called a TIG shot, tetanus immune globulin. This shot will actually give the child antibodies right now to go after the tetanus infection that the wound may have been inoculated with. The problem with a TIG injection is that there is a little bit more of a chance of having an allergic reaction to it.

JENNY: So bottom line, it is going to boil down to each parent's individual choice of which, if any, vaccines that they want to have administered to their child. In the states of Mississippi and West Virginia, it is entirely up to the state government to decide for you. There are some very good books on the subject that go much further in detail than we could provide here. The parents should be forewarned that vaccines, just like any medication or medical procedure, can and do have some very significant side effects. Some of these side effects may possibly be predicted by looking at the family tree for methylation defects. Again, vaccines do have a number of additives, preservatives, and adjuvants that can also modify how a patient is going to react to them. There are published studies demonstrating abnormal immune responses to vaccines that are exactly like what we see in our clinics. First day of life vaccination for a disease that our children are not at risk for (hepatitis B) is asinine!

Coming up in a few pages I put a shot list from www.generationrescue.org. Take special note of the autism rate increase with the INSANE increase of vaccinations.

On the next page is a shot list that pediatricians SHOULD hand to parents for EACH shot that contains possible side effects. I'm always amazed that we have to hear the laundry list of side effects in commercials for every paramedical drug they push on TV but parents are left in the dark as to what MIGHT happen with each shot. Not anymore. Thanks again to Generation Rescue, I bring it to you!

* A list of all vaccines and their ingredients can be accessed at: http://www.cdc.gov/vaccines/vac-gen/additives.htm (Updated April 2008).

Pediatric Vaccine Ingredients and Possible Side Effects		
Vaccines **by multiple manufacturers**	**Ingredients*** **partial list in one or more vaccines**	**Side Effects**** **including a partial list of reactions, events & reports***
DTaP (Diphtheria, Tetanus, Toxiods, and Acellular Pertussis) Vaccine Absorbed	Aluminum Phosphate, Ammonium Sulfate, Aluminum Potassium Sulfate, thimerosal [a vaccine preservative that is approximately 50% mercury by weight] Formaldehyde or Formalin, Glutaraldehyde, 2-Phenoxyethanol, Dimethyl-betacyclodextrin, Sodium Phosphate, Polysorbate 80.	Autism, fever, anorexia, vomiting, pneumonia, meningitis, sepsis, pertussis, convulsions, febrile, grand mal, afebrile and partial seizures, encephalopathy, brachial neuritis, Guillain-Barré syndrome, sudden infant death syndrome.
DTaP/HepB/IPV Combination Vaccine, Diphtheria and Tetanus Toxoids and Acellular Pertussis Adsorbed, Hepatitis B (Recombinant) and Inactivated Poliovirus Vaccine Combined	Aluminum Hydroxide, Aluminum Phosphate, Formaldehyde or Formalin, Glutaraldehyde, Monkey Kidney Tissue, Neomycin, 2-Phenoxyethanol, Polymyxin B, Polysorbate 80, Antibiotics, Yeast Protein.	Seizures, diabetes mellitus, asthma, sudden infant death syndrome, upper respiratory tract infection, abnormal liver function tests, anorexia, jaundice, shock, encephalopathy, Stevens-Johnson syndrome, brachial neuritis.
Flu Vaccine Influenza Virus Vaccine	Thimerosal [a preservative that is approximately 50% mercury by weight], Chick Kidney Cells, Egg Protein, Gentamicin Sulfate, Antibiotics, Monosodium Glutamate [MSG], Sucrose Phosphate Glutamate Buffer.	Significant respiratory and gastrointestinal symptoms, seizure, allergic asthma, decreased appetite, increased mitochondrial encephalomyopathy, partial facial paralysis, Guillain-Barré syndrome, Bell's palsy, Stevens-Johnson syndrome, herpes zoster [shingles].

Vaccines by multiple manufacturers	Ingredients* partial list in one or more vaccines	Side Effects** including a partial list of reactions, events & reports*
HepB Vaccine	Aluminum Hydroxyphosphate Sulfate, Amino Acids, Dextrose, Phosphate Buffers, Potassium Aluminum Sulfate, Formaldehyde or Formalin, Mineral Salts, Soy Peptone, Yeast Protein	Influenza, febrile seizure, anorexia, upper respiratory tract illnesses, herpes zoster, encephalitis, palpitations, arthritis, systemic lupus erthematosus (SLE), conjunctivitis, abnormal liver function tests, Guillain-Barré syndrome, Bell's palsy, multiple sclerosis, anaphylaxis, seizures.
HIB Vaccine Haemophilus b Conjugate Vaccine (Tetanus Toxoid Conjugate)	Ammonium Sulfate, Formaldehyde or Formalin, Sucrose.	Anorexia, seizures, renal failure, Guillain-Barré syndrome (GBS), diarrhea, vomiting.
HIB/HepB Vaccine (Recombinant) Haemophilus b Conjugate (Meningococcal Protein Conjugate) and Hep B	Aluminum Hydroxyphosphate Sulfate, Formaldehyde or Formalin, Sodium Borate, Soy Peptone, Yeast Protein, Amino Acids, Dextrose, Mineral Salts.	Anorexia, seizure, otitis media [ear infection], upper respiratory infection, oral candidasis [yeast infection], anaphylaxis [shock].
HIB/Meningococcal [Haemophilus b Conjugate Vaccine (Meningococcal Protein Conjugate)]	Aluminum Hydroxyphosphate Sulfate, Formaldehyde or Formalin, Phosphate Buffers.	Febrile seizures, early onset HIB disease, otitis media [ear infection], upper respiratory infection, Guillain-Barré syndrome.
MMR Vaccine Measles, Mumps, and Rubella Virus Vaccine Live	Chick Embryo Fibroblasts, Amino Acids, Bovine Albumin or Serum, Human Serum Albumin, Antibiotics, Glutamate, Phosphate Buffers, Gelatin, Sorbitol, Sucrose, Vitamins.	Atypical measles, arthritis, encephalitis, death, aseptic meningitis, nerve deafness, otitis media [ear infection].

Vaccines by multiple manufacturers	**Ingredients* partial list in one or more vaccines**	**Side Effects** including a partial list of reactions, events & reports***
Pneumococcal Pneumococcal 7-valent Conjugate Vaccine (Diphtheria CRM197 Protein)	Aluminum Phosphate, Yeast Extract, Amino Acids, Soy Peptone.	Febrile seizure, sudden infant death, anaphylactoid reaction including shock, decreased appetite.
Poliovirus Vaccine (IPV) Poliovirus Vaccine Inactivated	2-Phenoxyethanol, Formaldehyde or Formalin, Monkey Kidney Tissue, Newborn Calf Serum Protein, Antibiotics, Neomycin, Polymyxin B, Streptomycin.	Death, anorexia, Guillain-Barré syndrome.
Chicken Pox (Varicella) Virus Vaccine	Ethylenediamine-Tetracetic Acid Sodium (EDTA) [a metals chelation agent], Bovine Albumin or Serum, Antibiotics, Monosodium Glutamate [MSG], MRC-5 DNA and Cellular Protein, Neomycin, Potassium Chloride, Potassium Phosphate Monobasic, Sodium Phosphate Monobasic, Sucrose.	Febrile seizures, encephalitis, varicella-like rash, upper respiratory illness, lower respiratory illness, eczema, encephalitis, facial edema, cold/canker sores, aseptic meningitis, Guillain-Barré syndrome, Bell's palsy, pneumonia, secondary bacterial infections.

Downloaded Nov. 08 from: www.generationrescue.org/vaccine_information/
A partial ingredient list from Vaccine Excipient & Media Summary, Part 2, Excipients included in U.S. Vaccines, by Vaccine from:
www.cdc.gov/vaccines/pubs/pinkbook/downloads/appendices/B/excipient-table-2.pdf
**This list contains a combination of many adverse post-vaccination occurrences, and possible occurrences, that have been published in the manufacturers' documents. Any use of [brackets] is information added by the author. This list may not contain all the adverse occurrences; it may contain typographical errors, and obviously does not take the place of reading the most current manufacturer's document in its entirety.
The chart on the next page shows the amount of thimerosal and/or mercury that is in all the vaccines (pediatric and adult). This was updated in March 2008 and can be viewed at:
www.fda.gov/cber/vaccine/Thimerosal.htm#t3

Thimerosal and Expanded List of Vaccines (updated 3/14/2008)
Thimerosal Content in Currrently Manufactured U.S. Licensed Vaccines

Vaccine	Trade Name	Manufacturer	Thimerosal Concentration[1]	Mercury
Anthrax	Anthrax Vaccine	BioPort Corporation	0	0
DTaP	Tripedia[2]	Sanofi Pasteur, Inc	≤0.00012%	≤0.3 µg/0.5 ml dose
	Infanrix	GlaxoSmithKline Biologicals	0	0
	Daptacel	Sanofi Pasteur, Ltd	0	0
DTaP-HepB-IPV	Pediarix	GlaxoSmithKline Biologicals	0	0
DT	No Trade Name	Sanofi Pasteur, Inc	≤0.00012% (single dose)	≤0.3 µg/0.5 ml dose
		Sanofi Pasteur, Ltd[3]	0.01%	25 µg/0.5 ml dose
Td	No Trade Name	Mass Public Health	0.0033%	8.3 µg/0.5 ml dose
	Decavac	Sanofi Pasteur, Inc	≤0.00012%	≤ 0.3 µg mercury/0.5 ml dose
	No Trade Name	Sanofi Pasteur, Ltd	0	0
Tdap	Adacel	Sanofi Pasteur, Ltd	0	0
	Boostrix	GlaxoSmithKline Biologicals	0	0
TT	No Trade Name	Sanofi Pasteur, Inc	0.01%	25 µg/0.5 ml dose
Hib	ActHIB/OmniHIB[4]	Sanofi Pasteur, SA	0	0
	HibTITER	Wyeth Pharmaceuticals, Inc	0	0
	PedvaxHIB Liquid	Merck & Co, Inc	0	0
Hib/HepB	COMVAX[5]	Merck & Co, Inc	0	0

Vaccine	Trade Name	Manufacturer	Thimerosal Concentration[1]	Mercury
Hepatitis B	Engerix-B Pediatric/adolescent Adult	GlazoSmithKline Biologicals	 0 0	 0 0
	Recombivax HB Pediatric/adolescent Adult (adolescent) Dialysis	Merck & Co, Inc	 0 0 0	 0 0 0
Hepatitis A	Havrix	GlaxoSmithKline Biologicals	0	0
	Vaqta	Merck & Co, Inc	0	0
HepA/HepB	Twinrix	GlaxoSmithKline Biologicals	<0.0002%	<1 µg/1 ml dose
IPV	IPOL	Sanofi Pasteur, SA	0	0
	Poliovax	Sanofi Pasteur, Ltd	0	0
Influenza	Afluria	CSL Limited	0 (single dose) 0.01% (multi-dose)	0/0.5 ml (single dose) 24.5 µg/0.5 ml (multidose)
	Fluzone[6]	Sanofi Pasteur, Inc	0.01%	25 µg/0.5 ml dose
	Fluvirin	Novartis Vaccines and Diagnostics Ltd	0.01%	25 µg/0.5 ml dose
	Fluzone (no thimerosal)	Sanofi Pasteur, Inc	0	0
	Fluvirin (Preservative Free)	Novartis Vaccines and Diagnostics Ltd	<0.0004%	<1 µg/0.5 ml dose
	Fluarix	GlaxoSmithKline Biologicals	<0.0004%	<1 µg/0.5 ml dose
	FluLaval	ID Biomedical Corporation of Quebec	0.01%	25 µg/0.5 ml dose
Influenza, live	FluMist	MedImmune Vaccines, Inc	0	0

Vaccine	Trade Name	Manufacturer	Thimerosal Concentration[1]	Mercury
Japanese Encephalitis[7]	JE-VAX	Research Foundation for Microbial Diseases of Osaka University	0.007%	35 µg/1.0ml dose 17.5 µg/0.5 ml dose
MMR	MMR-II	Merck & Co, Inc	0	0
Meningococcal	Menomune A, C, AC and A/C/Y/W-135	Sanofi Pasteur, Inc	0.01% (multi-dose) 0 (single dose)	25 µg/0.5 ml dose
	Menactra A, C, Y and W-135	Sanofi Pasteur, Inc	0	0
Pneumococcal	Prevnar (Pneumo Conjugate)	Wyeth Pharmaceuticals Inc	0	0
	Pneumovax 23	Merck & Co, Inc	0	0
Rabies	IMOVAX	Sanofi Pasteur, SA	0	0
	Rabavert	Novartis Vaccines and Diagnostics	0	0
Smallpox (Vaccinia), Live	ACAM2000	Acambis, Inc	0	0
Typhoid Fever	Typhim Vi	Sanofi Pasteur, SA	0	0
	Vivotif	Berna Biotech, Ltd	0	0
Varicella	Varivax	Merck & Co, Inc	0	0
Yellow Fever	Y-F-Vax	Sanofi Pasteur, Inc	0	0

1. Thimerosal is approximately 50% mercury (Hg) by weight. A 0.01% solution (1 part per 10,000) of thimerosal contains 50 × of Hg per 1 ml dose or 25 × of Hg per 0.5 ml dose.
2. Sanofi Pasteur's Tripedia may be used to reconstitute ActHib to form TriHIBit. TriHIBit is indicated for use in children 15 to 18 months of age.
3. This vaccine is not marketed in the US.
4. OmniHIB is manufactured by Sanofi Pasteur but distributed by GlaxoSmithKline.
5. COMVAX is not licensed for use under 6 weeks of age because of decreased response to the Hib component.
6. Children under 3 years of age receive a half-dose of vaccine, i.e., 0.25 ml (12.5 × mercury/dose.)
7. JE-VAX is distributed by Aventis Pasteur. Children 1 to 3 years of age receive a half-dose of vaccine, i.e., 0.05 ml (17.5 × mercury/dose).

The rate of autism increased with the increase of vaccinations. Do we really need this many?

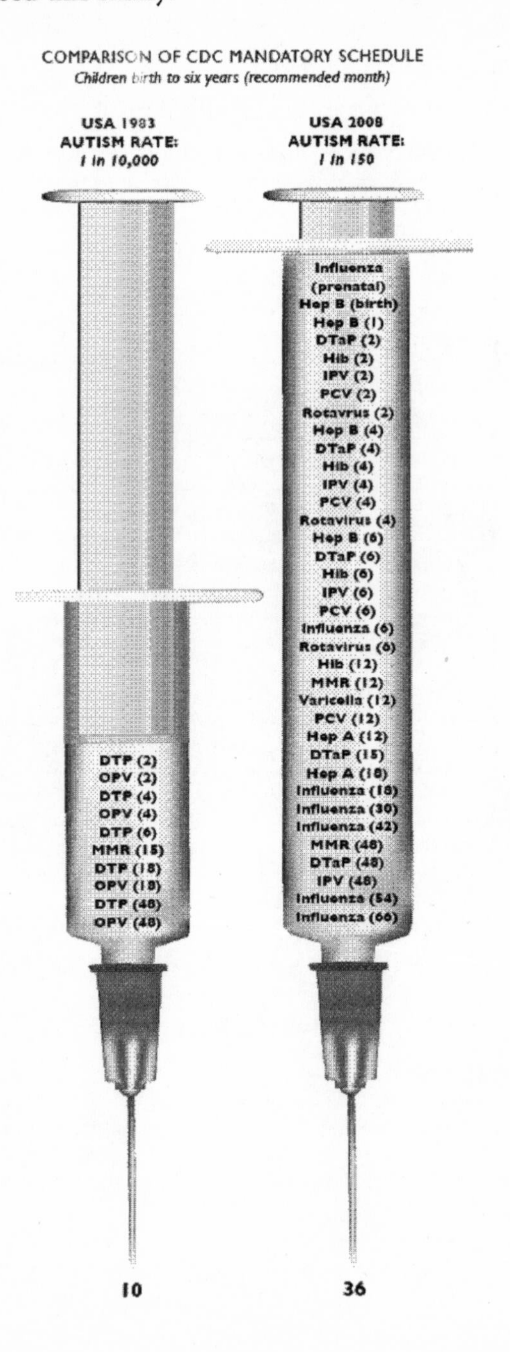

Reading List

The Vaccine Book, by Robert W. Sears, M.D., F.A.A.P.
Evidence of Harm, by David Kirby
A Shot in the Dark, by Harrison Coulter and Barbara Loe Fisher
What Your Doctor May NOT Tell You About Children's Vaccinations, by Stephanie Cave, M.D.

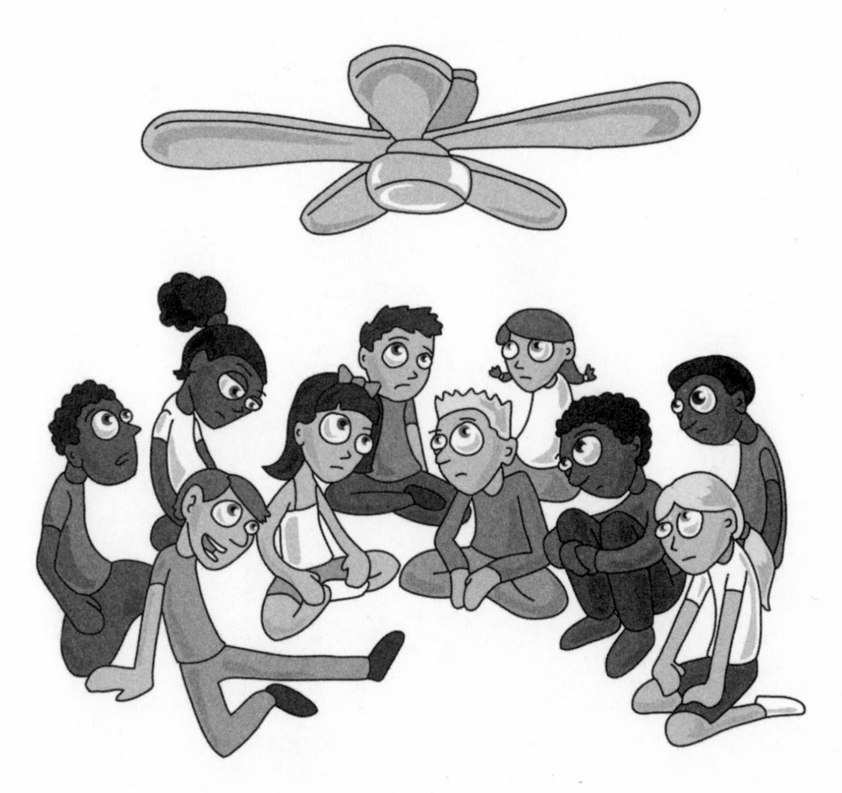

Vaccine Injured

17
RECOVERY

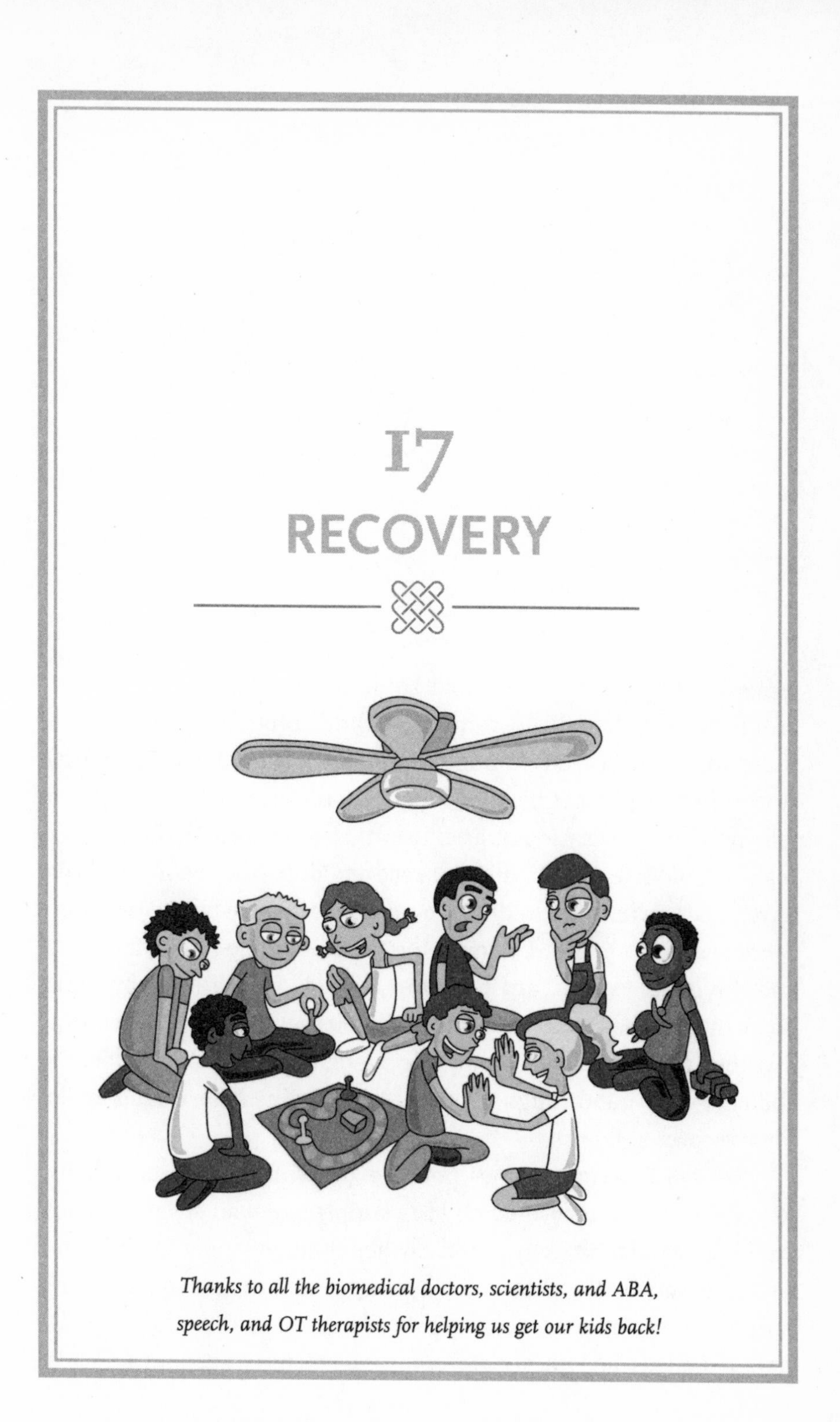

Thanks to all the biomedical doctors, scientists, and ABA, speech, and OT therapists for helping us get our kids back!

"Recovery" is a word that some parents have heard floating around within the autism community and some may not have. For those who have heard it, it might seem like a word that doesn't exist. A word that is just not possible when it comes to autism. I'm here to tell you that recovery is not an illusion. It is not a myth. Recovery is real. I would like to reiterate that recovery does not mean cured. We have no idea what our children would have been like before they were overloaded with toxins. I've used the "bus" example from Stan Kurtz and I'm going to use it again. Picture these kids getting hit by a bus. You can't say they were cured from the bus accident but you can say that they recovered from the bus accident. They might have lost the ability to walk, but through therapies they regained those skills again. They recovered them.

The word "recovery" does not have one simple definition. Some parents' idea of a recovered child is simply one who sleeps through the night. Another parent would say her child no longer qualified for any more services from the state by the age of four and considers her son recovered. Another mom might call her son recovered because he just integrated into typical classrooms but still has a shadow, a trace of odd behaviors that maybe only those closest to him would notice. Whatever the definition may be, the fact is, these kids can get better. And as we all know by now, some of them are what Dr. Jerry calls the lotto winners of autism, and others will have a much longer journey.

THE MEANING OF RECOVERY

JENNY: Many people in the media have mistaken the word "recovered" for "cured."

DR. JERRY: We look at each individual problem our children have. They can come in with a history of problems that include diarrhea, constipation, reflux, and immune system dysfunction. Can these complaints be cured or at least managed? Yes, and as physicians, it is our duty to. The medical community cannot be satisfied with allowing children to suffer with these diseases. They would not tolerate it in a child with cystic fibrosis, for example. But if the child comes in with the same problems but with the label "autistic," then it is okay to not treat. I don't think so.

JENNY: So the comorbid conditions can be cured. "Comorbid" meaning the conditions that exist sometimes with autism, such as candida, inflammatory bowel disease, and those types of things.

DR. JERRY: Autistic behaviors improve tremendously when infections are treated and metabolic and immune dysfunctions are addressed.

JENNY: And that is why we are seeing some of our children recover. Once we got rid of Evan's candida, he began to speak in conversations—candida being Evan's comorbid condition.

DR. JERRY: Most parents who use the word "recovered" actually do have children who are indistinguishable from their peer group. They may have certain quirks or oddities in their mannerisms, but for all intents and purposes, they no longer could be diagnosed with "autism." In fact, I had one mom tell me, "He is no longer autistic but is quirky just like Dad. Can you fix it?" I said, "No, you married Dad and he is *quirky*, now the rest is genetics!" So the children can be quirky but they can be indistinguishable from their peers.

MANAGED RECOVERY

JENNY: I've heard some parents talk about managed recovery. I consider Evan to be one of those. Can you explain it nicely?

DR. JERRY: "Managed recovery" is a term I use to explain the concept of requiring continued medical care in order to continue the gains made. In contrast, when the supplements are stopped or interrupted, the children regress. Another scenario may demonstrate a child who regresses every spring due to allergies. This springtime regression may include a return of obsessive-compulsive behaviors, an increase in impulsivity and loss of focus, or a return of clouded thinking. So these children require continued special diets, supplements, and medical management in order to maintain their higher functioning status. They can be so fragile that if allergies or a cold comes along, they will exhibit a dip in their performance. In addition, as we mentioned, they still may have some quirks that require some ironing out. Very often, as these children emerge from the autism, they commonly find themselves exhibiting one, two, or even three maladies that must be addressed: obsessive and compulsive behaviors accompanied by anxiety, attention and focus difficulties often accompanied with a hyperactivity component, and behaviors consistent with Tourette's syndrome. What this amounts to is some funny or quirky mannerisms.

JENNY: As in Evan's case, he wants to eat with his shoes on all of the time.

DR. JERRY: These children can demonstrate an endless number of behavioral variations. We can deal with them. At least now our children are learning, communicating, and they are enjoying life! It is a wonderful experience to see these children enjoying interacting with other children, whereas previously they had no regard for them at all.

JENNY: Is anyone ever completely satisfied? Do any parents of recovered patients say, "Doc, he's perfect, bye-bye!"

DR. JERRY: Parents always want more. So my job is never done. I have parents who say, "I'm really embarrassed at taking your time. I know there are a lot of kids out there who are far worse than my kid and I'm really embarrassed being here." And then I get the big "But . . ."

JENNY: BUT . . . I want more.

DR. JERRY: The bottom line is: Do we have previously autistic children who are now neurotypical and indistinguishable from their peers requiring no more medical management? Yes. Do we have children who are neurotypical and indistinguishable from their peers but continue to require medical management—in other words, do we have them on a lot of stuff to keep them on target? Yes. Do we have kids who are spending half the time in regular school and half the time in their special ed rooms? Do we have kids who are now sleeping through the night, potty trained, and more or less functioning like a five-year-old? Yes. Are the parents thrilled? Absolutely, because you look at where the starting point was—these children were incredibly difficult to manage. Some parents, in their "honest" moments, confided in me that there were times that they just wanted to drop-kick the child from here to the next county. Some parents may gasp when they hear this, but do not rush to pass judgment. Some of these children exhibited behaviors that are so violent that they even intimidate police.

JENNY: Is there hope for all kids? Even the ones who were hit hard?

DR. JERRY: Absolutely! I'm not done yet and thank God the physicians and researchers who work with these children are not done yet either. I think one of the reasons that my son is not totally recovered is to force me to keep looking. I'm not done with a lot of other people's children either. Just because they have not yet fully recovered does not mean we ever stop looking. Our goal in medicine must be to bring about as much restoration as possible.

JENNY: I know we talked about your son in the beginning of the book, but now that people got to know you more throughout this book, can you talk a little bit about where your son was and how far he came? What's actually left for you to try and recover?

DR. JERRY: Okay, In January 1996, our fourth son, Joshua, was born. Again, Josh was a full-term baby. Of course he received his vaccines, hep B at birth, followed by his hep B at one month, polio and DPT at two months, polio and DPT at five months, hep B, polio, and DPT at eight months. His growth and development the first year were typical and he met the basic milestones: rolling over, sitting, standing, playing with toys. At two months old Josh had double-hernia surgery. He then required numerous antibiotics for frequent ear infections. He developed fevers of no known origin and required a spinal tap to rule out meningitis at four months of age. Also at four months he developed bronchiolitis followed by pneumonia and an ear infection. Through these infections, he babbled and cooed, made great eye contact, and loved being with people. He was one of those babies everyone loved because he was so personable. His first Christmas (1996) followed closely by his first birthday (1/97) were memorable. He enjoyed presents, helped to open them, and smiled when he saw what he received! Shortly after his first birthday Josh began to walk and pointed well. However, he still had no words, only babbling. We even wondered if he was speaking a different language! The only "language" he developed was a particular quack, like a duck. He continued to play well with toys, look at books, and he loved to "read" books. At this point Josh had received all of the typical vaccinations and it was now time for his MMR. Again, I administered it to him.

Following that, we saw a gradual decline in his connectedness to the world around him, yet he was still doing some typical things, like trying to ride his tricycle at his second birthday. He could only ride backward, which his older brothers thought was funny. July 1997, Josh received his DTP and HIB vaccines. In November 1997 we moved into a brand-new home, new carpet, paint, and all the cabinets were constructed from pressboard. All, of course, were off-gassing and we didn't even know it! From then on, he slowly slipped completely into a self-interested autistic world. He was addicted to videos, "reading" the video jackets to pick out the right one. Then he would get stuck on watching one video over and over again. He would also act out the videos but he still had no language and even lost his babbling. His eating habits also declined, becoming severely self-limiting, preferring French fries, bacon, Fruit Loops, cookies, and a gallon of milk a day. He also quit using his silverware. At dinnertime he would quickly eat what he wanted and then spend the rest of dinnertime running around our island in the kitchen. He started lining up toys or objects, becoming very obsessive about how things were arranged. If one of his brothers moved an item, he would scream, throwing a major fit. His toxic load obviously became more than his little body could handle!

By Josh's second Christmas (1997), things were very different. He no longer had any interest in his presents or what we were all doing. He sat on the tile floor with our German shepherd, looking very detached. Donna ended up opening all of his presents, showing them all to him, but he had no interest. He received a Brio train set and table and all he wanted to do was sit on the table and throw the trains off of it. This became a big part of his life. He would tear things apart, throw toys especially down the stairs, and he dumped toys out of buckets. He seemed to like many things in disarray except his special toys.

On Josh's second birthday (1998), the only thing he enjoyed was blowing out the candles, which we had to relight numerous times. At this point he was very difficult to take places because he would no longer sit still and if he didn't get his way, he would scream and fuss. We would have to bribe him with Tic Tacs, which he would chew, not suck. We were constantly dispensing them in order to keep Josh from dropping to the floor and crawling under chairs at restaurants. During this time he also became a wanderer. He would open the door and leave, actually run off. We had to install extra locks on all of the doors and the boys had to be very careful when they left the house. Josh then began stacking the couch cushions and wanted to lie under them. He would also constantly play in the dog's water no matter how many times we removed him. He would only laugh at any punishment that was dealt him. He was also oblivious to pain and could walk on hot concrete in bare feet without discomfort. Josh then began having aversions to things like stickers, trimming of his fingernails, anything gooey, including Play-Doh, washing hair, etc.

We knew something was seriously wrong with Josh. We had used all of the excuses: youngest of four children, we moved, etc. . . . I finally figured out what was wrong with Joshua. He had autism. It was difficult to share with others, as it was still not very common. It was difficult to take Josh places because people would look at us like, "Why can't you control your kid!" At times, Donna wanted to hang a sign on Josh announcing that he was autistic and to please understand the difficulties that this incorporates.

Now, at age twelve, Josh is an absolute joy to be with. He is very independent and speaks in sentences. In full onset of puberty there are no behavioral problems. He is compliant and willing to please. We still struggle with recovering mental capacity and that is the next area of research I am going to explore.

POSSIBILITIES OF RECOVERY

JENNY: What percentage of your practice would you say you saw kids recovered?

DR. JERRY: Now we are talking about recovery that involves mainstream academics and social skills adequate for developing friendships. I think when you look at our kids a good 20 percent recover, but many are heavily managed with supplements and diets. About 5 percent recover entirely and require nothing more than a daily vitamin and some omega-3 fatty acids.

JENNY: That's so great.

DR. JERRY: I consider recovery to mean that the diagnosis of autism no longer applies to a child. They may have attention deficit disorder now, but not autism. Then, if we were to send the child to a neurologist, after a battery of testing, he would not be able to say the child has autism. I'd say 20 to 25 percent of our kids will eventually meet (or already have met) that goal.

JENNY: Wow.

DR. JERRY: I would probably say the next 30 percent of our children who undergo these interventions will have a much milder form of autism. These children tend to be an absolute joy to be with and there are very few negatives. They sleep well, enjoy school, and are well behaved, but their daily struggles include activities that require reading, math, and abstract thought. These children will be perceived as quirky. Many will get through school with a combination of medical interventions and multiple therapeutic interventions. They will always see things in a different way. And I celebrate them because they're going to visualize and experience our world differently and, in turn, teach *us*.

The next 20 percent or so of our children have a full grasp of eating, sleeping, toilet hygiene, and have adequate muscle tone and strength. There are obvious deficits with what I often refer to as "motor" systems: speech, math, language, and movement of gross and fine motor muscles. For example, some children have "hand motors" that do not work very well. They have trouble with buttoning or holding a pencil. They may not write well. In school, teachers tend to focus on writing. Instead of forcing them to spend so much time trying to write with broken "motors," we may have to think outside the box and allow them to write with a keyboard. The next thing we see is, not only are they able to type their names, but can start communicating with us.

Then there are about 20 percent of the kids who are still pretty tough. We've done the gluten-free, the dairy-free, the soy-free, and the corn-free diet. We've given them vitamins, minerals, and oils. We've worked on their yeast. We've worked on their allergies. We've worked on their immune system, and they're still just struggling. Jenny, you met Mary (not her real name) here at our office the other day and you could see her processing is still very slow. I tell her parents it's like she's got an old 386 computer processor trying to operate in the Pentium 5 world. She can process, but it just takes her a little longer. You can just see it in her eyes as she beckons you for patience.

JENNY: She was very sweet. How old was Mary?

DR. JERRY: She is thirteen and a half.

JENNY: I could tell she has a boy crush on your older son.

DR. JERRY: Oh, my—yes! These young teens have all of the feelings associated with puberty. She's an emerging young lady. She has all of the feelings and hopes and ambitions of a neurotypical girl.

VISIONS FOR THE FUTURE

JENNY: What is that dating world going to look like in a few years when this autism generation grows up?

DR. JERRY: We will have to be very careful. These teens are very trusting and truthful. Most (I said *most*) will not recognize deceit, danger, or understand consequences of behaviors (that covers most teens!).

JENNY: Isn't that interesting to think about?

DR. JERRY: Yes. I'm really concerned because there are only a few of us doctors biomedically working to get these children to function at their very best. The number of untreated children with autism is staggering. I'm worried about all the children who are severe, who are not getting biomedical treatment and are entering their teens. Some are very violent; they have untreated medical conditions that can be very painful. The parents are not going to be able to manage them at some point in their teens. We have no facilities for them.

JENNY: I know; it terrifies me.

DR. JERRY: This will be my opus. I want to build a model facility for the teens and adults who are not recovered. The kitchen will provide the specific diet each child requires. Supplements will be the major constituent of "medications," and only as a last resort will pharmaceutical agents be prescribed. Now we will have to keep this community active and those who can will tend the organic gardens, obtaining fresh produce for the kitchen. Others will be working in "housekeeping" using organic cleaning materials. Those who are my "TV guys" will be able to do that as well. Keeping them safe in this world will be the utmost priority. I hope that I'll be rocking in a chair out here taking care of them when I'm seventy-five and still tending to their supplements. We can make this community into a "blueprint" that can be replicated all over the country.

JENNY: You took the words right out of my mouth. When I have "Oprah" money, that's exactly what I plan on doing. I will be rocking in the rocking chair next to you because I'm going to build it for you someday.

DR. JERRY: I believe you. When you look at someone like Mary, what's going to happen to her? Someday her parents will not be able to care for her any longer. A facility like this will be a fabulous answer.

RECOVERY IN OLDER KIDS

JENNY: Let's talk a little bit more about recovery. I talked about there being a window of time to heal your child. I was clearly wrong about that, correct?

DR. JERRY: Can eight-, ten-, and twelve-year-olds recover? Yes.

JENNY: How about the severe ones?

DR. JERRY: Severe ones are tough. The older they are, the more medications they have been on. They can be very difficult. I saw Justin a few days ago. He is twenty years old and his mom and dad took him out of residential care because they wanted to give him one more chance. Here was his drug list last Monday:

Clonazepam 1 mg twice daily
Depakote 500 mg twice daily
Abilify 20 mg once daily
Paxil 20 mg once daily
Luvox 100 mg twice daily

I definitely have my work cut out for me! These drugs are "the big guns" that have some very severe potential side effects and can prove to be very difficult to wean. If I can get this young man off medications, find the source of his rages, I can bring him back home permanently and he may be able to complete his education and find work. Recovery may not be possible at this point, but marked improvement in his life quality is a distinct possibility.

The oldest we had in our clinic was a thirty-year-old man who was living in a group home. We started some interventions, and he came back in two weeks and thanked us because he had been waiting his whole life to talk. You can actually talk to some of the kids who will tell you what it's like not being able to talk. They have all of the thoughts in their head but until we do something, they can't get the thoughts out. And then they can say, "Thank you for allowing me to talk. I've been waiting to talk."

JENNY: How does that make you feel when they say that to you?

DR. JERRY: Oh, I love it. Does he still have to live in a group home? Yes. But at least now he can communicate. We have, as human beings, a tremendous need to talk.

WHAT DOES AUTISM FEEL LIKE?

JENNY: Evan just said to me recently, "Remember when I couldn't talk?" I said, "Yes, I do! Why couldn't you?" He said, "I don't know, I just couldn't get my words out." What do you think autism feels like? I always feel like—have you ever seen those movies where they say, "I'm buried alive" or "They were doing surgery on me and I was awake and couldn't speak"?

DR. JERRY: This is what continues to push the drive forward to figure out if we are doing everything we can for each child. Each system has to be examined thoroughly. It is amazing to see how illness in one part of the body (such as allergies or constipation) affects the brain. The brain is a fantastic system of electrical potentials and chemical neurotransmitters that are, indeed, affected by chemicals. As we know, alcohol can influence a whole variety of behaviors (some good, some not so good) and motor responses. Language continues to be a very difficult operation to start up in some children. I remember when my son was still in his screaming mode and I was trying to figure out "Are you hungry or what?" I'd hold him up and say, "Look, I'll give you anything you want, son. I'll move mountains, but you have to communicate with me. I don't know what you're telling me. I don't know what you want." Sometimes I'd say, "Well, he probably doesn't even know what he wants." But I absolutely think they do.

JENNY: Oh, absolutely, I think they do, too!

DR. JERRY: They know what they want; they just have tremendous difficulty communicating their thoughts. I think sometimes they're in such a state of frustration, that anxiety levels build so high, they just lose control of themselves. They're just screaming at the world.

HOPE OR FALSE HOPE

JENNY: Do you think you can give some words of advice to parents who are still wondering if we are giving false hope?

DR. JERRY: Well, there's no such thing as false hope. We all hope. We do cancer therapy not because it's false hope but because we're hoping that we're in the statistics that show recovery. As parents, our job is always to hope for the best for our kids. We always try to facilitate the life opportunities such as sports, academics, learning about life, or even teaching a teen how to drive. Autism is no different. Our job is to say, "How can I bring the best of academics to the child's world? How can I teach him to speak? What are the best interventions?" That's not false. That's being a parent.

JENNY: For the most part, whether it be diet or any of the other treatments you do, do you see at least a little improvement even in the hard, hard cases?

DR. JERRY: I haven't had a child who hasn't improved. The parents come in with a wish list and say, "Look, here are five things that need to happen." Usually on the top of the list is he needs to sleep the whole night. Number two is, he needs to not be in pain. Number three is, he needs to calm down. He is just running around the house nonstop from 7:30 in the morning until he drops literally at 10:30 or 11:00 at night. He is constantly on the go. Those are probably my top three things that have to stop. Number four would be he needs to not be sick all of the time.

And those are easy to fix. Oh, I have to apply some screws. I try to do things as naturally as possible, but sometimes I have to reach into my M.D. tool chest and say look, we need to put the child on this particular medicine. His body needs to be retrained how to sleep every night. So for forty-five days we need to show his body what it means to go to bed at 8:30 and wake up at 7:00 the next morning. If I have to use a drug to do that, I will use it. Once these emergent conditions are improved, language moves to the top of the list, followed by socialization.

JENNY: Why do you think there are still so many parents not into biomedical?

DR. JERRY: I have a family member who went to a leading research center in California and was told by the very best doctors at the institution that there was nothing left to do with this child. They wear white coats with their names beautifully embroidered above the left top pocket. They are the tops in their fields, and the parents believe them. As long as mainstream medicine does not embrace the concept of helping these children, many parents will go with what their physician recommends.

JENNY: It's people who haven't yet looked outside the box.

DR. JERRY: For a multitude of reasons, you are right. First and foremost, many remain in a state of denial for one to two years. Their physician may not make the diagnosis until their child is three to four years of age. Assured by the medical community, there are no biomedical interventions that are proven to be helpful and those that say they have something to offer must be preying on desperate parents. Then, there are those, I suppose, who are concerned about waiting on studies to demonstrate which treatments are effective and those who express concern over the long-term consequences of zinc usage. I think there's a group of parents who just feel that the rigors of some of the protocols are too inconvenient for their lifestyle. The list of excuses can go on and on. There is a group, though, of parents who really haven't heard about it yet. They are working families just trying to keep their heads above water and they just don't know about interventions that can radically change the lives of their children. It is exciting to see all of the television and media presentations currently being aired. The word is out and impossible to suppress: Autism is treatable!

JENNY: I'm sure there is a cost factor, too, because it can be so expensive.

DR. JERRY: Yes. The insurance companies do not pay for many of the interventions. Physicians will rarely take insurance payments for this kind of work. One way around this is to have a nonprofit support the work of the physician by providing scholarships to needy families. The added costs of the supplements, medications, and doctors' visits can be really tough on the families and their budgets.

JENNY: It breaks my heart.

DR. JERRY: So this is a partial list of why so many families do not go directly to biomedical interventions.

JENNY: I tell parents to get creative in raising money for biomedical treatment.

DR. JERRY: I had a grandpa who mowed lawns to see me. He thought my $20 an hour (I only charged him this much because I knew he would not take any charity!) was just way too much, but I was a good doc and he would continue to mow lawns for his grandson to be seen by me. I have other families who go around garage sales and they'll buy stuff and sell it on eBay. I have some families who will go to their local church or synagogue and talk to their clergy and say, "We need help. It's time for the church community to help us." Churches have sent us checks to cover the child's medical needs for that year and have told us to let them know if we need more. They don't give the family the money. But we apply the money to their account. From that account, we pay for their supplements, their labs, and our physician's time, whatever they need. Some parents are accustomed to punching down roadblocks. I have one mom who had some pretty gnarly biker dudes do a bike ride for her child to get IVIG (intravenous immunoglobulin therapy used to strengthen the immune system by transferring antibodies to another person. The cost is sometimes covered by insurance: $1,500 per treatment.). So you've got these really scruffy-looking dudes doing a biker thing to raise money. She was going to ask anybody and everybody she could to get help for her child.

JENNY: Well, to close up this recovery section, I would like to end by saying that many families I have talked to who have gone down this road and who have NOT recovered their child have said to me, "Well, when life used to be impossible with my son, it's now manageable."

DR. JERRY: And everyone needs to know there are many doctors and scientists who will not give up trying to recover these children, and neither should they!

RESOURCES

VITAMINS AND SUPPLEMENTS

Kartner Health

High-quality vitamins formulated by Dr. Jerry Kartzinel and Dr. Bo Wagner. Specializes in supplements for children with autism. Investor, Jenny McCarthy

866-960-9251

www.kartnerhealth.com

Stan Kurtz's MB_{12} Lollipop

Methyl-B_{12} that works in an all-natural lollipop. Available without a prescription.

www.mb12pop.com

Kirkman Labs

www.kirkmanlabs.com

PROBIOTICS

ThreeLac from GHT
www.ghthealth.com

EDUCATIONAL VIDEOS

Teach2Talk
Teach2Talk, LLC, produces educational resources for children that target core speech and language, play and social skills such as teaching understanding and proper usage of nouns, verbs, forming questions, conversations, pronouns, and many more, using techniques including video modeling.
www.teach2talk.com

AUTISM SCHOOLS

Teach2Talk Academy—Los Angeles, California
Teach2Talk Academy is an intensive early intervention program for the treatment of preschool-aged children aged two to six with autism spectrum disorders and other development disorders. Working in small classrooms featuring a one-to-one instructor-to-child ratio, the academy's multidisciplinary team of professionals implements unique instructional plans for each child, combining evidence-based practices and current research with clinical best practices, and incorporating behavioral therapy (utilizing Applied Behavioral Analysis and discrete trial training principles), speech and language therapy, occupational therapy, play therapy, and socials skills.
www.t2tacademy.com, 888-LA-T2T-ACADEMY

HYPERBARIC OXYGEN CHAMBERS

Oxy Health LLC
877-789-0123
www.oxyhealth.com

INFRARED SAUNA

Heavenly Heat
800-697-2862
www.heavenlyheatsaunas.com

GFCF SUGAR-FREE COOKIES

Nana's Cookies
www.nanascookiecompany.com

GFCF DELIVERED MEALS TO YOUR DOOR

GF Meals
www.gfmeals.com

GENERATION RESCUE

Generation Rescue is Jenny McCarthy's autism organization. The author will donate a portion of the proceeds from this book to Generation Rescue, an international movement of scientists, physicians, and parent-volunteers researching the causes and treatments for autism, ADHD, and chronic illness, and whose volunteers mentor thousands of families in recovering their children from autism.

Please visit www.GenerationRescue.org for more information about how to receive help or to donate to help other families.

APPENDIX

BEHAVIOR AND REMEDY CHART

When I first found out about biomedical interventions I was so excited to learn that MOST of Evan's behaviors had a reason AND a possible remedy. I had wished there was a simple chart that listed behaviors with causes and remedies to make it easy on moms. Well, Dr. Jerry and I just made it for you! Again, please note the word "possible"—as in POSSIBLE reasons and POSSIBLE remedies—doesn't mean we are stating that we know for a fact that these will work. This is only a list of common traits that the biomedical community has been treating for years (with great success, of course!).

Behavior/symptom	Possible causes	Possible remedies
Arm/Hand flapping	Toxins, foods, deficiencies in omega-3s, yeast	Correct deficiencies and remove toxins, antifungal
Tiptoe walking	Yeast, constipation, pain/irritation in the bowels	Detox yeast with antifungal, specific antibiotics, laxatives
Spinning in circles, rocking back and forth	Pain related. Infection, dietary issues, heavy metals	Anti-virals. Treat infection. Anti-inflammatories, dietary modifications, chelation.
Head banging, self-injury	Pain that could be anywhere. Could be ulcers, reflux, bowel disease, anxiety. Brain structural abnormalities, migraines.	Test for inflammation, treat ulcers, treat infection, treat anxiety with Xanax. If Xanax works, it confirms anxiety and then TAKE OFF Xanax and treat with natural remedies. If Xanax doesn't work, look and treat for other causes. Motrin. MRI of brain.
Looking out of corner of eye	Low in the natural form of vitamin A	Cod liver oil (mercury-free), urocholine, vision therapy
Bloated belly	Yeast, constipation, gas	Antifungal, laxative
Loss of muscle tone	Starvation of food and nutrients, metabolic problems	Supplement calories, protein, vitamins, minerals, and oils. Supplement with carnitine, creatine, as well as mitochondrial support supplements
Pale skin	Vascular instability, bacterial infection. Immune dysfunction, neurologic dysfunction.	Treat underlying disorder(s)
Diarrhea	Too much juice, infectious disease such as yeast, decreased digestive enzymes, inflammatory bowel disease, constipation	Remove and eliminate certain foods, isolate and treat infectious disease such as yeast, give digestive enzymes, treat inflammatory bowel disease. Treat underlying constipation
Dark circles under eyes	Allergies	IgG food test, treat chronic sinus infection, eliminate allergens. Treat with allergy medications
Mouthing, eating abnormal things like clothing, dirt	Overall untreated autism, yeast, nutritional deficiencies, mineral deficiencies	Vitamins, minerals, oils, kill yeast, treat overall autism
Constipation	Inflammatory bowel disease. Infectious disease such as yeast, a methylation defect	Find the right laxative, kill the yeast, treat inflammatory bowel disease

Behavior/symptom	Possible causes	Possible remedies
Teeth grinding	Parasites, inflammatory bowel disease, pain, anxiety, yeast	Treat for parasite, treat inflammatory bowel disease, kill yeast, treat overall autism
Obsessive-compulsive disorder	Dysbiosis (imbalance in gut such as candida), streptococcus, low serotonin, methylation defects, PANDAS, inflammation	Treat dysbiosis such as candida, antibiotic for strep, 5-HTP supplementation to increase serotonin, B_{12} shots, TMG, folic acid, cysteine, glutathione
Gas	Constipation, candida	Laxative, antifungal
Acid reflux	Food allergies, environmental allergies, constipation	IgG test, Claritin, Singular, gastrochrom, laxative
Rashes	Virus, bacteria, eczema, allergy, methylation pathway defects	Antibiotic for bacteria, antifungal for eczema, Claritin for allergy, methylation support such as B_{12} shots
Aggression	Inflammatory bowel disease, anxiety, obsessive compulsive disorder, pain, bacterial infection, allergies. Hormone imbalances	Treat inflammatory bowel disease, treat bacterial infection with antibiotic, Claritin or Singulir for allergies. Androgen panel (LabCorp) for evaluation of hormones
Undigested food in stool	Yeast, lacking digestive enzymes	Antifungal, digestive enzymes
Vomiting	Allergies, constipation, severe sensory integration disorder	IgG test, laxative, feeding programs
Constant fevers	Inflammation, infection	Immune system evaluation, bowel evaluation. Infectious disease evaluation. Autoimmune evaluation.
Exhaustion, tired all the time	Virus, nutritional deficiencies, mitochondrial poisoning, allergies, yeast. Thyroid dysfunction. Heavy metal poisoning.	Nutrition, supplements, hyperbaric chamber, IgG test, Claritin, antifungal. Thyroid evaluation. Mitochondrial evaluation, chelation.
No pain, sensory dysfunction	Gluten/dairy	Go GF/CF!
Not sleeping through the night	Eating wrong foods, reflux, bowel pain, decreased melatonin production, constipation, sleep cycle dysfunction, anxiety	IgG test, 5-HTP, melatonin, antacid, investigate bowel pain, removal of wheat and dairy

Behavior/symptom	Possible causes	Possible remedies
Loss of eye contact	Center vision switched off and using only peripheral vision	Cod liver oil, bethanechol, vision evaluation
Sound sensitivity	Inappropriate response to sound stimuli as part of their autism, heavy metal poisoning, viral infection	Detox and sound therapy
High pain tolerance	Opiate from wheat and dairy is a pain blocker	Removal of wheat and dairy, deep pressure and joint compression
Don't want to be touched	Abnormal perception to everyday stimuli, hypersensitivity, pain	Overall autism healing
Screaming tantrums	Pain, anxiety, OCD, sights, sounds, triggerable offense	Remove from offending place/ situation. Treat overall autism

LIST OF RECOMMENDED PRODUCTS AND WHERE TO BUY THEM

Food

Recipes and informational sites for the Gluten-Free Casein-Free Diet:

- TACA—http://gfcf-diet.talkaboutcuringautism.org/
- GF Meals, by Your Dinner Secret—www.gfmeals.com
- The Official GFCF Diet Web site—www.gfcfdiet.com
- Applegate Farms lunch meat is nitrate-free (available at Whole Foods—www.wholefoodsmarket.com)
- GFCF Breads (health food stores)
  - —Kinnikinnick—(www.kinnikinnicks.com)
  - —Glutino—(www.glutino.com)
- Good for Dessert Mixes—www.namastefoods.com

Recipes and informational sites for the Specific Carbohydrate Diet:

- www.scdrecipe.com/home
- www.scdiet.org

Supplements—Vitamins and Minerals

- Multivitamins, Digestive Enzymes
  - —Kartner Health—www.kartnerhealth.com or call 866-960-9251
  - —Klaire Labs: VitaSpectrum—www.klaire.com
  - —Kirkman Labs: Super Nu-Thera line—www.kirkmanlabs.com
  - —Brainchild Nutritionals (www.brainchildnutritionals.com)
- Mercury-Free Fish Oils (Cod Liver Oil, Omega-3s, and Omega-6s)
  - —Kartner Health—www.kartnerhealth.com or call 866-960-9251
  - —Nordic Naturals—www.nordicnaturals.com or call 800-662.2544 x3
  - —Carlson—www.carlsonlabs.com or call 888-234-5656
- Probiotics (Dairy-Free)
  - —Kartner Health—www.kartnerhealth.com or call 866-960-9251
  - —Global Health Trax's ThreeLac—www.ghthealth.com or 760-542-3000
  - —Klaire Labs: VitaSpectrum—www.klaire.com or call 888-488-2488
  - —Kirkman Labs: Super Nu-Thera line—www.kirkmanlabs.com

Supplements	
MindLinx	NRG Solutions www.nrgsolutions.net Phone: 630-853-8383 Nature's Choice www.natureschoicetn.com Phone: 417-889-4184 Rockwell Nutrition (United Kingdom) www.rockwellnutrition.com Phone: +44 207 742 6700
Therbiotic	Klaire Labs www.klaire.com Phone: 888-488-2488
Primal Defense	Garden of Life www.gardenoflifeusa.com Phone: 800-819-6742 or 810-281-5507
Healthy Trinity	Organic Pharmacy www.organicpharmacy.org Phone: 800-819-6742 or 828-232-2842 Natren (United Kingdom) www.natren.com Phone: +44 134 231 2811 The Vitamin Store (contact via Web site only) www.shopthevitaminstore.com

Digestive Enzymes: Many to Choose From	
Kartner Health	www.kartnerhealth.com Phone: 866-960-9251
Creon 10	A prescription enzyme which is very good and can save you some money (if you have pharmacy coverage) Informational Web site (contact via Web site only): www.revolutionhealth.com/drugs-treatments/creon-10 Purchasing Web site: www.drugstore.com Phone: 800-378-4786
TriEnza	Houston Enzymes www.houstonenzymes.com Phone: 866-757-8626
Enzyme Complete with DPPIV (DPP4)	Kirkman Labs www.kirkmanlabs.com Phone: 503-694-1600 or if outside of Oregon 800-245-8282

Products for Your Home

No-VOC glues and paint for your home:

- Green Planet Paints—www.greenplanetpaints.com
- Fresh Aire Choice Paint—www.freshairechoicepaint.com
- Ecos Paints—www.ecospaints.com

Organic Recommendations and Nontoxic Household Products	
Location	**Web site**
Whole Foods Market	www.wholefoodsmarket.com
Wild Harvest Organic, found in many major grocery stores	www.wildharvestorganic.com
Listings (by state), food co-ops, health food stores, and natural food stores	Green People www.greenpeople.org/healthfood.htm Organic Consumers Association www.organicconsumers.org/foodcoops.htm
Seventh Generation	www.seventhgeneration.com
Earth-friendly products	www.ecos.com
Organic Valley Family of Farms	www.organicvalley.coop

Hyperbaric Oxygen Chambers

*Insurance coverage depends on your plan, but please look into it because it has been covered for some people.

Where you can Buy or Rent a Hyperbaric Oxygen Chamber:

OXYHEALTH
877-789-0123
www.oxyhealth.com
3224 Hoover Avenue
National City, CA 91950

PRICES TO RENT ($ PER MONTH):

(Small $1,500)
(Medium $2,000)
(Large $3,000)

PRICES TO BUY:

(Small $10,500)
(Medium $16,900)
(Large $20,900)

HYPERBARIC SUPPORT
866-937-9755
www.hyperbaricsupport.com
6015 University
Cedar Falls, OH 50613

PRICES TO RENT ($ PER MONTH):

(Small $1,895)
(Medium $2,395)

PRICES TO LEASE:

(Small $200 per session)
(Medium $400 per session)

PRICES TO BUY:

(Small $7,998)
(Medium $13,995)

GENOX INC
678-957-0156
www.genoxinc.com

PRICES TO RENT ($ PER MONTH):

(Large $2,500)

PRICES TO BUY:

(Small $9,450)
(Medium $15,210)
(Large $18,810)

PERFORMANCE HYPERBARICS
888-456-4268
www.performance-hyperbarics.com
372 Hopalua Drive
Pukalani, HI 96768

PRICES TO RENT ($ PER MONTH):

(Small $2,000)
(Large $2,650)

PRICES TO BUY

(Small $12,900)
(Large $16,900)

Treatment Centers Where You Can Go for Hyperbaric Oxygen Chamber Sessions:
To find out where you can go for hyperbaric oxygen treatment, visit www.geocities.com/aneecp/hbocent.htm for a great list, arranged alphabetically by state for centers in the United States.

Stevia Sugar Information, Products, and Cookbooks

- www.stugar.com/home.asp
- www.stevia.com
- www.steviacafe.net
- www.healthyshopping.com/SweetLeaf/
- Miss Roben's: www.allergygrocer.com

Nontoxic Clothing

- Hanna Andersson organic line—www.hannaandersson.com

Nontoxic Bedding and Furniture

- Nirvana Safe Haven—www.nontoxic.com

Mercury-Safe Fish Sources

- Safe Harbor—www.safeharborfoods.com/stores/

MEDICAL ARTICLES TO SHOW TO YOUR DOCTOR AND WHAT EACH ARTICLE PROVES

#1

For an article that examines the role of sugars, see A. Sanchez et al., "Role of Sugars in Human Neutrophilic Phagocytosis," *American Journal of Clinical Nutrition*, 26: 1180–84. Copyright © 1973 by The American Society for Clinical Nutrition, Inc.

2

ALUMINIUM AS AN ADJUVANT IN VACCINES AND POST-VACCINE REACTIONS

Fiejka M, Aleksandrowicz J., Zakladu Badania Surowic, Warszawie. Rocz Panstw Zakl Hig. 1993;44(1):73–80. PMID: 8235346 [PubMed—indexed for MEDLINE]

Aluminium compounds have been widely used as adjuvants in prophylactic and therapeutic vaccines. Adjuvants are able to stimulate the immune system in a nonspecific manner, i.e. high antibody level can be obtained with minimal dose of the antigen and with reduced number of inoculations. Adjuvants use has been mostly empirically determined by such factors as efficacy and safety. The mechanism of action of the aluminium adjuvants is not completely understood and is very complex. The basic factors of the mode of action: 1) the complex of antigen and aluminium gel is more immunogenic in structure than free antigen, 2) effect "depot"—The antigen stimulus lasts longer, 3) the production of local granulomas. Vaccines adsorbed onto aluminium salts are a more frequent cause of local post-vaccinal reactions than plain vaccines. 5-10% those vaccinated can develop a nodule lasting several weeks at the injection site. In some rare cases the nodules may become inflammatory and even turn into an aseptic abscess. The nodules persisting more than 6 weeks may indicate development of aluminium hypersensitivity. **Finally aluminium adjuvant immunogens induce the production of IgE antibodies.**

#3

The table below is courtesy of Environmental Working Group's study "Body Burden: The Pollution in Newborns" on July 14, 2005. The entire study and results can be found at www.ewg.org.

Chemicals and pollutants detected in human umbilical cord blood

Mercury (Hg)—tested for 1, found 1
Pollutant from coal-fired power plants, mercury-containing products, and certain industrial processes. Accumulates in seafood. Harms brain development and function.

Polyaromatic hydrocarbons (PAHs)—tested for 18, found 9
Pollutants from burning gasoline and garbage. Linked to cancer. Accumulates in food chain.

Polybrominated dibenzodioxins and furans (PBDD/F)—tested for 12, found 7
Contaminants in brominated flame retardants. Pollutants and by-products from plastic production and incineration. Accumulate in food chain. Toxic to developing endocrine (hormone) system

Perfluorinated chemicals (PFCs)—tested for 12, found 9
Active ingredients or breakdown products of Teflon, Scotchgard, fabric and carpet protectors, food wrap coatings. Global contaminants. Accumulate in the environment and the food chain. Linked to cancer, birth defects, and more.

Polychlorinated dibenzodioxins and furans (PBCD/F)—tested for 17, found 11
Pollutants, by-products of PVC production, industrial bleaching, and incineration. Cause cancer in humans. Persist for decades in

the environment. Very toxic to developing endocrine (hormone) system.

Organochlorine pesticides (OCs)—tested for 28, found 21
DDT, chlordane, and other pesticides. Largely banned in the U.S. Persist for decades in the environment. Accumulate up the food chain, to man. Cause cancer and numerous reproductive defects.

Polybrominated diphenyl ethers (PBDEs)—tested for 46, found 32
Flame retardant in furniture foam, computers, and televisions. Accumulates in the food chain and human tissues. Adversely affects brain development and the thyroid.

Polychlorinated Naphthalenes (PCNs)—tested for 70, found 50
Wood preservatives, varnishes, machine lubricating oils, waste incineration. Common PCB contaminant. Contaminate the food chain. Cause liver and kidney damage.

Polychlorinated biphenyls (PCBs)—tested for 209, found 147
Industrial insulators and lubricants. Banned in the U.S. in 1976. Persist for decades in the environment. Accumulate up the food chain, to man. Cause cancer and nervous system problems.

#4

This article was published on January 18, 2006 at 12:00 am and can be viewed at: www.post-gazette.com/pg/06018/639721.stm.

DRUG ERROR, NOT CHELATION THERAPY, KILLED BOY, EXPERT SAYS

By Karen Kane, *Pittsburgh Post-Gazette*.

One of the nation's foremost experts in chelation therapy said she has determined "without a doubt" that it was medical error, and not the therapy itself, that led to the death of a 5-year-old boy who was receiving it as a treatment for autism.

Dr. Mary Jean Brown, chief of the Lead Poisoning Prevention Branch of the Atlanta-based Centers for Disease Control and Prevention, said yesterday that Abubakar Tariq Nadama died Aug. 23 in his Butler County doctor's office because he was given the wrong chelation agent.

"It's a case of look-alike/sound-alike medications," she said yesterday. "The child was given Disodium EDTA instead of Calcium Disodium EDTA. The generic names are Versinate and Endrate. They sound alike. They're clear and colorless and odorless. They were mixed up."

Both types of EDTA are synthetic amino acids that latch onto heavy metals in the bloodstream.

Dr. Brown said she obtained the child's autopsy report on behalf of the CDC after reading an article about the death in the *Pittsburgh Post-Gazette*. She said it didn't take long to figure out what had happened.

Essentially, Tariq died from low blood calcium. Without enough calcium—a metal—in the blood, the heart stops beating.

Dr. Brown said the Disodium EDTA the child was given as a chelation agent "acted as a claw that pulled too much calcium" from his blood.

"The blood calcium level was below 5 [milligrams]. That's an emergency event," she said.

Officials from the state police, the district attorney's office and the coroner's office will meet soon to decide whether to hold an inquest into the child's death and whether it should remain listed as accidental.

Dr. Brown said the same mix-up happened in two other recent cases: a 2-year-old girl in Texas who died in May during chelation for lead poisoning and a woman from Oregon who died three years ago while receiving chelation for clogged arteries.

Dr. Brown said that in each case, the blood calcium level was below 5 milligrams. Normal is between 7 and 9.

The correct chelation agent—Calcium Disodium EDTA—would not have pulled the calcium from the bloodstream, she said.

The Butler County coroner's office confirmed last week that Tariq had died as a result of his chelation treatment, but the findings that were released didn't indicate whether the treatment had been improperly administered.

Dr. Brown said chelation was once a common and necessary therapy that was used on children and adults alike for lead poisoning. Chelation means administering an agent into the bloodstream that causes heavy metals in the body to cling to it and then be excreted in urine.

Though its only approved use, according to the U.S. Food and Drug Administration, is for lead poisoning, Dr. Brown said she is aware that it is used by some people for other medical problems, ranging from clogged arteries to autism.

She said there have been no reputable medical trials demonstrating the effectiveness of chelation as a therapy for anything but lead poisoning. But if it were administered accurately, the procedure would be harmless.

She said it is well known within the medical community that Disodium EDTA should never be used as a chelation agent. She quoted from a 1985 CDC statement: "Only Calcium Disodium EDTA should be used. Disodium EDTA should never be used . . . because it may induce fatal hypocalcemia, low calcium and tetany."

"There is no doubt that this was an unintended use of Disodium EDTA. No medical professional would ever have intended to give the child Disodium EDTA," Dr. Brown said.

Tariq was brought to the United States from England last spring by his mother, Marwa, for the chelation therapy. He was in the Portersville, Butler County, office of Dr. Roy Eugene Kerry when he went into cardiac arrest.

In recent months, chelation treatments of a wide variety ranging from IV to oral to topical have been gaining popularity for autistic children due to anecdotal information from parents indicating a reduction in symptoms. The underlying belief is that autism is caused by a sensitivity to heavy metals in the bloodstream.

Howard Carpenter, executive director of the Advisory Board on Autism and Related Disorders—the largest autism advocacy group in the region—said the determination by Dr. Brown clears up the mystery surrounding Tariq's death but not the uncertainty over chelation itself.

"Since this child died, there have been parents who are pro-chelation who have been very angry that there's talk against it. On the other side, they say the death was a natural consequence of a dangerous activity. Maybe what happened to [Tariq] is explained, but we still don't have a conclusion about whether chelation is an effective treatment for autism," he said.

Tariq's father is a medical doctor who practices in England.

Dr. Kerry could not be reached for comment. A board-certified physician and surgeon, he advertises himself as an ear, nose and throat doctor who also specializes in allergies and environmental medicine.

* Karen Kane can be reached at kkane@post-gazette.com

#5

GASTROINTESTINAL ABNORMALITIES IN CHILDREN WITH AUTISTIC DISORDER

Horvath K, Papadimitriou JC, Rabsztyn A, Drachenberg C, Tildon JT. J Pediatr 1999 Nov;135(5):559-63. Department of Pediatrics, University of Maryland School of Medicine, Baltimore, USA. PMID: 10547242 [PubMed—indexed for MEDLINE]

OBJECTIVES: Our aim was to evaluate the structure and function of the upper gastrointestinal tract in a group of patients with autism who had gastrointestinal symptoms. STUDY DESIGN: Thirty-six children (age: 5.7 +/- 2 years, mean +/- SD) with autistic disorder underwent upper gastrointestinal endoscopy with biopsies, intestinal and pancreatic enzyme analyses, and bacterial and fungal cultures. The most frequent gastrointestinal complaints were chronic diarrhea, gaseousness, and abdominal discomfort and distension. RESULTS: Histologic examination in these 36 children revealed grade I or II reflux esophagitis in 25 (69.4%), chronic gastritis in 15, and chronic duodenitis in 24. The number of Paneth's cells in the duodenal crypts was significantly elevated in autistic children compared with non-autistic control subjects. Low intestinal carbohydrate digestive enzyme activity was reported in 21 children (58.3%), although there was no abnormality found in pancreatic function. Seventy-five percent of the autistic children (27/36) had an increased pancreatico-biliary fluid output after intravenous secretin administration. Nineteen of the 21 patients with diarrhea had significantly higher fluid output than those without diarrhea. **CONCLUSIONS: Unrecognized gastrointestinal disorders, especially reflux esophagitis and disaccharide malabsorption, may contribute to the behavioral problems of the non-verbal autistic patients.** The observed increase in pancreatico-biliary secretion after secretin infusion suggests an upregulation of secretin receptors in the pancreas and liver. Further studies are required to determine the possible association between the brain and gastrointestinal dysfunctions in children with autistic disorder.

6

This study looks at the Hepatitis B Vaccine in adults:

CHRONIC ADVERSE REACTIONS ASSOCIATED WITH HEPATITIS B VACCINATION.

David A Geier, Mark R Geier M.D., Ph.D. *The Annals of Pharmacotherapy*, 2002: Vol. 36, No. 12, pp. 1970–1971. PMID: 12452762 [PubMed—indexed for MEDLINE]

In conclusion, our study demonstrates that adult HBV is statistically associated not only with acute neuropathy, neuritis, myelitis, vasculitis, thrombocytopenia, gastrointestinal disease, multiple sclerosis, and arthritis, but some of these patients go on to develop chronic adverse reactions that persist for at least 1 year following HBV. These types of chronic adverse reactions following adult HBV should be discussed with patients contemplating being immunized with HBV and should be included in the differential diagnosis of those who develop them following adult HBV.

#7

CLUSTERING OF CASES OF INSULIN DEPENDENT DIABETES (IDDM) OCCURRING THREE YEARS AFTER HEMOPHILUS INFLUENZA B (HIB) IMMUNIZATION SUPPORT CAUSAL RELATIONSHIP BETWEEN IMMUNIZATION AND IDDM

Classen JB, Classen DC. Classen Immunotherapies Inc., 6517 Montrose Avenue, Baltimore, MD 21212, USA. classen@vaccines.net *Autoimmunity*, 2003 May;36(3):123. PMID: 12482192 [PubMed—indexed for MEDLINE]

OBJECTIVE: The hemophilus vaccine has been linked to the development of autoimmune type 1 diabetes, insulin dependent diabetes (IDDM) in ecological studies. METHODS: We attempted to determine if the Hemophilus influenza B (HiB) vaccine was associated with an increased risk of IDDM by looking for clusters of cases of IDDM using data from a large clinical trial. All children born in Finland between October 1st, 1985 and August 31st, 1987, approximately 116,000 were randomized to receive 4 doses of the HiB vaccine (PPR-D, Connaught) starting at 3 months of life or one dose starting after 24 months of life. A control-cohort included all 128,500 children born in Finland in the 24 months prior to the HiB vaccine study. Non-obese diabetic prone (NOD) mice were immunized with a hemophilus vaccine to determine if immunization increased the risk of IDDM. RESULTS: The difference in cumulative incidence between those receiving 4 doses and those receiving 0 doses is 54 cases of IDDM/100,000 ($P = 0.026$) at 7 years, (relative risk = 1.26). Most of the extra cases of IDDM appeared in statistically significant clusters that occurred in periods starting approximately 38 months after immunization and lasting approximately 6-8 months. Immunization with pe-

diatric vaccines increased the risk of insulin diabetes in NOD mice.
CONCLUSION: Exposure to HiB immunization is associated with an increased risk of IDDM. NOD mice can be used as an animal model of vaccine induced diabetes.

#8

Generation Rescue funded a study, simply asking if there were more cases of autism, ADHD, and neurological disorders in the vaccinated group of children compared to unvaccinated children. Let's look at the results:

ALL VACCINATED BOYS, COMPARED TO UNVACCINATED BOYS:

- Vaccinated boys were 155 percent more likely to have a neurological disorder (RR 2.55).
- Vaccinated boys were 224 percent more likely to have ADHD (RR 3.24).
- Vaccinated boys were 61 percent more likely to have autism (RR 1.61).

OLDER VACCINATED BOYS, AGES 11–17 (ABOUT HALF THE BOYS SURVEYED), COMPARED TO OLDER UNVACCINATED BOYS:

- Vaccinated boys were 158 percent more likely to have a neurological disorder (RR 2.58).
- Vaccinated boys were 317 percent more likely to have ADHD (RR 4.17).
- Vaccinated boys were 112 percent more likely to have autism (RR 2.12).

Granted, in this study, only autism, ADHD, and neurological disorders were queried. I think the next study, asking about infectious disease (ear infections, allergies, asthma, etc.) would be most telling.

For more information on the Generation Rescue study, go to: www.generationrescue.org

9

For an article that examines the ileum as being a target issue, see "Persistent Ileal Measles Virus in a Large Cohort of Regressive Autistic Children with Ileocolitis and Lymphonodular Hyperplasia: Revisitation of an Earlier Study," by S. Walker, K. Hepner, J. Segal, A. Krigsman of the Wake Forest University School of Medicine.

BOOKS AND WEB SITES

Books

A Shot in the Dark, by Harris Coulter and Barbara Loe Fisher

Breaking the Vicious Cycle, by Elaine Gloria Gottschall

Caring for Children with Autism Spectrum Disorders: A Resource Toolkit for Clinicians, by the American Academy of Pediatrics

Evidence of Harm, by David Kirby

Healing Foods: Cooking for Celiacs, Colitis, Crohn's and IBS, by Sandra Ramacher

Louder Than Words, by Jenny McCarthy

The Low Oxalate Cookbook: Book 2, edited by Joanne Yount and Annie Gottlieb

Mother Warriors, by Jenny McCarthy

The Vaccine Book, by Robert W. Sears, M.D., F.A.A.P.

What Your Doctor May NOT Tell You About Children's Vaccinations, by Stephanie Cave, M.D.

The Yeast Connection, by Dr. William G. Crook

Web sites

Air Purifiers
Nirvana Safe Haven: www.nontoxic.com

Allergen-Free Food
www.allergygrocer.com

Colostrum
Kirkman Labs: www.kirkmanlabs.com

Constipation
www.oxypowder.com

Digestive Enzymes
Creon 10: www.revolutionhealth.com/drugs-treatments creon-10; www.drugstore.com
Houston Enzymes: www.houstonenzymes.com
Kartner Health (Dr. Jerry's supplements line): www.kartner health.com
Kirkman Labs: www.kirkmanlabs.com

Food Dye Information
www.cfsan.fda.gov/~dms/col-toc.html
www.thealmightyguru.com/Pointless/FoodDye.html

Fruit Juice
http://gfcfdiet.com/beverages.htm

GFCF Breads
Glutino: www.glutino.com
Kinnikinnick: www.kinnikinnicks.com

Glutathione and Cysteine Tests
Genova Diagnostics: www.genovadiagnostics.com
Vitamin Diagnostics/European Laboratory of Nutrients: www .europeanlaboratory.com

Gluten-Free, Casein-Free Resources
GFMeals, by Your Dinner Secret: www.gfmeals.com
The Official GFCF Diet Web site: www.gfcfdiet.com
TACA: http://gfcf-diet.talkaboutcuringautism.org/
Miss Roben's: www.allergygrocer.com

Healthy Paint
Earth Friendly Products: www.ecospaints.com
Fresh Aire Choice Paints: www.freshairechoicepaint.com
Green Planet Paints: www.greenplanetpaints.com

Hyperbaric Oxygen Treatment/Chambers
Information/products:

- Genox Inc: www.genoxinc.com
- Hyperbaric Support: www.hyperbaricsupport.com
- Oxyhealth: www.oxyhealth.com
- Performance Hyperbarics: www.performance-hyperbarics.com

List of Treatment Centers by State:
- www.geocities.com/aneecp/hbocent.htm

IgG and IgE Tests
Within Your HMO:

- LabCorp: www.labcorp.com
- Quest Diagnostics: www.questdiagnostics.com

Out of Network:

- Alletess Medical Laboratory: www.foodallergy.com
- Immunolabs: www.immunolabs.com

Magnesium Citrate
Informational site: www.drugs.com/ppa/magnesium-citrate.html
Purchasing site: www.organicpharmacy.org

Mercury Food Risks Information
www.cfsan.fda.gov/~frf/sea-mehg.html

Mercury-Safe Fish Sources
Safe Harbor: www.safeharborfoods.com/stores

Milk of Magnesia
www.magnesiumdirect.com

Nontoxic Bedding and Furniture
Nirvana Safe Haven: www.nontoxic.com

Nontoxic Clothing
Hanna Andersson's organic line: www.hannaandersson.com

Organic Recommendations and Nontoxic Household Products
Earth Friendly Products: www.ecos.com
Green People: www.greenpeople.org/healthfood.htm
Organic Consumers Association: www.organicconsumers.org/foodcoops.htm
Organic Valley Family of Farms: www.organicvalley.coop
Seventh Generation: www.seventhgeneration.com
Whole Foods Market: www.wholefoodsmarket.com
Wild Harvest Organic: www.wildharvestorganic.com

Probiotics
The Body Ecology Diet: www.bodyecologydiet.com
Garden of Life: www.gardenoflifeusa.com
Kartner Health (Dr. Jerry's supplements line): www.kartnerhealth.com
Klaire Labs: www.klaire.com
Natren: www.natren.com
Nature's Choice: www.natureschoicetn.com
NRG Solutions: www.nrgsolutions.net
Organic Pharmacy: www.organicpharmacy.org

Rockwell Nutrition: www.rockwellnutrition.com
The Vitamin Store: www.shopthevitaminstore.com

Seizure Control
Depakote (divalproex sodium): www.depakoteer.com
Lamictal (lamotrigine): www.lamictal.com
Neurontin (gabapentin): www.pfizer.com

Specific Carbohydrate Diet
www.scdiet.org
www.scdrecipe.com/home

Stevia Sugar Information, Products, and Cookbooks
www.healthyshopping.com/sweetleaf
www.stevia.com
www.steviacafe.net
www.stugar.com/home.asp

Stool Diagnostics
LabCorp: www.labcorp.com
Quest Diagnostics: www.questdiagnostics.com

Vitamins, Minerals, Supplements
Brainchild Nutritionals: www.brainchildnutritionals.com
Carlson Labs: www.carlsonlabs.com
Kartner Health (Dr. Jerry's supplements line): www.kartnerhealth.com
Kirkman Labs: www.kirkmanlabs.com
Klaire Labs: www.klaire.com
Nordic Naturals: www.nordicnaturals.com
NutriBiotic: www.nutribiotic.herbsmd.com
Phyto Pharmica: www.phytopharmica.com

Yeast Testing
Doctors Data: www.doctorsdata.com

Stool Cultures: Genova Diagnostics, www.genovadiagnostics.com
Urine Organic Acid: The Great Plains Lab, www.greatplainslaboratory.com

Biomedical Doctors

Clinicians Who Treat Individuals with Autism
A list of clinicians is listed on the Autism Research Institute Web site: www.autismwebsite.com/practitioners/us_lc.htm. Please contact Generation Rescue to find out which of these doctors they work closely with and support the *Rescue Family* Program.

Naturopaths and Homeopaths
Many naturopaths and homeopaths do not require a license to practice in their state—do your research! A list of naturopathic physicians and homeopathic physicians can be found on the Autism Research Institute Web site: www.autismwebsite.com/practitioners/us_nl.htm

International Nutritionists
Nutritionists, listed alphabetically by country, are available to you on the Autism Research Institute Web site: www.autismwebsite.com/practitioners/foreign_nt.htm.

Generation Rescue's Lead Nutritionist
Bo Wagner Ph.D., D.N.M.
Dean and Professor at the University of Natural Medicine
Member of the University's Scientific Advisory Board
Universal Life Force, Inc.
269 S. Beverly Drive Suite #1153
Beverly Hills, CA 90212
Ph: (877) 277-2216
Ph: (310) 281-8387
staff@drbowagner.com
www.drbowagner.com

ONLINE VACCINE RESOURCES

A list of all vaccines and their ingredients:
www.cdc.gov/vaccines/vac-gen/additives.htm

Excipients included in U.S. vaccines, by vaccine:
www.cdc.gov/vaccines/pubs/pinkbook/downloads/appendices/B/excipient-table-2.pdf

The amount of thimerosal and/or mercury that is in all the vaccines (pediatric and adult):
www.fda.gov/cber/vaccine/Thimerosal.htm#t3

PROTOCOLS

Supplements

Zinc and Selenium:

Zinc: 20 mg per day to start

Selenium: depending on weight, can be added anywhere from 50 mcg to 100 mcg per day. Monitor blood levels.

Digestive Enzymes:

1/2 to 1 capsule with each meal and snack.

Calcium and Magnesium:

Since most of our children need to be dairy-free, alternative sources for calcium are necessary for proper growth and development. We typically recommend 500–1,000 mg of calcium citrate (not Tums) daily. Magnesium should be given with calcium to enhance absorption. Calcium and magnesium blood levels should be checked regularly. Remember, we need to be on a vitamin D supplement as well.

Chromium:
If this is revealed to be low on blood level tests, we recommend 50–100 mcg daily.

Protein:
Many children do not consume protein, or if they do, it's in very small amounts. We recommend supplementation with a rice-protein powder put directly into their drink. NutriBiotics makes a very clean product; 1 tablespoon typically is equal to 14 g of protein. The amount of protein our children require usually depends on age: If under three years, supplement with 1 g of protein per 2 pounds of body weight. Ages four to six years, 1 tablespoon daily; seven to ten years of age, supplement with 1 3/4 tablespoons daily. Older boys and girls require 2 tablespoons daily. This protein powder can easily mix into any fluid since it contributes only a very bland flavor. It does have "texture" that some of our kids can detect. This can be minimized if mixed into juice, rice milk, etc., with a blender.

Cod Liver Oil/EFA:
Just about all children will require omega-3 fatty acids. When using cod liver oil, we recommend starting with the RDA of vitamin A. Usually this is 1/2 tsp of cod liver oil for children ages two to five years; 1 tsp for children who are older. A blood test, called an Essential Fatty Acid Profile, will reveal other possible fatty acid deficits that can be supplemented. Some children react poorly to cod liver oil and can get very hyper and aggressive. This will resolve one to two days after discontinuing.

Vitamin D3:
Also known as cholecalciferol, this vitamin regulates absorption and deposition of calcium and phosphorus. It can be found in some fish oils (think omega!), and our body can generate vitamin D with exposure to sunlight. We recommend supplementing from 600 IU to

2,000 IU of vitamin D_3 daily, depending on the child's weight and measured 25-hydroxy vitamin D levels (blood test).

Vitamin E:
This is another potent antioxidant. The recommended dosage for children is in the range of 100–400 IU daily, depending on their weight.

Detox

- TMG or DMG is taken orally.
- Start with 250 mg twice daily. Some children do better with TMG, others with DMG. Side effects, if seen, are hyperactivity and more emotional behaviors.
- Methyl B_{12} usually injected by parents every other night; we start dosing at 1,250 mcg of methyl B_{12} per injection.
- We tend to start the trio methyl B_{12}, folinic acid, and N-acetyl-cysteine all in one injection.
- Here is the formula we have compounded at the pharmacy: Methyl B_{12} 12.5 mg/folinic acid 50 mg/NAC 50 mg per ml. We then start with 0.1 ml subcutaneously every other day.
- Folinic acid is usually placed in the methyl B_{12} injections but can be taken orally. It, too, can cause some hyperactivity. If taken orally, 400 mcg daily is a good starting dose. This is a really safe vitamin, and toxicity is rare.
- Cysteine can be taken orally but, in some children, can cause yeast to grow. Cysteine can be applied transdermally (as a cream that allows the cysteine to enter the body) and if given this way (not in an injection), we recommend starting with 100–200 mg twice daily.
- Glutathione, transdermally or IV: This is so crucial for many children. This is one of the end products of the methylation pathway. When given orally it, too, like N-acetyl-cysteine, can cause yeast to bloom. Children do very well with IV infusions (where we stick a small

catheter in the arm and infuse the glutathione directly into the vein) of glutathione—but they rarely like the procedure/needle stick! We can give anywhere from 300 mg to 1,000 mg of glutathione IV once or twice monthly. Glutathione can also come in a transdermal preparation, and we recommend 200 mg twice daily. One other route to administer glutathione would be to inhale it. Using a special "nebulizing" machine (about $50–$70), glutathione can be aerosolized and breathed "in" by the child. We recommend 100 mg–200 mg once or twice daily if given by this method.

Enhancing Cognitive Abilities

- B vitamins: Many children really respond to the B vitamins, especially B_6, B_{12}, and magnesium.
- Essential fatty acids: Children usually have such a poor dietary intake, and the "good" fats are no exception. We will often get a blood test, a "Fatty Acid Profile," and will supplement according to the results. It is safe to assume the children will need omega-3 fatty acids. That is why we start with cod liver oil. In addition:

1. Minerals: Because of dietary limitations, many minerals are lacking
2. CoQ10
3. NADH
4. TMG/DMG
5. EFA
6. Grape seed extract (GSE)
7. Antioxidants in general: Vitamins C and E and grape seed extract (just to name a few)
8. Chelation in selected cases
9. Removal of nitrites (cured meats)

Reducing Autistic Behaviors

- Normalize neurotransmitter levels. Supplement with:

  —Tyrosine, TMG, GABA, NADH, Cerefolin, Deptin

- Improve receptor site activity. Supplement with:

  —TMG
  —NADH (maybe)

- Remove substances that can interfere with normal function.

  —Digestive enzymes: 1 capsule with each meal
  —Remove MSG, NutraSweet, aspartame, hydrolyzed vegetable proteins, excitotoxins, soda
  —Food dyes
  —Reduce high-phenol-containing foods (blueberries, strawberries, etc.)

- Protect from excitotoxins. Supplement with:

  —Vitamin C 500–1,000 mg daily
  —Vitamin E 100–200 IU daily
  —Magnesium 2 mg per pound daily
  —Grape seed extract (50–100 mg/day—PhytoPharmica)

- Increase the seizure threshold (stabilization of neuronal cell membrane potentials). Supplement with:

  —EFA
  —Taurine 250–500 mg daily
  —Vitamin B_6

- Improve gastrointestinal function.
- Improve motility.
- Secretin: This hormone is normally released by specialized cells in the duodenum (the channel that directly follows the stomach outlet) that tells the pancreas to secrete bicarbonate (neutralizes the acidic stomach content). Given through IV or transdermally, this has had profound positive effects on many of the children we see. It can normalize bowel function with respect to the child having formed brown, one- to twice-daily stools that smell like regular bowel movements. Secretin can also have profound effects on autistic behaviors, with some of the children responding remarkably. The children who tend to benefit most from secretin have loose stools and have very limited to no language. Unfortunately, secretin needs a physician's involvement and prescription.
- Fiber: Fiber has always been helpful for developing regular stooling behavior. We currently are using Miracle Fiber and Fibersure.
- Calcium: As previously discussed, calcium HAS to be supplemented in our dairy-free kids. We follow general RDA guidelines, 500–1,000 mg daily, given with magnesium.
- Magnesium (avoid magnesium oxide)
- Probiotics

Nutritional Pharmacology for Specific Issues

- Hyperactivity

    —Suspect gluten/casein leaks, consider specific carbohydrate diet
    —GABA (500–1,000 mg three times daily)
    —Taurine (500–1,000 mg three times daily)
    —EFA (1,000–2,000 mg once daily)
    —Calcium/magnesium (doses vary)
    —TMG (125 mg twice daily and work the dose up slowly to 500 mg twice daily)

—DMSA (chelation by protocol in selected cases only)
—No refined sugars
—Elimination of artificial colors
—Magnesium glycinate (200–400 mg twice daily)
—Glycine (start with 250 mg twice daily)

- Inattention

—Suspect gluten/casein leaks
—Tyrosine (500 mg twice daily)
—EFA (up to 2,000 mg once daily)
—CoQ10 (25–50 mg twice daily)
—NADH (2.5–5 mg twice daily)
—TMG (125–250 mg twice daily)
—DMAE
—Theanine
—DMSA (by protocol)
—Ginkgo biloba

- Self-abusive behaviors and rage, impulsivity, disinhibition: This is often linked to disturbances in serotonin metabolism.

—Suspect gluten/casein leaks
—Inositol (1–6 g three times daily)
—Chromium (100–200 mcg daily)
—Taurine (up to 10,000 mg total daily)
—GABA (up to 10,000 mg total daily)
—Low-carbohydrate diet (no refined sugars)
—Elimination of artificial colors
—Often improve with chelation (DMSA)
—Naltrexone (by prescription)
—Consider Risperdal (Rx)

- Poor Sleep

    —Melatonin (1–3 mg at bed); Taurine (1,000–4,000 mg at bedtime)
    —GABA (1,000–5,000 mg at bedtime)
    —DMSA (by protocol)
    —TMG (250–500 mg once or twice daily)
    —Magnesium (400–800 mg at bedtime)
    —5HTP (50–100 mg at bedtime)
    —Naltrexone transdermal (1–4 mg at bedtime)

- Diarrhea: We often obtain an X-ray of the abdomen, because sometimes diarrhea is a sign of constipation.

    —Colostrum (variable dosing)
    —Probiotics (as discussed)
    —Digestive enzymes (food sensitivity—malabsorption—osmotic)
    —Lauricidin (1/4 teaspoon three times daily and increase as needed to get normal stool consistency)
    —Echinacea
    —Aloe extracts
    —EFA
    —Specific Rx meds:
    - antibiotics such as metronidazole benzoate and vancomycin
    - antifungals such as fluconazole, ketoconazole, and itraconazole
    - antiparasitics such as Alinia and Yodoxin

- Constipation: Get an X-ray of the abdomen (called a "KUB" X-ray)

    —Soluble fiber is easily mixed in a drink and has no flavor
    —Xprep (prune concentrate)/Fruit Eze
    —Senna: Smooth Move TEA!
    —Mineral oil
    —Aloe resin (leaf, not gel) can be harsh

—PediFleets (daily if necessary, until the plug is out)
—MiraLAX (1/2 or 1 teaspoon daily as needed, up to a tablespoon)
—HIGH-dose vitamin C
—Magnesium
—Colon cleanser from oxypowder.com

Immune System

Ask for an IgG food allergy panel test and an IgE test from your doctor.

Within Your HMO:

LabCorp (www.labcorp.com or call 504-838-8250)
Quest Diagnostics (www.questdiagnostics.com or call 610-454-4158)

Out of Network:

Alletess Medical Laboratory (www.foodallergy.com or call 800-225-5404)

Immunolabs (www.immunolabs.com or call 800-231-9197 or 954-691-2500)

Make the home environment as allergy-free as possible:

- Stay away from VOC paint.
- Use organic cleaning products that do not contain ammonia or chlorine.
- Do not install new carpeting or padding; if you have it, remove it.
- Use laundry detergent, dishwashing detergent, and cleaners from brands such as Planet, Ecover, Seventh Generation, EcoFriendly.

Give an antihistamine to relieve symptoms, such as Claritin RediTabs: Break in half (for small children) and put directly into the mouth (it melts like cotton candy) or in a drink.

The Best Antifungals and Course

Diflucan, and the generic form is called fluconazole

Diflucan is best given once a day, and somewhere between fourteen and twenty-one days. It's not a five-day course and it's definitely not a one-day dose. Some of these kids actually need thirty days of treatment. Some children are on an antifungal treatment for a year.

After treatment I will switch to Nystatin or oral amphotericin, which are nonsystemic. "Nonsystemic" is a term used to mean that it does not leave the digestive tube. In addition to lowering sugar, I always recommend probiotics (see the supplement recommendations on page 67). These are healthy bacteria that help make the gut less favorable for fungal growth. There are some wonderful natural antifungals like caprylic acid, monolaurin, oregano, and olive leaf extract.

Yeast and Die-Off Reactions

Cut in half whatever you're using to kill the yeast.
Epsom salt baths. One cup of Epsom salts in a tub of water.

Activated charcoal two or three times a day, orally. Charcoal absorbs everything in the digestive tract. It'll absorb our zinc supplements. It'll absorb our selenium supplements. It'll absorb seizure medication, if the kids are on these things. So be careful not to give the charcoal with something. It should be given by itself, but at least an hour or two before or after something that we needed to get in there is in there. Keep in mind that charcoal will turn the stools black. So don't be shocked if you see that. But it'll absorb the toxins, too, and that's what we want, and they'll poo that out. During this period, which we call "die-off," the children may be experiencing headaches or bowel cramps. It may be a good idea to add some ibuprofen (Motrin or Advil). Look for dye-free or obtain some compounded dye-free, sugar-free ibuprofen. Bottom line: When your child is in distress, think charcoal, Epsom salt baths, and ibuprofen.

In the cases of rash or hives or extreme behaviors, stop the drug and call the doc.

ADVICE

If Positive for yeast:

- Fluconazole: 4–6 mg per 2 pounds of body weight once daily
- Ketoconazole: 4–6 mg per 2 pounds of body weight once daily
- Itraconazole: 4–6 mg per 2 pounds of body weight once daily
- Amphotericin B: For ages two to five, 100 mg given three to four times a day (four times per day is better, but for some parents it is very difficult to get in that fourth dose)
    —For five-year-olds and older, 250 mg given three to four times per day

- Nystatin

    —Infants: 200,000 units four times daily
    —one-to-four-year-olds: 500,000 units four times daily
    —five-year-olds and older: 1,000,000 units four times daily

Natural antifungals can be very effective as well. Their use can be limited in children who are not able to swallow capsules due to the very pungent aromas and flavors. A short list follows that has been very helpful to some of the children I treat. Dosing depends on concentration, which varies from one manufacturer to another, so just follow the package's instructions.

Caprylic acid
Garlic
Grapefruit seed extract
Olive leaf extract
Oregano
Probiotics

- Be sure the child is not constipated. A laxative may be required during the yeast killing. (See the "poop" chapter on page 217.)
- Get activated charcoal, Epsom salt, and dye-free ibuprofen (e.g., Motrin) to lessen behavior.
- Stay away from sugar, and lower the carbohydrate intake.
- Yeast thrives on sugar! That's it, plain and simple. In fact, yeast does not care about the source of sugar—be it organic honey from California or pure maple syrup from Vermont. Pure fruit juice is loaded with sugar. Remember, sugar is sugar. In fact, carbohydrates and starches (complex forms of sugar) are rapidly metabolized to sugar, and feed yeast as well. So, we have children who crave sweets and we have children who are carbo-junkies! One way to decrease the number of yeast colonies thriving is to limit their food availability. This means decreasing the source of sugars in a child's diet and replacing them with vegetables and proteins.

Viral and Bacterial Infections

Chronic viral and bacterial infections should be considered in every child with autism. The laboratory workup should include:

- CBC with differential
- Viral infections

    —Viral IgG and IgM titers to: HHV-1, HHV-2, HHV-6, CMV (cytomegalovirus), and an Epstein-Barr viral panel. Consider Lyme disease panel.

- Bacterial infections
- Inflammatory markers: erythrocyte sedimentation rate, C-reactive protein, platelet count
- Streptococcus markers: ASO titers, Anti-DNase antibodies
- Stool cultures

- Urine cultures
- Urine organic acid testing

Seizures

- Get an EGG
- If seizure activity starts, consider antiseizure medication. Common ones (not listed by favorite, but maybe they are, hee hee):

    —Lamictal
    —Depakote
    —Neurontin

- During a fever, rotate:

    —Tylenol and Motrin (ONLY DYE-FREE) every THREE hours
    —Fluids to ensure adequate hydration

- Keep up on vitamins B_6 and B_{12}.
- Hyperbaric oxygen chamber (www.oxyhealth.com)

Glutathione

- Support for the methylation pathway is support for the production of glutathione, one of our body's most important antioxidants
- Methyl B_{12} injections
- Raise glutathione: intravenous, transdermal, nebulized
- Folic acid (See page 72 in the supplements chapter for dosage)
- TMG or DMG
- N-acetyl-cysteine
- Oxidative Stress Reducer (OSR) is a great antioxidant and may increase glutathione levels as well

Poop

- Constipation: Bowel movements must be daily and complete. Many children need daily help (not just "once in a while"). Consistency is the name of the game if you're looking for improvements in language, behavior, and ability to connect socially.
- Dietary considerations: Removal of gluten and casein.

—For more information, go back to the diet chapter (page 29).

1. Daily laxatives may be needed to enhance motility
   —GlycoLax/MiraLAX available at a pharmacy
   —Sold over-the-counter at most major and small pharmacies, drugstores, and health food stores

2. Oxy-Powder
   —www.oxypowder.com

3. Fleet enemas (one daily for about five days)
   —Sold over-the-counter at most major and small pharmacies, drugstores, and health food stores

4. May need an X-ray to determine the extent of the problem
   —Ask your doctor for one

5. May need a "blast" from magnesium citrate, also a laxative (given over two days)
   —Informational site: www.drugs.com/ppa/magnesium-citrate.html
   —Purchasing site: www.organicpharmacy.org

6. May try a short course of MOM (milk of magnesia)
   —Sold over-the-counter at most major and small pharmacies, drugstores, and health food stores
   —Purchasing site: www.magnesiumdirect.com

7. Expect to be vigilant for six months to a year

- Fiber:
  —Fibersure (1–2 teaspoons daily) http://us.fibersure.com/index_flash.shtml
  —You can also place your order at www.drugstore.com

- Nutritional healing

1. Zinc
   —20–40 mg daily
   —Zinc supplements are available for purchase, without a prescription, at almost all major and small drugstores, pharmacies, health food stores
   —Fact Sheet—http://ods.od.nih.gov/FactSheets/Zinc.asp
   —Dosing information—http://www.lenntech.com/recommended-daily-intake.htm
   —General information—http://www.mayoclinic.com/health/drug-information/DR602313

2. George's Aloe
   —2–6 ounces per day
   —Warren Laboratories—www.warrenlabsaloe.com, 254-580-9990
   Online purchasing also available at Natural Nirvana
   http://store.naturalnirvana.com

- Probiotics

    —Kartner Health (Dr. Jerry's supplements)
    www.kartnerhealth.com or call 866-960-9251
    —Kirkman Labs
    www.kirkmanlabs.com or call 800-245-8282
    —Klaire Labs
    www.klaire.com or call 888-488-2488

- Diarrhea

    —Remove offending foods
    - Most common are juices/fruits/dairy products.

    —Treat bacterial infections
    - Antibiotics depend on bacteria. Have to get stool studies as outlined.

    —Treat parasitic infections
    - Antiparasitic agents such as Alinia or metronidazole are excellent choices. Since parasites may be hard to discern on stool cultures, may have to treat empirically (as a "trial").

    —Nutritionally—much the same way as constipation
    - Zinc
    - Fiber
    - George's Aloe
    - Probiotics
    - Digestive enzymes

BEFORE HYPERBARIC TREATMENT

Begin the diet and supplement protocol, and help your child detox first. Be aware of all the risks (you can check out www.genoxinc.com, www.hyperbaricsupport.com, www.oxy health.com, or www.performance-hyperbarics.com for some good information).

Here are the supplements to focus on:
Antioxidants:
Vitamin C (1,000 mg per day)
Vitamin A (5,000 IU per day minimum)
N-acetyl-cysteine (600 mg daily)
Selenium (100 mcg daily)
Glutathione (transdermally 100–200 mg twice daily)
Melatonin (1 mg per day)

Pediatric Autoimmune Neuropsychiatric Disorders Associated with Streptococcus (PANDAS)

Dietary changes

- Markedly reduce sugars, juices, carbohydrates (pastries, French fries, sweetened cereals, "healthy waters" that have flavorings/sugar, pancakes, waffles). Each meal and snack should consist of a protein, carbohydrate, and a fat. Meat is a nice combination of protein and fat.
- Follow a gluten-free and dairy-free diet.
- Completely remove food colors and dyes from all food, supplements, and medication sources.

—To find out about food dyes, go to:
www.cfsan.fda.gov/~dms/col-toc.html
www.thealmightyguru.com/Pointless/FoodDye.html

- Organic diet
- Antifungal therapy (see "The Best Antifungals and Course" on page 160 in the yeast chapter)

Supplements

(Please note that this is a separate set of recommendations for the conditions discussed in this chapter. The supplement recommendations on page 53 also work. This is in addition.)

- Vitamins: www.kartnerhealth.com or call 866-960-9251
  www.kirkmanlabs.com or call 800-245-8282
  www.klaire.com or call 888-488-2488

  —High-quality multivitamin, vitamin D3 (see page 70)
  —Vitamin B_{12} in methyl form (injected subcutaneously every other night)

- Minerals: (Kartner Health, Kirkman Labs, Klaire)

  —Calcium (see page 67)
  —Magnesium (see page 67)
  —Zinc (see page 67)

- Oils: Omega-3 fatty acids (Kartner Health, Kirkman Labs, Klaire)

  —Omega-3 fatty acids (see page 71)

- Short-term medications, such as Ritalin, are a great Band-Aid until the cause of the inability to focus/concentrate is discovered.

Preventing and Dealing with Regression

1. Start one new supplement at a time, giving three to four days before adding another supplement/intervention.
2. Start with 1/2 the target dose for one to two days to see how it is tolerated.
3. Keep a diary.
4. Look for patterns of behavior changes:
   —Before or after bowel movements
   —Before or after eating
   - After a supplement starts
   - When starting or stopping a medication
   - Changes in school performance
   - Increase or decrease in tantrums
   - An improvement in sleep, or changes in sleep
   - More language
   - More or less flexibility/OCD/perseverations/anxiety

ACKNOWLEDGMENTS

Thanks to Dr. Jerry, Brian Tart, Amy Hertz, Ed Ormandy, and Lauren Auslander (you rock, girl!). What an amazing team of angels to help deliver this message to the world!

INDEX

Note: Page numbers in **bold** indicate chapter subjects. Page numbers in *italics* indicate charts and illustrations.

ABOUT THE AUTHOR

Jenny McCarthy is the *New York Times* bestselling author of *Belly Laughs: The Naked Truth About Pregnancy and Childbirth*, *Baby Laughs: The Naked Truth About the First Year of Mommyhood*, *Louder Than Words: A Mother's Journey in Healing Autism*, and *Mother Warriors: A Nation of Parents Healing Autism Against All Odds*. She lives in Los Angeles with her son, Evan, and Jim Carrey.

Jerry Kartzinel, M.D., is one of the top doctors in the country treating children's medical conditions associated with autism. In addition to his private practice in Florida, he speaks at autism conferences around the country and frequently appears on television and in print. He is the father of a son with autism and lives with his family in Ponte Verda, Florida.